METABOLIC BONE DISEASE

Volume I

List of Contributors

LOUIS V. AVIOLI

OLAV L. M. BIJVOET

PAUL D. BYERS

CORALIE CORNISH

C. E. DENT

MICHAEL KLEEREKOPER

SOLOMON POSEN

EDWIN L. PRIEN

LAWRENCE G. RAISZ

T. C. B. STAMP

HIBBARD E. WILLIAMS

METABOLIC BONE DISEASE

Volume I

Edited by

LOUIS V. AVIOLI, M.D.

Department of Medicine
Bone and Mineral Metabolism
Washington University School of Medicine
and The Jewish Hospital of St. Louis
St. Louis, Missouri

STEPHEN M. KRANE, M.D.

Department of Medicine
Harvard Medical School
and Medical Services (Arthritis Unit)
Massachusetts General Hospital
Boston, Massachusetts

ACADEMIC PRESS   New York   San Francisco   London   1977

A Subsidiary of Harcourt Brace Jovanovich, Publishers

LOM J [LSP W]

ACADEMIC PRESS, INC.
111 Fifth Avenue, New York, New York 10003

United Kingdom Edition published by
ACADEMIC PRESS, INC. (LONDON) LTD.
24/28 Oval Road, London NW1

Library of Congress Cataloging in Publication Data

Main entry under title:

Metabolic bone disease.

    Includes bibliographical references and index.
    1.   Bones–Diseases.   2.   Calcium metabolism
disorders.   3.   Phosphorus metabolism disorders.
I.   Avioli, Louis V.   II.   Krane, Stephen M.
[DNLM: 1.   Bone diseases.   2.   Metabolic diseases.
3.   Bone and bones–Metabolism.   WE200 M587]
RC930.M46   616.7'1   76-27431
ISBN 0–12–068701–1

Contents

4   The Diagnostic Value of Bone Biopsies

PAUL D. BYERS

5   Vitamin D, Rickets, and Osteomalacia

C. E. DENT AND T. C. B. STAMP

6   Osteoporosis: Pathogenesis and Therapy

LOUIS V. AVIOLI

7   Nephrolithiasis

HIBBARD E. WILLIAMS AND EDWIN L. PRIEN, JR.

Index

List of Contributors

Numbers in parentheses indicate the pages on which the authors' contributions begin.

Louis V. Avioli, M.D. (307), Department of Medicine, Bone and Mineral Metabolism, Washington University School of Medicine, and The Jewish Hospital of St. Louis, St. Louis, Missouri

Olav L. M. Bijvoet, M.D. (49), Department of Clinical Endocrinology and Metabolism, University Hospital, Leiden, The Netherlands

Paul D. Byers, M.D. (183), Department of Morbid Anatomy, The Institute of Orthopaedics, Royal National Orthopaedics Hospital, London, England

Coralie Cornish (141), Department of Medicine, University of Sydney, Sydney, New South Wales, Australia

C. E. Dent, C.B.E., M.D., Ph.D., F.R.C.P., F.R.S.* (237), Department of Human Metabolism, University College Hospital Medical School, University of London, London, England

Michael Kleerekoper, M.D.† (141), Department of Medicine, University of Sydney, Sydney, New South Wales, Australia

Solomon Posen, M.D. (141), Department of Medicine, Sydney Hospital, Sydney, New South Wales, Australia

Edwin L. Prien, Jr., M.D. (387), Department of Medicine, Harvard Medical School, and Medical Services (Arthritis Unit), Massachusetts General Hospital, Boston, Massachusetts

Lawrence G. Raisz, M.D. (1), Department of Medicine, Division of Endocrinology and Metabolism, University of Connecticut, Health Center, Farmington, Connecticut

* Deceased.

† Present address: Bone and Mineral Research Laboratory, Henry Ford Hospital, Detroit, Michigan.

T. C. B. Stamp, M.D. (237), Royal National Orthopaedic Hospital, London, England

Hibbard E. Williams, M.D. (387), Medical Services, San Francisco General Hospital, and Department of Medicine, University of California School of Medicine, San Francisco, California

Preface

Is this the poultice for my aching bones?

Romeo and Juliet II, 5, 65

In 1948, a textbook entitled "The Parathyroid Glands and Metabolic Bone Disease, Selected Studies" appeared for the first time. The authors, Fuller Albright and Edward C. Reifenstein, prefaced the text with

> We are not content merely to present data; we attempt, where possible, to develop an hypothesis upon which to hang the observations. The hypotheses—it almost follows—are subject to change without notice.

Although this monograph simply represented the collective experiences of Drs. Albright and Reifenstein with a variety of metabolic bone diseases, it still remains the classic textbook of its kind, offering house officers, postdoctoral fellows, medical students, professors, and practicing physicians a clear and most concise approach to a variety of disorders of mineral metabolism.

It should be emphasized that the book by Albright and Reifenstein was written nearly 30 years ago. At that time the fruits of technology developed during the second world war were just beginning to be applied to clinical problems. In 1977 many of our readers might not be aware that the titration methods for determining serum calcium levels in 1948 were tedious and unavailable in more than a few laboratories, that parathyroid hormone preparations were crude, and that there were no suspicions that calcitonin existed or that the kidney and liver were essential for vitamin D bioactivation. Although there were many considerations of bone matrix, collagen, which comprises 90–95% of the organic material of bone, was never mentioned. Albright and Reifenstein's book nevertheless contained a wealth of material, and many of the observations made then, such as clinical descriptions and aspects of pathophysiology, are still pertinent now, a fact largely attributable to the uncanny wisdom of Doctor Albright.

The book was based on personal experience and copiously illustrated with detailed case reports and metabolic studies from which generalizations were derived. We are delighted that one of our contributors, Eleanor Pyle, is currently preparing a biography of the late Fuller Albright, which should be of great interest to our readers.

It was our intention that both volumes of this treatise provide detailed clinical information concerning metabolic bone diseases and consider their pathophysiology. These volumes are multiauthored and, although as editors we have reviewed each contribution in detail, the emphasis and style of each chapter are those of the individual author or authors. The approach to each subject is different. Some have preferred to review critically the relevant literature and not to include work based on personal experience. Others have emphasized their own views. This is particularly true in the chapter on osteomalacia by Professor Dent and Dr. Stamp. We consider it a special privilege to have this contribution in this treatise. Charles Dent, like Fuller Albright, was one of those unique individuals who had an extraordinary talent for deciphering clinical problems. The chapter on osteomalacia coauthored by Professor Dent and Dr. Stamp was updated just before Professor Dent's death last year. In a few other chapters details of documented personal experience and previously unpublished metabolic and biochemical studies have been used to illustrate or explain problems of pathophysiology in a manner somewhat reminiscent of the Albright and Reifenstein treatise. Many authors tend to emphasize their own point of view when different opinions exist concerning a particular problem. Consequently interpretations of pathophysiology may vary when the same point is considered in different chapters.

Although it may be disconcerting to some to read books in which style and approach differ, this must be expected in multiauthored volumes and perhaps is not too important in what we intend as a detailed treatise. We also recognize that the contributions vary markedly in length, not necessarily in proportion to what generally might be considered the clinical and pathophysiological importance of the subject matter. Some authors felt "cramped" by restrictions imposed on the size of their contributions since they wished to present a critical review of what they considered pertinent material. Our publisher has been unusually tolerant in this regard.

There are disorders that some classify as metabolic bone diseases, such as the bone dysplasias, that are not considered at all in either volume. As the planned volumes grew in size, we considered it prudent to publish the contributions included in the two volumes and to consider alterations in size, style, scope, and format for possible future editions.

We extend our grateful appreciation to the many medical students, trainees, and house staff who indirectly contributed to these volumes by offering constructive criticism regarding form and content. It would also have been impossible to complete the text without the whole-hearted cooperation of Ms. Linda Graf who single-handedly accomplished the enormous task of retyping all the chapters and, with the assistance of the library staff at Washington University and the Jewish Hospital of St. Louis, reviewed and confirmed the mass of references submitted. Thanks are also due Ms. Eleanor Pyle who generously offered her time and energy during the editing process.

Louis V. Avioli, M.D.
Stephen M. Krane, M.D.

Contents of Other Volumes

1

Bone Metabolism and Calcium Regulation

LAWRENCE G. RAISZ

I. INTRODUCTION

More than a quarter century ago, Albright and Reifenstein (1948) were able to summarize briefly the fragmentary and conflicting information then available on bone metabolism and its role in calcium regulation. Ten years later, the physicochemical background against which biological regulation

1

must play its part was described by Neuman and Neuman (1958). Since that time the problem appears to have received more than its share of fallout from the information explosion in biomedical science of the 1950's and 1960's. These 25 years have seen the following:

1. A clear definition of the feedback system which maintains serum calcium concentration constant by changes in parathyroid hormone secretion mediated through control of bone resorption as well as renal and intestinal calcium transport

2. Chemical characterization of parathyroid hormone and the beginning of studies on its complex metabolism

3. The identification of early effects of parathyroid hormone on production of cyclic 3',5'-adenosine monophosphate (cAMP) and on mineral translocation in kidney and bone

4. The discovery of calcitonin and the remarkably rapid elucidation of its chemistry and of an entirely new feedback system, regulating calcium and affecting bone. Except in the area of mechanism of action, our knowledge of calcitonin is at least as extensive as that for parathyroid hormone

5. The discovery of the activation of vitamin D by multiple-step metabolic transformation, which has led to the concept that vitamin D is really a third calcium-regulating hormone

6. Analysis of the chemical composition, biosynthesis, and degradation of bone and cartilage matrix, particularly collagen. In the description of bone matrix in Albright and Reifenstein's book the word *collagen* does not appear.

Thirty years ago, Albright left open the question of whether parathyroid hormone acts primarily on bone or on kidney in regulating serum calcium; we can answer that question only with a thunderingly equivocal *both!* Now we must reevaluate the relative importance of parathyroid hormone and active metabolites of vitamin D in physiologic calcium regulation, and we still do not know the physiological function of calcitonin. Moreover, the processes of bone formation and resorption are understood only in general descriptive terms; the cellular and chemical events involved are largely unknown.

II. GENERAL PROBLEM OF CALCIUM REGULATION

In this section, the most salient features of calcium regulation and the roles of the major regulatory hormones, parathyroid hormone, calcitonin, and the active metabolites of vitamin D, are briefly reviewed. A more detailed discussion of the regulatory hormones is presented in Volume II, Chapters 1–4.

The maintenance of a constant calcium ion concentration in extracellular fluid plays a central role in the control of bone metabolism. Bone is also important in the regulation of magnesium, phosphate, sodium, and hydrogen ions, and under certain circumstances the control systems may depend on these ions as well as on calcium. Even though feedback control appears to be exerted largely by *extracellular* calcium ion concentration, this is not the only purpose of regulation. Parathyroid hormone can increase the entry of calcium into the cells, and its earliest effect is a transient lowering of serum ionized calcium concentration (Parsons *et al.,* 1971). Thus, the hormone could help maintain intracellular calcium, which is essential for secretion, muscular contraction, and many other cell functions. The subsequent increase of serum calcium concentration because of calcium mobilization from the skeleton and increased transport across the renal tubule or the intestinal mucosa is necessary to maintain this calcium supply. Moreover, extracellular regulation is essential because neuromuscular excitability depends on the concentration of calcium ion at the cell surface.

Calcitonin and vitamin D may be more important for maintaining calcium mass than concentration. Calcitonin secretion can be stimulated by calcium ingestion, with little increase in serum calcium concentration, and the formation of the most active metabolite of vitamin D—1,25-dihydroxycholecalciferol—may not be regulated by changes in serum calcium concentration itself but by intracellular ion concentration or indirectly by other regulatory hormones.

Parathyroid hormone (see Volume II, Chapter 1) is initially synthesized as a larger prohormone, which is probably cleaved intracellularly to the classical 84 amino acid molecule prior to secretion. The secreted hormone is rapidly degraded to fragments that may be biologically active or inactive. These fragments can react with antibodies to bovine parathyroid hormone (PTH). Thus, immunoreactive PTH and biologically active PTH concentrations are not necessarily the same.

Calcium ion concentration is largely responsible for feedback control of parathyroid hormone synthesis and secretion. Magnesium has a similar acute effect on the release of preformed hormone, but low magnesium is less effective than low calcium in stimulating hormone synthesis and gland hyperplasia. Impairment of both hormone secretion and end organ response may be responsible for the hypocalcemia that occurs in magnesium deficiency. There are few factors other than calcium and magnesium which have been shown to influence PTH synthesis and secretion directly. Phosphate loading stimulates the gland, but this is probably entirely mediated by the associated decrease in serum calcium ion concentration. The role of hydrogen ion, catecholamines, and other factors is currently under study.

The discovery of *calcitonin* (Copp *et al.*, 1962) was followed by a re-markably rapid elucidation of the chemistry, effects, and metabolism of this new hypocalcemic hormone secreted by cells of ultrabranchial origin located parafollicularly in the mammalian thyroid (see Volume II, Chapter 4). Unlike PTH, which is largely under direct divalent cation control, calcitonin secretion is stimulated not only directly by high calcium but also by gastrointestinal hormones, particularly gastrin (Cooper *et al.*, 1972). The latter response may be the most important physiological mechanism for calcitonin secretion in mammals, and may explain why young, rapidly growing animals deficient in calcitonin develop hypercalcemia and hyper-calciuria after oral calcium loading, whereas normal animals do not. The major direct effect of calcitonin in mammals is inhibition of bone resorp-tion, although there are also effects on renal and intestinal ion transport. Calcitonin-secreting cells may have still other functions, which could ex-plain why parafollicular cell secretory granules also contain serotonin and why calcitonin is found in such high concentrations in fish and birds, species in which it has little demonstrable effect on calcium metabolism. The role of calcitonin in human physiology and disease is also puzzling. Calcitonin deficiency appears to cause little difficulty, and an enormous excess of calcitonin in medullary carcinoma of the thyroid may not impair calcium regulation (Volume II, Chapter 4).

Twenty-five years ago *vitamin D* was considered essential for intestinal calcium absorption, and there was little evidence for other physiological effects. The subsequent recognition that vitamin D was an important regu-latory hormone in calcium metabolism could have been predicted from the early observations that vitamin D excess could cause hypercalcemia and that deficiency could result in hypocalcemia and impaired response to PTH. These changes indicated a direct effect of vitamin D on bone. The substantial time lag between administration of vitamin D and its effects suggested that some activation process might be required. The active metabolites, particularly 1,25-dihydroxycholecalciferol, have only re-cently been identified, and there may still be other, unidentified active forms. We have considerable data on synthesis and secretion of active metabolites but do not yet know the exact mechanisms of control. Both calcium deficiency and phosphate deficiency can increase the synthesis of 1,25-dihydroxycholecalciferol in the kidney, which seems appropriate teleologically if we consider vitamin D as a mineralizing or bone growth hormone. Since PTH affects calcium and phosphate transport by the kid-ney, it is not surprising that vitamin D metabolism also depends on the parathyroid status of the animal. 1,25-Dihydroxycholecalciferol is a po-tent direct stimulator of intestinal calcium transport and bone resorption. Since phosphate supply is also increased by these direct effects, more mineral is made available for new bone formation. Other metabolites can affect these processes at higher concentration. Direct effects on bone matrix formation or mineralization have been postulated but not yet demonstrated.

Humoral factors other than parathyroid hormone, calcitonin, and vitamin D probably do not regulate serum ionized calcium concentration directly, but sex hormones, glucocorticoids, thyroxine, growth hormone, glucagon, and other agents do affect mineral metabolism and may thus indirectly affect regulation. One special regulatory system occurs in egg-laying vertebrates. Under estrogen control, calcium is stored in new medullary bone, mobilized via a calcium binding protein in the serum, phosvitin, and transported to the developing egg. This system has been studied largely in birds and appears to be vestigial in mammals.

Finally, there are factors that are most important for their local effects on skeletal metabolism but may also affect calcium regulation. Local changes in pH, oxygen tension, or mechanical stress can alter bone formation and resorption. Humoral agents that do not ordinarily circulate at sufficiently high concentrations could affect bone locally. Prostaglandins stimulate bone resorption (Klein and Raisz, 1970) *in vitro* but do not produce hypercalcemia on injection probably because they are so rapidly destroyed. In inflammation and neoplasia, prostaglandins may be released locally or in very large amounts and produce bone lesions and hypercalcemia (Tashjian *et al.,* 1972; Goldhaber *et al.,* 1973: Raisz *et al.,* 1974). No physiological role for prostaglandins in bone metabolism has been identified. Heparin can enhance the response to PTH (Avioli, 1974; Goldhaber, 1965) and increase the activity of collagenase (Sakamoto *et al.,* 1973). Mast cells, which produce heparin, are found in the bone marrow, but their role in bone metabolism is not clear. Recently a new bone-resorbing factor, named osteoclast activating factor (OAF), was found in supernatants of cultured normal human leukocytes stimulated by antigens or mitogens (Horton *et al.,* 1972; Luben *et al.,* 1974b). This factor could also affect bone in chronic inflammation and neoplasia (Raisz and Horton, 1973; Mundy *et al.,* 1974).

III. GENERAL DESCRIPTION OF SKELETAL STRUCTURE AND FUNCTION

The mammalian skeleton has evolved to serve two sets of needs, which are not necessarily compatible. One function is to provide a structural support that is strong, mobile, capable of orderly growth, and able to protect vital organs. At the same time, the skeleton must serve as a reservoir for almost all the body calcium and most of the phosphorus and magnesium and as an additional source of sodium, carbonate, and hydroxyl ions. The skeleton is never metabolically at rest. Bone is constantly being renewed by endosteal and haversian remodeling. The patterns of skeletal renewal and loss (Harris and Heany, 1969) have been well characterized in gross morphological terms, but little is known about changes in skeletal ultrastructure or chemical composition with age.

The pattern of skeletal development appears to be similar for long bones and vertebrae. The embryologic anlage is a condensation of mesenchymal cells to form a cartilage rudiment. This rudiment develops the basic shape ultimately characteristic of that particular bone before bone formation itself begins. In long bones, the shaft begins to form as a collar of periosteal new bone around the cartilaginous rudiment. The cartilage in the shaft becomes hypertrophic, calcifies, and is then resorbed. An epiphyseal growth plate develops at each end of the bone shaft, with characteristic zones of resting, proliferative, and hypertrophic cartilage. Calcification begins in the hypertrophic zone. Below the hypertrophic zone, the cartilage condenses and calcifies further in the primary spongiosa of the metaphysis, which consists of trabeculae of calcified cartilage with a superimposed calcified bone matrix. These trabeculae are resorbed and replaced by completely bony trabeculae in the secondary spongiosa. The cortical bone of the shaft, or diaphysis, initially enlarges by periosteal new bone formation of woven and lamellar bone, but in man and many other mammals, it begins to undergo haversian remodeling late in fetal development, converting the lamellar bone to a system of osteons. These are formed by vessels that penetrate behind a cutting cone of osteoclasts to form a tubular cavity in which osteoblasts lay down concentric layers of new bone to form the cylindrical osteon. As the shaft grows, the medullary cavity is enlarged by endosteal resorption. The cartilaginous epiphyses develop ossification centers and are gradually converted to bone.

Humans show a characteristic pattern of overall skeletal growth (Frisancho et al., 1970; Garn, 1972). In childhood, linear growth occurs at the epiphyseal plate, and the controlling step is probably cartilage cell proliferation. In utero and in early childhood, the cortex becomes larger without becoming much thicker because endosteal resorption almost keeps pace with periosteal apposition, and the controlling steps are osteoblastic matrix synthesis and osteoclastic bone resorption. Later in childhood and during adolescence, there is a linear growth spurt followed by closure of the epiphyses and cessation of linear growth. Net endosteal resorption is no longer seen in some bones, and there may be considerable endosteal apposition so that the cortex becomes substantially thicker. As described in detail in Chapter 6, thickening of the bones continues in adults, and bone mass can continue to increase into the third, and even the fourth, decade. Thereafter, there may be a steady state period during which bone formation equals resorption and mass is constant. However, the length of this phase, or even its existence, is uncertain because we have no precise longitudinal data on changes in bone mass in the same individual; it may be so brief as to be considered a transitional phase rather than a distinct period of skeletal development. Thereafter, there is a long phase of progressive bone loss in humans and in some other mammals. The loss of long bone mass appears to be due largely to increased endosteal resorption, which increases the size of the marrow cavity of the long bones; the outside diameter of the long bones does not ordinarily decrease and may even increase slightly. Formation of new osteons also fails to keep pace with resorption in haversian remodeling, so that the cortex develops resorption cavities. Finally, there is extensive loss of trabecular bone, particularly in the vertebrae, which may be accompanied by thickening of some of the remaining trabeculae.

A. Bone Histology

Bone formation and resorption have been fairly completely described at the cellular level. Mesenchymal precursor cells differentiate into osteoblasts (Owen, 1970), which are highly active in protein synthesis and have a characteristic large Golgi zone and abundant granular endoplasmic reticulum. The osteoblasts synthesize a matrix that consists largely of collagen but also contains glycoprotein, protein polysaccharides, and some lipid. The matrix does not become calcified immediately, but is laid down as a thin layer of osteoid between the active osteoblasts and the calcification front. As the bone grows, the osteoblasts become surrounded by matrix and develop into osteocytes. These osteocytes continue to lay down a small amount of matrix, which ultimately becomes calcified, reducing the size of the lacunae in which they rest (Baylink and Wergedal, 1971). The osteoblasts and osteocytes remain connected with one another by a series of cytoplasmic processes that extend radially from each cell in canaliculae. Electron microscopic observations indicate that these processes are connected with one another by intercellular junctions that could form a communication network in bone (Fig. 1) (Holtrop and Weinger, 1972). It has also been suggested that nutrients circulate in the extracellular fluid between the cells and the bone, since labeled extracellular proteins can penetrate into this space. Once the osteocyte has become fully enveloped in mature mineralized bone, it usually shows electron microscopic and histochemical evidence of decreasing cellular activity (Doty and Schofield, 1972). However, it is possible that these cells may develop

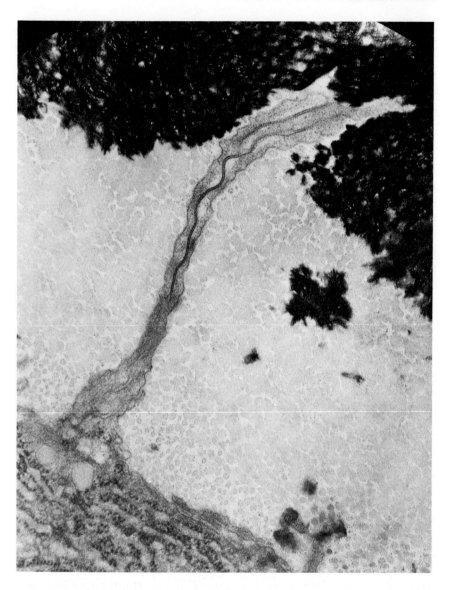

Fig. 1. Electron micrograph of the bone-forming surface. A portion of osteoblast cytoplasm on the upper left shows extensive rough endoplasmic reticulum. Between the cell and the calcified bone at lower left, there is a layer of collagen fibers that appear to form aggregates of increasing size toward the bone. There is cytoplasmic extension from the osteoblast which shows a long, tight junction, presumably connecting it to a cytoplasmic extension from an underlying osteocyte within the bone. ×29,250. (From Holtrop and Weinger, 1972. Reprinted by permission of the publisher.)

a new activity and become resorbing osteocytes. The main evidence for osteocytic osteolysis is morphological. Enlarged lacunae are seen around osteocytes in circumstances when resorption is increased, such as hyperparathyroidism (Bélanger, 1969). Large lacunae are sometimes subjacent to surfaces undergoing osteoclastic resorption. Estimates of the magnitude of osteocytic osteolysis suggest that it ordinarily accounts for only a small proportion of total bone resorption (Liu *et al.,* 1974).

The cell responsible for most of the resorption of bone is the multinucleated osteoclast (Fig. 2). Despite extensive study, we know little about this cell. Its precursor may be an undifferentiated progenitor cell in bone, but it is possible that a specific preosteoclast exists (Scott, 1967; Rasmussen and Bordier, 1973). Osteoclasts may be formed from osteoblasts (Tonna, 1960) or macrophages (Jee and Nolan, 1963). Osteoclasts are distinguishable morphologically by their abundant mitochondria and scant endoplasmic reticulum, with many of their ribosomal particles present in clusters. The osteoclast does not appear to resorb unmineralized collagen, but acts on calcified matrix of both cartilage and bone. The nonresorbing bone surface is normally covered with active or inactive osteoblasts, which may in turn be connected with the osteocytes. This covering has been termed the bone membrane (Neuman and Ramp, 1971). This membrane is broken at the site of osteoclastic resorption. Intercellular junctions between osteoclasts and other bone cells have not been demonstrated. The active osteoclast is closely apposed to the surface of mineralized bone but can move around on that surface. A portion of the osteoclast apposed to the bone surface shows an active ruffled border, which appears to be the site of resorption. Around this, there is a clear zone in which the cytoplasm is devoid of subcellular particles, but the cell membrane is still closely apposed to the bone. The relative proportions of ruffled border and clear zone vary with the state of osteoclastic activity (Holtrop *et al.,* 1974). It is assumed that the osteoclast initiates resorption by removing mineral because mineralized collagen is resistant to enzymatic degradation (Stern *et al.,* 1970), but the manner in which this mineral is transported is not known. Free apatite crystals and demineralized collagen can be seen in the spaces between cell processes in the ruffled border. However, little of this material is identifiable within the osteoclast cytoplasm or its vacuoles, suggesting that extensive dissolution of mineral and degradation of matrix takes place in the ruffled border area.

The cellular pattern of cartilage formation and calcification is strikingly different from that of bone. Cartilage calcification normally occurs in the hypertrophic zone. There are no structural elements comparable to the osteoid seam, lamellar bone, or the osteon. From electron microscopic

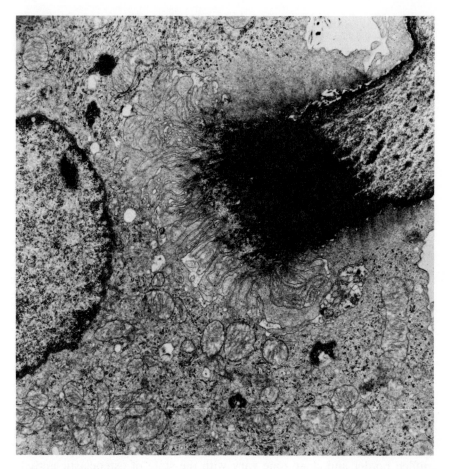

Fig. 2. Electron micrograph of a portion of an osteoclast from a fetal rat bone cultured with PTH. The osteoclast is seen enveloping a spicule of bone. The clear zone, free of subcellular particles, is closely adherent to the sides of the spicule, while at the end an active ruffled border appears to be engaged in removing mineral and matrix. The cell contains many mitochondria, ribosomes in small aggregates as well as associated with endoplasmic reticulum, and both clear and dense vacuoles. ×9100. (From Holtrop *et al.*, 1974; reprinted with permission of the publisher).

evidence, the initial step in cartilage calcification may be the extracellular deposition of cytoplasmic vesicles that contain calcium (Anderson, 1969). Such vesicles may also play a role in initiating calcification of embryonic bone (Anderson and Reynolds, 1973). In the primary spongiosa, the calcified spicules of cartilage are resorbed, often together with the bone that had been laid down upon their surface. The resorbing cell is sometimes called a chrondoclast but does not appear to be different from the osteoclast.

B. Bone Chemistry

The major constituents of bone are collagen, which comprises the bulk of the inorganic matrix, and calcium phosphate, largely in the form of small crystals of hydroxyapatite. Other components include glycoproteins, acid mucopolysaccharides, lipids, calcium phosphate salts other than hydroxyapatite, and ions, such as magnesium, carbonate, sodium, and fluoride, which are associated with the mineral phase. These components, although small in quantity, can have powerful effects on the metabolism and physical characteristics of bone.

1. Collagen—Composition and Synthesis

Collagen is deposited as extracellular fibers made up of smaller fibrils that are many collagen molecules in length and perhaps 5 to 7 collagen molecules thick. Electron micrographs of these fibrils show characteristic cross-striations at intervals of 640 to 700 Å. These striations are due to changes in charge density resulting from the arrangement of the collagen molecules, which are packed in an overlapping fashion staggered at approximately one-quarter of their length. This arrangement can be predicted from the primary structure of collagen, since it is the one that results in the maximum attraction between molecules by noncovalent forces (Hulmes *et al.*, 1973). The linear arrangement of the collagen molecules is such that there is a gap of about 400 angstroms between the end of one molecule and the beginning of the next. These "holes" may be important in mineralization (see Fig. 3). The collagen molecules that make up the fibrils are long, thin, relatively rigid rods, approximately 14×3000 Å, made up of three polypeptide chains coiled around each other in a unique triple helix. Both the triple helix and the fibrils can be assembled by noncovalent forces, but covalent cross-links (see below) are important in making them more stable and less soluble. Collagen molecules in bone, as well as in skin and tendon, consist of two α_1 chains that have identical amino acid sequences and one α_2 chain that shows considerable homology (Piez *et al.*, 1972) but has a different amino acid sequence. The amino acid composition and much of the sequence of these chains have been determined for several species (Miller, 1972; Hulmes *et al.*, 1973) and are nearly identical for bone and skin collagen (Table I). Human bone and skin collagen probably also have similar amino acid sequences (Miller and Lunde, 1973). The α_2 chains that comprise one-third of the collagen molecule, have different amino acid composition, but show a high degree of homology so that the distribution of charge density is similar to that of α_1 chains (Piez *et al.*, 1972). The amino acid composition of α chains is unusual in that every third amino acid residue is glycine and almost one-quarter of the amino acid residues are either proline or hydroxyproline, properly called imino acids. Collagen also contains about 35 lysine residues per

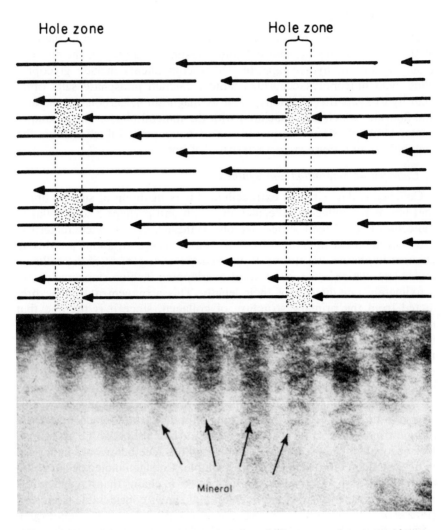

Fig. 3. The packing of molecular collagen in polymeric fibers occurs in a staggered array, with the formation of hole zones between the "head" of one molecule and the "tail" of the next. In the sample of bone collagen (bottom), the early deposition of crystals has occurred in the hole zones. (From Glimcher and Krane, 1968. Reprinted with permission of the publisher).

chain, some of which are hydroxylated. Hydroxyproline and hydroxyly-sine are almost unique to collagen; only a few other proteins, such as elastin and the C1q component of complement, contain these residues. When the imino acid is immediately after glycine, it is most often proline,

TABLE I

Amino Acid Composition of α Chains of Chick Bone Collagen, $[\alpha_1(I)]_2\alpha_2$, and Cartilage Collagen, $[\alpha_1(II)]_3$[a]

Amino acid	$\alpha_1(I)$	$\alpha_1(II)$	α_2
3-Hydroxyproline	1	2	1
4-Hydroxyproline	110	106	102
Aspartic acid	43	43	49
Threonine	19	27	22
Serine	28	27	32
Glutamic acid	81	89	73
Proline	128	118	116
Glycine	342	336	338
Alanine	132	106	110
Valine	14	16	31
Isoleucine	7	7	18
Leucine	21	27	31
Tyrosine	2	2	2
Phenylalanine	13	15	14
Hydroxylysine	6	24	10
Lysine	30	13	23
Histidine	2	2	7
Arginine	53	51	53
Methionine	9	12	5
	1041	1023	1037

[a] Values are calculated for a molecular weight of 95,000 and rounded off to the nearest whole number (Miller *et al.*, 1969; Lane and Miller, 1969; Miller, 1971).

whereas hydroxyproline is usually located just before glycine. Hydroxyproline is probably important in providing stability to the triple helix through hydrogen bonding between α chains, while the relative rigidity of the imino acids are important in enabling collagen molecules to form extended triple helices as opposed to the more tightly coiled α helical structure of other proteins, in which hydrogen bonding occurs between loops of the same helix rather than between different chains. Hydroxylysine is important as the site of glycosylation of collagen, and both lysine and hydroxylysine are involved in cross-linking.

To consider in more detail how these and other modifications of the collagen molecule affect its properties, particularly in the collagen of bone, it is useful to review the steps in collagen biosynthesis (Fig. 4). Collagen is synthesized as large pro-α chains with a molecular weight of about 150,000. Although it is generally believed that there is a separate

SYNTHESIS

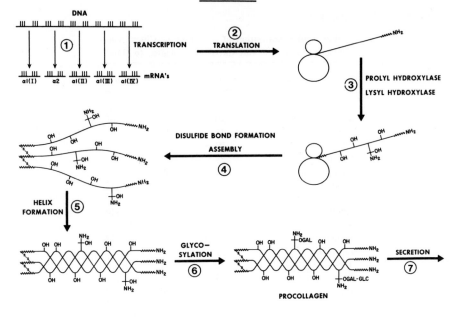

EXTRACELLULAR MATURATION

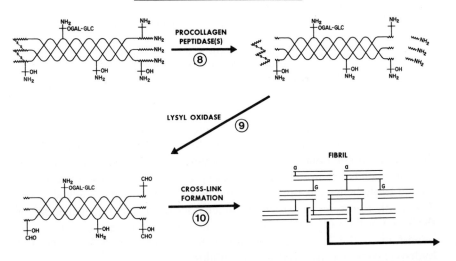

Fig. 4. An outline of the major steps in collagen synthesis and fibril formation. The steps shown represent a minimal number of control points. For example, several processes are involved in forming collagen from procollagen; some may be intracellular and some extracellular, and different enzymes are probably required to remove the amino + carboxy terminals of procollagen (Step 8). There are several enzymatic and nonenzymatic processes involved in the formation of cross-links, which include many different chemical species (Step 10). Note that the collagen molecule is drawn with the amino terminal on the right and the carboxy terminal on the left, opposite to the more usual presentation. (Figure kindly provided by Dr. Richard A. Salvador).

messenger for each chain, the possibility of a large polycistronic messenger that codes for several α chains and intermediate pieces has been suggested (Church *et al.*, 1971). The pro-α chains have additional sequences at both the amino and carboxy terminus (Tanzer *et al.*, 1974; Church *et al.*, 1974; Park *et al.*, 1975). The amino terminal sequence contains some helical sequences (Gly-Pro-Hyp) as well as nonhelical portions. It probably does not contain any disulfide bonds. The carboxy terminal portion is nonhelical and has a high content of cysteine. Selected lysyl and prolyl residues of the procollagen chains are hydroxylated, perhaps while the chains are still attached to the polyribosomes (Diegelmann *et al.*, 1973; Olsen *et al.*, 1973). These hydroxylations are catalyzed by two separate enzymes, peptidyl prolyl hydroxylase and peptidyl lysyl hydroxylase. The prolyl hydroxylase acts on the 4 position (there may be one or two 3-hydroxyprolines in collagen) and only on proline residues immediately preceding glycine and not those following glycine. Lysine is hydroxylated at the 5 position, usually on residues preceding glycine in the chain. Although about half the proline residues are usually hydroxylated, less than one-fifth the lysine residues are hydroxylated in bone and skin collagen. Both the lysyl and prolyl hydroxylases use α-ketoglutarate and molecular oxygen as substrates, and one molecule of succinate is formed on hydroxylation. Ferrous ion and ascorbic acid are required for activity. After release from the polyribosomes and hydroxylation, some of the hydroxylysine residues are glycosylated. Initially a galactose residue is added by a UDP galactosyltransferase. Glucose is added to some of the galactosylhydroxylysyl residues by the action of another enzyme, UDP glycosyltransferase. It is not known whether this addition of sugars occurs before or after the assembly of the procollagen molecules into a triple helix. It is possible that these residues are added to helical molecules, since the transferases can act on triple helical molecules *in vitro*. Glycosylation is thought to occur in the Golgi region or at the cell membrane and to be important in facilitating the transport of collagen out of the cell. Triple helix formation is probably initiated by noncovalent forces, but the formation of disulfide bridges between the cysteine residues in the nonhelical carboxy terminal procollagen sequence should accelerate this process and help place the helical portion of the α chain in register (Byers *et al.*, 1975). The helix is subsequently stabilized by noncovalent forces, chiefly hydrogen bonding, for which hydroxyproline is particularly important. Procollagen molecules are then extruded from the cell by a process that is probably active, since it can be inhibited by drugs such as colchicine (Ehrlich and Bornstein, 1972). After extrusion, the procollagen portion is cleaved from the main body of the molecule by procollagen peptidase. It is probable that this cleavage involves several enzymes and occurs in steps. Once the extra procollagen portion is removed, most of the collagen molecule is in the form of a triple helical structure with glycine in every third position, but a small nonhelical amino acid sequence remains at the amino terminal end of the molecule, and there is also a small nonhelical carboxy terminal portion. These may be important in cross-linking. The intramolecular cross-linking of collagen molecules and the intermolecular cross-linking of molecules in collagen fibrils is initiated by the oxidation of certain lysyl and hydroxylysyl residues through the action of an enzyme lysyl oxidase. This enzyme requires copper and is inhibited by the lathyrogen, β-aminopropionitrile. The residues formed, α-aminoadipic acid semialdehyde and 5-hydroxyaminoadipic acid semial-dehyde, can then interact with each other as well as with ϵ-amino groups of lysyl and hydroxylysyl residues to form cross-links. Glycosylated hy-droxylysine residues are probably involved in some cross-links (Eyre and Glimcher, 1973). A wide variety of cross-links can be formed, some of which have been identified as Schiff bases and aldol condensation prod-ucts (Tanzer, 1973). Initially, single cross-links are formed between two adjacent α chains of the same or neighboring molecules. Later more com-plex cross-links, involving three or four α chains, may be formed. Some of these could involve the addition of histidine or the formation of complex ring structures such as demosine, which is found in elastin.

Bone collagen does not differ from skin collagen in primary amino acid sequence, but does differ in posttranslational modifications, hydroxylation of lysine, glycosylation, and the distribution of cross-links. One striking difference is in the ratio of diglycosylated to monoglycosylated hy-droxylysine. About one-third of hydroxylysyl residues are glycosylated in both skin and bone, but the ratio of glucosylgalactosylhydroxylysine to galactosylhydroxylysine is 2.06 in skin and 0.47 in bone (Pinnell *et al.,* 1971). Bone and skin collagen also differ in the relative proportion of different specific cross-links. For example, the most abundant reducible cross-link in bone is probably dihydroxylysinonorleucine, a Schiff base formed from two hydroxylysine residues, one of which has been oxidized to 5-hydroxy-α-aminoadipic semialdehyde. In skin, there is an abundant reducible cross-link formed between aldohistidine and hydroxylysine, termed histidinohydroxymerodesmosine. These different cross-links are undoubtedly important in determining some of the physical properties of skin and bone collagen. Bone collagen is less soluble, more densely packed, and less hydrated than skin. If peptides containing these specific cross-links are resistant to breakdown and quantitatively excreted in the urine, then these might also serve as useful indicators of the relative rates of bone and skin matrix collagen degradation.

One of the major recent advances in collagen chemistry has been the discovery that there are several genetically distinct forms of collagen in different tissues. The collagen in cartilage has a different primary sequence of amino acids from the collagen in skin and bone (Miller and Lunde, 1973). Moreover, the cartilage collagen molecule consists of three identical α chains. These have been designated α_1 (II) for type II collagen. Cartilage collagen differs from that of bone and skin in having the greater portion of lysine residues hydroxylated and more of the hydroxylysyl residues glycosylated. The pattern of intermolecular cross-linking of cartilage collagen also differs from that of either skin or bone. Two other forms of collagen have been identified. One of these, type III collagen, is characteristically found in blood vessel walls and has also been found in skin, particularly in young animals (Byers *et al.*, 1974). It now appears more likely to represent a specialized form of collagen for elastic tissue, and a deficiency of type III collagen has been found in form of Ehlers–Danlos syndrome in which vascular lesions are prominent (Pope *et al.*, 1975). Type III collagen has three α_1 chains and has the unique feature that the extracellular fibrillar form contains disulfide bonds. Basement membrane or type IV collagen is the least well characterized. It is complex and may be heterogeneous. One unique property that separates it from other collagens is the presence of a large proportion of 3-hydroxyproline. In other collagens, 4-Hyp predominates and 3-Hyp represents at most one residue per thousand amino acids. In the basement membrane collagen there may be up to twenty 3-Hyp residues per thousand.

2. Fate of Collagen Breakdown Products

The mechanisms for initial degradation of collagen are discussed in Section VI,A. Collagen breakdown occurs not only by degradation of previously deposited extracellular collagen but also involves the breakdown of newly synthesized collagen. The proportion of newly formed collagen that is jettisoned is probably small. It has been suggested that α_1 and α_2 chains are synthesized at the same rate and that the excess α_2 is rapidly degraded, but this has not yet been demonstrated *in vivo*. A variety of fractions containing hydroxyproline have been identified in blood and urine. The materials in blood have not been intensively studied. Protein-bound hydroxyproline could represent not only large collagen fragments but also a hydroxyproline-containing component of complement, C1q. There is some evidence that non-protein-bound hydroxyproline in blood may reflect the rate of collagen breakdown, since there is some correlation between this value and osteolytic bone disease (Bishop and Smith, 1971).

The hydroxyproline-containing compounds in urine have been studied much more extensively. The nondialyzable fraction of urinary hydroxyproline is thought largely to represent products of newly synthesized collage that has been rapidly degraded rather than being deposited in extracellular matrix. The nondialyzable peptides are heterogeneous, their average molecular weight is about 5000, they have an amino acid composition typical of collagen, and they are susceptible to cleavage by bacterial collagenase (Krane *et al.*, 1970). Although they differ somewhat in average composition from bone collagens, it seems likely that a substantial portion of these polypeptides is derived from bone, since the amount increases when bone turnover is increased, as in Paget's disease. These peptides may reflect degradation of some of the newly formed collagen. In tracer studies with labeled proline, these peptides have much higher specific activity shortly after injection than the dialyzable peptides in urine.

Dialyzable hydroxyproline-containing peptides comprise over 90% of the total urinary hydroxyproline (Meilman *et al.*, 1963; Kivirikko, 1970). These consist primarily of the dipeptide prolylhydroxyproline and its diketopiperazine and the tripeptide glycylprolylhydroxyproline. These sequences are consistent with those in mammalian collagen and are presumed to represent products of collagen degradation. This material still represents only a small fraction of total collagen breakdown. Most of the amino acids released from bone are degraded into small carbon fragments (Adams, 1970; Kivirikko, 1970). The oxidation of hydroxyproline in the liver may be carried completely to CO_2 and water (Kuttan and Radnakrishnan, 1973), but a small amount of hydroxyproline is oxidized and excreted in the urine as pyrrole-2-carboxylic acid (Yamanishi *et al.*, 1972). Nevertheless the proportion of hydroxyproline in the oligopeptide which is excreted in the urine appears to be sufficiently constant so that the rate of excretion is a useful rough index of the rate of collagen degradation, and the amount in urine does reflect alterations in bone breakdown in a variety of diseases. The ratio of proline to hydroxyproline in urine may also serve as an index of bone turnover. This ratio is lower in growing children than in adults, largely because children excrete relatively more hydroxyproline (Nusgens and Lapiere, 1973). In addition to urinary hydroxyproline, the urinary excretion of other products may serve as useful indices of bone breakdown. Hydroxylysine excretion generally parallels that of hydroxyproline (Nagant de Deuxchaisnes and Krane, 1967), and, in particular, the glycosylated hydroxylysines may be useful indices, since the relative proportion of glucosylgalactosylhydroxylysine and galactosylhydroxylysine may reflect the relative contributions of skin and bone, respectively, to the excreted material because skin collagen has a relatively higher content of the dissacharide than bone collagen.

3. Other Bone Matrix Components

These noncollagenous organic components of bone are not fully characterized. A number of glycoproteins are present, one of which is an acidic sialoprotein (Herring *et al.*, 1971). Some of the proteins in bone may contain covalently linked phosphate (Spector and Glimcher, 1972). Both types of molecule could play a role in mineralization. There is recent evidence that bone takes up serum proteins, including a glycoprotein less acidic than Herring's sialoprotein, and albumin and incorporates them into bone matrix (Triffit and Owen, 1973). Sulfated acid mucopolysaccharides are present, and these may be concentrated in the uncalcified osteoid, since a decrease in sulfur content has been described at the calcification front (Baylink *et al.*, 1972). Phospholipids are present, and there is also evidence for a concentration of these at the calcification front (Wuthier, 1971). Hyaluronic acid synthesis is stimulated by PTH and appears to be associated temporally and quantitatively with increased bone resorption (Luben *et al.*, 1974a).

4. Chemistry of Bone Mineral

Bone mineral is quite different from pure hydroxyapatite, which is a macrocrystalline mineral of the composition $[Ca_{10}(PO_4)_6(OH)_2]$. Calcium and phosphate may be deposited initially not as hydroxyapatite but as amorphous calcium phosphate salts that are gradually transformed to hydroxyapatite crystals (Posner, 1973). These bone crystals are small and impure, and many ions other than the calcium, phosphate, and hydroxyl of pure synthetic hydroxyapatite are incorporated or adsorbed on their surfaces. There are substantial quantities of carbonate, sodium, potassium, and magnesium in bone mineral, mainly in the hydration shell; sodium is also incorporated in the crystal lattice. Pryophosphate can replace phosphate in the crystal surface and alter exchange properties (Jung *et al.*, 1973). Depending on the fluoride intake, some of the bone crystal is not hydroxyapatite but fluoroapatite, and this may also affect crystal size and solubility.

The small apatite crystals, with their hydration shells, provide an enormous surface for exchange, which can rapidly take up limited quantities of a variety of bone-seeking elements. These include not only the normal constituents of bone but also toxic elements such as strontium, lead, plutonium, uranium, and radium. The amount of amorphous calcium phosphate, of imperfect crystals, and of incompletely mineralized bone tends to decrease with the age of the bone and the age of the animal. With maturation, the exchange of various ions between bone and extracellular fluid, as well as the ability to take up bone-seeking elements, decreases (Vaughan, 1973).

5. Control of Mineralization

The mechanisms by which mineralization of bone is initiated and maintained remain an unsolved problem, although many possible factors have been identified (Howell, 1971) as discussed below.

a. Changes in Calcium Phosphate Activity Product at the Mineralizing Site. Alkaline phosphatase is very active in osteoblasts, and its activity in serum is increased when bone formation is increased. An attractive theory, which has been neither proved nor disproved in 50 years of study, is that alkaline phosphatase specifically increases phosphate concentration at the mineralizing site and initiates calcium phosphate salt deposition (Robison, 1923). Other calcium- or phosphate-binding substances, such as sialoprotein, phosphoproteins, or lipids, might release these ions and raise the local ion product. One difficulty with these concepts is that the calcium phosphate activity product in serum is already supersaturated with respect to initiation of mineralization of bone (or nonbone) collagen (Neuman and Neuman, 1958).

b. Membrane Function of Bone Cells. As noted above, the bone-forming surface is covered by a layer of osteoblasts that are connected to each other and to the underlying osteocytes. This would provide a barrier to the free movement of ions into bone, and there is evidence that ion concentrations on the bone surface are different from that of the extracellular fluid (Neuman and Ramp, 1971). Thus, mineralization could be controlled by selective transport of ions across cell membranes. The cells could not only regulate the calcium concentration at the bone surface but also affect mineralization by changing concentrations of other ions, particularly hydrogen and magnesium. A low concentration of either of these ions can enhance mineral deposition. A bone cell transport system could not explain why mineralization begins some distance from the initial site of matrix deposition.

c. Collagen Nucleation. The structure of the collagen fiber probably determines the initial localization of mineral deposition in bone. Mineral is first deposited in the hole zones produced by the characteristic staggered spacing of collagen molecules in the fiber (Fig. 2). This initial deposition may be related to binding of phosphate or calcium to some of the amino acid residues of collagen (Glimcher and Krane, 1968). X-Ray diffraction studies show that the gaps between collagen molecules are larger in bone and dentin, which mineralize, than in tendon, which does not mineralize (Katz and Li, 1972). In addition to localizing the initial deposits, the amount of collagen probably determines the amount and type of mineralization that ultimately develops. Some of the smaller holes in collagen may limit mineral deposition to an amorphous form of calcium phosphate (Katz and Li, 1973). In enamel, which has little collagen, there are high concentrations of hydroxyapatite in the form of large crystals, whereas in the adjacent dentin, which has much more collagen, the concentration of hydroxyapatite is lower and the crystals are smaller.

d. Noncollagenous Components of Matrix. As noted above, calcification may be affected by the glycoproteins, acid mucopolysaccharides, and lipids present in the osteoid and at the calcifying front. These substances could act to carry calcium and phosphate (Cotmore *et al.*, 1971) as bound ions, which could be released for deposition on partially mineralized bone or act as crystal nucleators. Their addition or removal could also affect collagen spacing and cross-linking.

e. Transport in Calcium "Packets." A variety of morphological studies suggest that bone cells may concentrate calcium in mitochondria (Matthews *et al.*, 1971) or other specialized vesicles. "Packets" containing calcium could be formed in the cells and transported to the calcifying site. The best evidence for membrane-bound vesicles containing mineral has been obtained in cartilage or fetal bone (Anderson, 1969; Ali *et al.*, 1970; Anderson and Reynolds, 1973). In all of these studies, the possibilities of artifactual translocation of calcium during fixation or processing make interpretation uncertain.

f. The Role of Inhibitors of Calcification. Calcification of collagen can be inhibited by adding serum or serum ultrafiltrates (Fleisch and Neuman, 1960). One inhibitory component that is effective in artificial systems is pyrophosphate. It is possible that the calcification requires the removal of pyrophosphate, since there is evidence that pyrophosphatase activity is increased at some calcifying areas of cartilage and bone (Alcock, 1972). However, pyrophosphate may accelerate calcium uptake in cultures of embryonic bone (Anderson and Reynolds, 1973). There are also organic inhibitors of calcification, probably peptides, whose removal may be required to initiate calcification. Rather than playing their major role in bone mineralization, these substances could be responsible for the fact that mineralization does not ordinarily occur in the collagen of skin, tendon, and other tissues which can be calcified *in vitro* with the calcium phosphate activity products found in extracellular fluid. In cartilage, there is evidence that a specific protein polysaccharide component can inhibit calcification and that the concentration of this component decreases at calcifying sites (Pita *et al.*, 1970; Cuervo *et al.*, 1973).

IV. DISTRIBUTION AND TRANSPORT OF CALCIUM AND PHOSPHATE

A. Distribution

1. Calcium

Although 98% of the total body calcium is in bone, largely in the form of hydroxyapatite crystals, which are relatively insoluble and inaccessible, there is a substantial amount of calcium in the body which undergoes rapid exchange. This exchange has been studied extensively by using tracer doses of radioactive calcium and by examining their distribution curves (Harris and Heaney, 1969). From these curves a variety of compartmental models can be deduced, but these are only theoretical and require simplifying assumptions by which a large number of slightly different exchanging systems are combined into a few groups.

The most rapidly exchanging pool is extracellular calcium, which is present in at least three forms—free calcium ions, calcium ions that are ionically bound but ultrafiltrable. and calcium bound to plasma protein. The serum contains several chelators of calcium, including citrate, and there is also probably some interaction between calcium and phosphate or carbonate, which decreases the calcium ion activity. Thus, the calcium ion activity in the plasma is about 1.1 to 1.2 mM (4.4 to 4.8 mg per 100 ml) while the ultrafiltrable calcium is about 1.4 to 1.5 mM (5.6 to 6 mg per 100 ml) normally. In serum the calcium that is not ultrafiltrable is bound to plasma protein. Most of the binding occurs on serum albumin, and in hypoalbuminemia the total serum calcium concentration will be decreased by about 0.8 to 1.0 mg per 100 ml for each 1 gm per 100 ml reduction in albumin concentration. When total serum proteins are altered by hemodilution or concentration and the albumin to globulin ratio is normal, a corrected total serum calcium concentration can be obtained from measured total calcium and total protein concentrations as follows (Husdan *et al.,* 1973):

$$\text{Corrected total Ca (mg/100 ml)} = \frac{\text{measured total Ca (mg/100 ml)}}{0.6 + [\text{total protein (gm/100 ml)}]/19.4}$$

This corrected value can then be compared with the normal range in a given laboratory. The various forms of extracellular calcium are in equilibrium with each other and exchange is almost instantaneous.

Total cell calcium concentrations are usually in the range of 1–2 mM, but this is not homogeneously distributed. The cells probably bind calcium to their surfaces, mainly on the acidic glycoproteins and possibly also on phospholipids. This calcium is also in rapid equilibrium with the extracellular calcium ion concentration. Intracellular calcium is highly compartmentalized. Only a small amount is present as free calcium ion, probably less than 10^{-6} M. The mitochondria are probably the major intracellular compartment for calcium, and this calcium can be sequestered so that it is not rapidly exchangeable (see Section VII). Some calcium is bound to proteins in the cytosol and to various components of the nucleus.

The calcium in bone can probably also be divided into multiple compartments with varying rates of exchange with extracellular calcium. Several methods of analysis have been proposed (Marshall, 1969). A small proportion of bone calcium is rapidly exchangeable and probably represents calcium not yet in the hydroxyapatite crystals but in the hydration layer of bone mineral. Exchange can also occur in newly formed crystals that are incomplete or during the conversion of amorphous calcium phosphate to hydroxyapatite. It is likely that much of the bone mineral does not represent perfect hydroxyapatite crystals and that because of this there is a component of diffuse exchange that can be extensive anatomically but so slow that in kinetic studies its contribution is relatively small.

Kinetic analysis of calcium exchange using tracers has been widely employed as a method for studying calcium metabolism in the skeleton. After the readily exchangeable compartments have equilibrated, the rate of loss of tracer calcium from the extracellular fluid can be equated with skeletal accretion of calcium; however, this is not identical with bone formation because of the intracrystalline exchange component noted above. Moreover, after a variable period of time in different species and in different metabolic states, some of the labeled calcium that has entered the skeleton will be returned to it by resorption. This will not be a problem with cortical haversian systems, which are formed and resorbed relatively slowly. However, in some trabecular bone there may be sufficiently rapid turnover that even early after the administration of tracer some of the isotope that was deposited is resorbed and returned to the circulation.

Despite these drawbacks the compartmental model has been widely used in assessing skeletal metabolism and can indicate marked changes in mineral accretion rate, such as might occur with large areas of rapid turnover in Paget's disease or with diminution in bone turnover or mineralization in osteomalacia or osteopetrosis.

2. Phosphate

The body content of phosphate is not concentrated in the skeleton to as great an extent as calcium. While only 1 or 2% of the body phosphate is in the extracellular fluid, about 20% is present in the cells, largely as organic phosphate bound to nucleotides and sugars. Unlike serum calcium, negligible amounts are bound to plasma protein, and less than 10% of serum inorganic phosphate is complexed by divalent cations. The remainder is ionized, and at normal body pH this is present largely as HPO_4^{2-}, with about 20% as $H_2PO_4^-$ and a trace of PO_4^{3-}. In addition to inorganic phosphate, there is normally a small amount of pyrophosphate in blood (3.5 μM), which may be important in regulating phosphate transport (Russell *et al.*, 1971).

In man the serum concentrations range between 3 and 6 mg of inorganic phosphorus per 100 ml, or 1 to 2 mM. Higher concentrations are found in children and are associated with rapid growth. Although calcium concentration in the blood of different mammals is constant, phosphate concentration varies widely. In young rats, phosphate concentration is normally 4 mM. As noted elsewhere, there does not appear to be any precise homeostatic regulation of serum phosphate concentration, and large changes can occur with loading or deprivation, with increases or decreases in cellular uptake as well as in disease. For example, the administration of insulin and glucose leads to increased entry and phosphorylation of glucose in cells and a sharp decrease in serum phosphate concentration.

Serum phosphate concentration does generally reflect the state of cellular phosphate. In uremia, changes in serum phosphate concentrations are accompanied by parallel changes in red blood cell ATP (Lichtman and Miller, 1970). Intracellular phosphate is present in many different molecular forms, and probably very little is not bound to nucleotides, sugars, or proteins. The plasma contains relatively little organic phosphate, although marked increases in concentration of phosvitin, a calcium-binding phosphoprotein, occur in egg-laying animals. Most of the phosphate in mineralized tissue is in the form of calcium phosphate salts, particularly hydroxyapatite. However, as noted above, phosphoproteins have been found in bone and enamel matrix, and phospholipids may also play a role in mineralization. Because of the complexity of phosphate metabolism and the much larger proportion in soft tissue compared with calcium, tracer studies with phosphate are not generally used for compartmental analysis and measurements of skeletal turnover.

B. Factors Controlling Entry and Exit of Calcium and Phosphate

The entry and exist of calcium and phosphate from the body are subject to tight hormonal regulation, and the amounts of calcium and phosphate in the extracellular fluid, cells, and bone are generally dependent on the amounts absorbed in the intestine and excreted by the kidney. There is controversy over the relative importance of kidney, bone, and intestine in minute-to-minute and day-to-day calcium regulation. Although this controversy cannot be settled, there are certain points upon which there is general agreement: (1) When dietary intake of calcium is low, serum calcium levels can be maintained by bone resorption, although this will occur at the expense of the structural function of the skeleton (Jowsey and Raisz, 1968). (2) When dietary phosphate is low or when phosphate deficiency occurs because of decreased intestinal absorption or excessive renal excretion, phosphate concentrations fall and phosphate supply for cellular metabolism decreases (Silvis and Paragas, 1972). The ability of the bone to provide needed phosphate is limited by the development of osteomalacia (Baylink *et al.,* 1971). (3) When calcium and phosphate supply are adequate, the intestine controls calcium entry by selective absorption. In individuals in calcium balance, who are neither adding calcium to nor losing it from the skeleton, the kidney excretion of calcium is equal to the amount absorbed. Rapid changes in renal tubular reabsorption of calcium can be used to adjust serum calcium concentration. Similarly, in patients in balance, renal excretion of phosphate is equal to the amount ingested, and rapid changes in tubular reabsorption can regulate serum concentrations. (4) When calcium intake is excessive, the intestine normally serves as a barrier to excessive absorption, although there is often transient hypercalcemia. When phosphate intake is excessive, the kidney is able to excrete the load quite rapidly, but prolonged phosphate loading can lead to secondary hyperparathyroidism and bone lesions (Laflamme and Jowsey, 1972). The mechanisms for this are discussed below.

These homeostatic responses depend on the normal functioning of three organ systems: intestine, kidney, and skeleton. Abnormalities in these systems or in the hormones that regulate them are the basis for the development of metabolic bone disease and disorders of calcium regulation. These systems are discussed elsewhere in this treatise. The following sections will summarize the major exit and entry controls for intestine and kidney. The controls for exit and entry in the skeleton will be discussed in detail subsequently, in terms of regulation of bone formation and resorption. It is important to recognize, however, that while long-term changes in mineral homeostasis are probably related to changes in net bone formation and resorption, the skeleton may also contribute substantially to short-term changes in serum calcium and phosphate concentration through transient alterations in entry of mineral into bone cells, the initiation of calcification, or the discharge of mineral from bone-resorbing cells (Neuman, 1972). The importance of such rapid changes in mineral homeostasis is much debated, and, despite strong theoretical arguments for such a role, the mechanisms involved are more speculated upon than understood.

1. The Role of Intestinal Absorption and Secretion in Mineral Metabolism

Changes in the intestinal absorption of calcium are important in the pathogenesis of metabolic bone disease (Avioli, 1972). At normal dietary intakes (600–1000 mg/day) less than half the dietary calcium is absorbed (Irwin and Kienholtz, 1973). Calcium is also secreted by the small intestine; some of this represents the calcium content of saliva and normal gastrointestinal secretions. The amount is small but fairly constant (about 100 mg/day, of which half is reabsorbed) and has not been shown to be under regulatory control.

Calcium is absorbed in the small intestine by a combination of facilitated diffusion and active transport. Active transport is greatest in the duodenum, but the duodenum is not the most important site of absorption. Under normal conditions the transit time through the duodenum is short, and the more distal segments absorb most of the calcium.

The major physiological regulations of calcium absorption are associated with changes in growth and dietary intake (Ireland and Fordtran, 1973). In young growing animals a larger proportion of dietary calcium is absorbed. In low calcium diets, the proportion absorbed is increased regardless of growth rate. Decreased absorption in high calcium diets reduces the likelihood of absorbing toxic amounts of calcium. Nevertheless, transient hypercalcemia can occur in otherwise normal individuals fed large amounts of calcium salts (Rushton et al., 1971). The way in which percent absorption is changed is not clear, but evidence suggests that it may be achieved by altering the metabolism of vitamin D (Omdahl and DeLuca, 1973; DeLuca, 1973).

Phosphate deficiency can also stimulate calcium absorption, but it is not established whether this is because of altered vitamin D metabolism (Bar and Wasserman, 1973).

Vitamin D is the major hormone controlling the intestinal absorption of calcium and probably also of phosphate (Wasserman and Taylor, 1973). Many features of vitamin D action on calcium transport have been identified. In the absence of vitamin D, both active and passive transfer of calcium across the intestinal mucosa are impaired. Enzyme activities that can be measured either as alkaline phosphatase- or as a calcium-dependent ATPase (Haussler et al., 1970) are dependent on vitamin D and are believed to be concerned with active calcium transport. Vitamin D stimulates the synthesis of a specific calcium-binding protein (Wasserman et al., 1971; Emtage et al., 1973) which appears to be localized in the brush border of the mucosal cells and in the cytoplasm of goblet cells. This calcium-binding protein may be important in facilitating diffusion as well as active transport. Vitamin D may also interact directly with lipids in the cell membrane and alter their permeability to calcium (Wong et al., 1970). Vitamin D can affect the transport of other ions, but this may be related to changes in calcium transport or may reflect general impairment of cell metabolism in vitamin D-deficient intestinal mucosa, which is morphologically altered (Spielvogel et al., 1972).

Many other agents affect calcium transport in the gut. Growth hormone, thyroxine, estrogens, and androgens can enhance calcium transport. Glucocorticoids inhibit calcium transport and oppose the effect of vitamin D. This appears to be a direct effect that occurs regardless of the amount or metabolism of the vitamin (Kimberg, 1969; Lukert et al., 1973). The role of PTH is controversial. In vivo studies suggest that the presence or absence of parathyroids has little effect on overall calcium absorption (Clark and Rivera-Cordero, 1970). *In vitro* studies show that large doses of PTH can increase intestinal calcium transport (Olson *et al.,* 1972), but since PTH may enhance 1,25-dihydroxyvitamin D_3 [1,25-$(OH)_2D_3$] synthesis, an increase in absorption might not necessarily be a direct effect. Calcitonin may have an inhibitory effect on calcium transport in the gut (Olson *et al.,* 1972), although this effect is not sufficient to impair absorption clinically. Large doses of calcitonin can also increase intestinal secretion of water and salts (Gray *et al.,* 1973).

There are many complex interactions between various ions in absorption. Strontium can impair calcium absorption markedly, and there is evidence that this effect is mediated by decreased production of 1,25-$(OH)_2D_3$ in the kidney (Omdahl and DeLuca, 1972). A similar mechanism may obtain for the impaired intestinal absorption that occurs with chronic administration of diphosphonates (Hill *et al.,* 1973). Magnesium and phosphate absorption can certainly occur independently of calcium, but there are important interactions. Deficiency of either ion is associated with impaired calcium absorption. Excesses have also been reported to impair calcium absorption, but the only well-documented effect is when large amounts of organic phosphate compounds or polyphosphates are administered.

2. Renal Regulation of Mineral Metabolism

A large number of factors can influence the renal excretion of calcium and phosphate (Massry *et al.,* 1973), and the kidney may be the most important organ regulating serum calcium concentration in certain species. The hamster, for example, has been shown to respond to changes in PTH largely by altering the renal excretion of calcium (Biddulph, 1972). Renal regulation of phosphate excretion also provides an indirect mechanism for regulating calcium. As Albright pointed out years ago (Albright and Reifenstein, 1948), the phosphaturic effect of PTH, by lowering blood serum phosphate concentration, can enhance calcium removal and impair calcium deposition in bone and thus increase serum calcium concentration.

As noted in greater detail in Chapter 2, the renal effects of PTH are complex. PTH has been shown to alter renal blood flow and glomerular filtration rate and to affect the transport of several different ions in the proximal and distal tubules. The increase in renal blood flow produced by PTH is transient and part of a general increase in the splanchnic blood flow (Charbon, 1969). In the proximal tubules, PTH stimulates adenyl cyclase to increase production of cyclic AMP. Because this effect precedes the effect of PTH on phosphate excretion and other ion changes and because many of the electrolyte transport effects of PTH can be mimicked by infusion of dibutyryl cyclic AMP (Agus et al., 1971), it has been assumed that the change in cyclic AMP concentration is responsible for the observed changes in transport in the proximal tubules. Not only the proximal tubular reabsorption of phosphate but also the reabsorption of sodium, calcium, magnesium, and bicarbonate are all decreased (Agus et al., 1973). Although this effect resembles the response to plasma volume expansion, changes in urinary excretion are quite different. The sodium rejected proximally under the influence of PTH is not accompanied by chloride, but is accompanied by phosphate and bicarbonate. As a result, chronic hyperparathyroidism is sometimes associated with systemic hyperchloremic acidosis.

Hyperparathyroidism increases the urinary excretion of calcium, largely because of an increase in filtered load resulting from increased serum calcium concentration. At any given filtered load, the urinary excretion of calcium is lower in the presence of PTH than in its absence, probably because PTH increases distal tubular calcium reabsorption (Agus et al., 1973).

The active vitamin D metabolites $25\text{-}OHD_3$ and $1,25\text{-}(OH)_2D_3$ have recently been found to increase tubular reabsorption of phosphate in parathyroidectomized, volume-expanded dogs (Puschett et al., 1972a,b). Earlier studies, however, suggested that massive doses of vitamin D might have a late phosphaturic effect in parathyroidectomized animals (Ney et al., 1968), so that the response may not be consistent. The direct effect of vitamin D on renal calcium transport is not known. Since hypercalciuria at normal serum concentration has been observed in patients with hypoparathyroidism maintained on vitamin D, this agent may not enhance tubular reabsorption of calcium as PTH does. The overall result of the direct and indirect effects of vitamin D on kidney, intestine, and bone is to increase both the calcium and phosphate concentration in the serum, thus increasing their product and enhancing mineralization of bone. An excess of vitamin D may produce pathological mineral deposits in soft tissue, including kidney. Thus, vitamin D acts as a mineralizing hormone, whereas PTH affects calcium ion regulation itself. The phosphaturic effect of PTH enhances the hypercalcemic effect and decreases the risk of soft tissue deposition.

The renal effects of calcitonin vary with different forms of the hormone, different modes of administration, and different species (see this volume, Chapter 2 and Volume II, Chapter 2). Calcitonin can increase the urinary excretion of phosphate, calcium, sodium, and magnesium (Paillard et al., 1972). The increase in sodium excretion, accompanied by chloride, can decrease extracellular fluid volume. Calcitonin has been shown to activate adenyl cyclase in the kidney and to increase cyclic AMP concentration, but there is evidence that the receptor is in a different location from that for PTH (Marx *et al.,* 1972a,b). These effects suggests a role for calcitonin in renal regulation of ion transport, but there is not enough information to determine the physiological importance of this role.

Many other hormones can affect calcium and phosphate transport in the kidney. Growth hormone administration is associated with an increase in calcium and a decrease in phosphate excretion in the urine. Thyroxine and glucocorticoids produce an increase in the excretion of both ions. These effects may be in part an indirect result of changes in intestinal absorption or changes in extracellular fluid volume which affect proximal tubular sodium reabsorption.

The kidney can regulate mineral metabolism not only by changing ion transport but also by altering the metabolism of the major humoral regulators themselves. As noted above, PTH is inactivated in the kidney and vitamin D is activated; moreover, these two processes may be related. Hence, it is not surprising that renal disease is associated with abnormalities of bone metabolism.

3. Other Routes of Mineral Transport

Calcium can be lost from the body through the skin. The amount of calcium in sweat is quite variable, usually it is less than 100 mg/day, but in a hot environment the value may increase to more than 1000 mg/day. Trace amounts of calcium are also lost in hair (Irwin and Kienholz, 1973). Calcium requirement increases greatly during pregnancy and lactation. Up to 1 gm of calcium per day may be required for fetal growth in late pregnancy, and 200 to 400 mg are secreted in milk by nursing mothers. Little is known about calcium transport in placenta and breast, but a binding protein has been identified in mammary tissue, and vitamin D could play a regulatory role. Estrogen, as well as prolactin, is clearly important in mammary development and milk production, but mammals do not appear to have the elaborate estrogen-dependent calcium transport and storage systems found in egg-laying animals.

V. REGULATION OF BONE FORMATION

Much of the growth and development of the skeleton is determined genetically and is not mediated by differences in the output of hormones; thus, the short stature of pygmies is due to a genetically determined rate of tissue growth and not to a deficiency in growth hormone. Some of the skeletal determinants appear to be sex linked, and abnormal height is often associated with abnormalities of the X or Y chromosomes. Evidence for the importance of genetic factors in determining total bone mass has recently been obtained from studies of bone density in twins (Smith *et al.*, 1973).

The size and shape of the skeleton are further modified by stress. Trabecular pattern, cortical thickness, and even bone length can be altered by changes in muscular tension or weight bearing. The mechanism by which stress determines skeletal remodeling may involve development of small electric currents in bone in response to changes in pressure (Bassett, 1968). This piezoelectric effect can result from stress upon the collagenous matrix, rather than on mineral (Marino *et al.*, 1971).

There are probably numerous humoral determinants of skeletal growth and development (Raisz and Bingham, 1972). Although many hormones take part, we know remarkably little about their mechanism of action. It is likely that bone growth is regulated by alteration of matrix formation, since matrix is laid down first and calcification follows. However, the rate of calcification may be a hormonally controlled system in which events at the calcification front are fed back to the matrix-forming cells; when calcification is rapid, osteoid formation keeps pace; when calcification is slowed, osteoid formation also gradually slows. Anatomically this feedback is feasible, since the osteoblasts are in communication with the calcified matrix through their processes and tight junctions with osteocytes. Such a control would explain the close correlation between serum calcium and phosphate concentration and bone growth (Stauffer *et al.*, 1973; Wergedal *et al.*, 1973; Baylink *et al.*, 1971) and the apparent cessation of new matrix formation when the osteoid seams become wide in rickets or osteomalacia (Baylink *et al.*, 1970). Restoration of calcification may restore growth. This can be observed in experimental animals even when vitamin D deficiency is used to produce the rickets, and phosphate is used to cure it.

Among the humoral agents, only growth hormone is considered to increase linear growth specifically, but thyroxine may play an important role (Thorngren and Hansson, 1973). Thyroxine has been shown to enhance bone turnover, and growth is accelerated in hyperthyroidism (Schlesinger *et al.*, 1973) and impaired in hypothyroidism. Thyroxine has recently been shown to stimulate bone resorption directly (Mundy *et al.*, 1976).

Cortisol probably has an important permissive role in skeletal growth. Growth is impaired with both deficiency and excess of glucocorticoids. The latter effect is probably due to a direct inhibition of the development of osteoblasts from their precursors (Jee *et al.*, 1972; Dietrich *et al.*, 1976).

Androgens and estrogens may affect skeletal growth by altering maturation of the epiphyses, by stimulating bone formation, by inhibiting bone resorption, or, indirectly, by altering muscular development. While an excess of these hormones accelerates growth in preadolescents, final height is often below normal. Large doses of estrogen can impair growth in laboratory animals. There are probably other skeletal growth factors that have not been identified. It has been suggested that vitamin D can enhance bone matrix formation directly (Cañas *et al.*, 1969), but it is also possible that impaired growth in vitamin D deficiency is due to inadequate calcium or phosphate supply for bone cell function and calcification (Wergedal *et al.*, 1973).

Parathyroid hormone could regulate growth directly or indirectly. In tissue culture, active osteoblasts disappear in the presence of high concentrations of PTH, and the incorporation of proline into collagen is decreased (Raisz, 1970b). PTH could also impair growth indirectly by lowering serum phosphate concentration. However, since in clinical and experimental hyperparathyroidism the number and activity of osteo- blasts often increases, the effects of PTH on bone formation *in vivo* may differ from those observed in tissue culture. Increased bone forma- tion in hyperparathyroidism could be an indirect effect mediated by hypercalcemia or increased bone resorption. Clearly, the changes in bone resorption and formation are linked in some way; the mechanism is unknown but could be related to changes in stress.

Growth hormone may have a direct effect on the skeleton, but it also has an indirect effect mediated by sulfation factor or somatomedin (Daughaday, 1971). Somatomedin is produced by the liver (and possibly the kidney) in response to growth hormone. It stimulates growth in carti- lage and probably also in muscle, but has not been shown to act on bone itself. Growth hormone also increases serum phosphate concentration. There is a rough correlation between serum phosphate concentration and growth rate not only within a given species but also among different species of mammals. In organ culture, increased phosphate concentration not only enhances mineralization of bone but also increases the amount of bone matrix produced (Bingham and Raisz, 1974). Bone growth is im- paired not only when the supply of minerals is deficient but also in protein-deprived animals (LeRoith and Plimstone, 1973). Ascorbic acid deficiency greatly impairs bone growth (Chen and Raisz, 1975) because collagen cannot be hydroxylated normally, and this impairs both triple helix formation (Jimenez *et al.*, 1973) and cross-linking.

The role of calcitonin in bone growth is disputed (Hirsch and Munson, 1969). In most experiments, calcitonin administration has not increased growth, and in the few experiments that suggest that bone growth is increased by calcitonin, the changes are small (Dietrich *et al.*, 1976).

Other bone growth factors undoubtedly exist and may include some component of the bone matrix itself. Decalcified bone matrix causes new bone formation when implanted into the skin (Urist, 1970). The presence of an "inductive principle" has been postulated to explain this phenomenon, but no specific compound has been isolated. Certain cell types may be inducible to osteogenesis including bone marrow and thymus cells (Friedenstein and Lalykina, 1972). Pyrophosphate (Fleisch and Russell, 1970) and organic inhibitors of calcification (Howard *et al.*, 1967) may be important in regulating bone mineralization and growth, although a more likely physiological role would be to prevent the calcification of nonbone collagen exposed to extracellular fluid in tendon, skin, and other tissues.

VI. REGULATION OF BONE RESORPTION

The regulation of bone resorption has been more intensively studied than bone formation, perhaps because bone resorption is important not only for growth but for calcium regulation, or because it is easier to study experimentally. One result of this has been an increasing emphasis on the role of factors influencing bone resorption in the pathogenesis of metabolic and inflammatory bone disease (Raisz and Horton, 1973).

It is important to differentiate between true bone resorption, which involves the net removal of both mineral and matrix, and any transfers of mineral alone, in which no net resorption takes place. Such transfers could be important in the minute-to-minute regulation of calcium and phosphate homeostasis. However, it is not known whether such net transfers represent movement on and off bone matrix or in and out of bone cells. True bone resorption is probably a function of both osteoclasts and osteocytes, but quantitatively osteoclasts account for most bone breakdown (Liu *et al.*, 1974).

A. Parathyroid Hormone and Bone Resorption

Parathyroid hormone has several effects on bone cells which occur in a few minutes, including activation of adenyl cyclase to produce an increase in cellular cyclic AMP concentration (Chase and Aurbach, 1970), increased entry of calcium into cells (Parsons and Robinson, 1968; Robertson *et al.*, 1972), increase in the uptake and incorporation of uridine (Peck *et al.*, 1972), and both increases and decreases in the uptake of different amino acids (Phang *et al.*, 1970). *In vivo*, PTH causes a transient decrease in serum calcium and phosphate concentration, which is followed in 1 or 2 hours by an increase, due presumably to removal of calcium and phosphate from bone (Fig. 5). A similar pattern has been

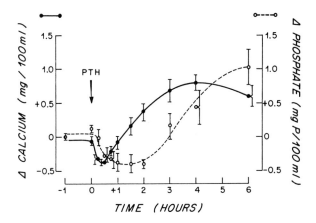

Fig. 5. Early effects of PTH on serum calcium and phosphate concentration in the dog. Twenty USP units per kg of PTH were given intravenously in unanesthetized dogs. The points are means and the vertical lines standard errors for eight experiments in three animals. (From Parsons *et al.*, 1971. Reprinted with permission of the publisher).

found in organ culture (Robertson *et al.*, 1972). It is not certain which, if any, of these early effects of PTH is related to bone resorption. Since the majority of cells in bone are not osteoclasts or resorbing osteocytes, there may be effects on the rest of the bone cell population that may have little to do with the resorptive response. However, some acute effects of PTH on osteoclasts have been identified. Osteoclasts can be divided into two populations by differences in their membrane potential (Mears, 1971); one population has a potential higher than 20 mV and the other a low potential of around 10 mV. After PTH, all the osteoclasts were found to have the lower potential. Moreover, by autoradiography, the incorporation of uridine into osteoclasts was found to be increased within 1 hour after PTH administration (Bingham *et al.*, 1969).

Early calcium mobilization by PTH could be due to activation of existing osteoclasts or resorbing osteocytes, but further stimulation of bone resorption, which takes place over many hours or days after the administration of large doses of PTH, requires cell transformation and the formation of new osteoclasts. Hence it is not surprising that this effect can be blocked by inhibitors of RNA and protein synthesis (Raisz, 1965). In fact, the delivery of calcium from bone to blood is so sensitive to such inhibitors that hypocalcemia is one of the earliest toxic effects of agents such as actinomycin D, mithramycin, and puromycin.

An important question that remains unanswered is the relation of PTH stimulation of adenyl cyclase to the late effect on bone resorption. Supporting a direct connection are the observations that some other agents that increase cyclic AMP levels can enhance bone resorption *in vitro* and *in vivo*. These include dibutyryl cyclic AMP, theophylline, and prostaglandins (Klein and Raisz, 1970, 1971). These agents, however, do not completely mimic the effects of PTH (Herrmann-Erlee and van der Meer, 1974). For example, they are not as effective in inducing the formation of osteoclasts after brief application (Raisz *et al.*, 1972b). Application of PTH for 8 hours or less in organ culture produces prolonged osteoclastic resorption, which continues until the bone mineral and matrix are completely removed. This response cannot be obtained or enhanced with dibutyryl cyclic AMP or theophylline, but vitamin D metabolites, which have not been shown to increase cyclic AMP concentrations in bone, can induce osteoclastic resorption. These results may be complicated by the fact that calcitonin also increases cyclic AMP concentration in bone (Heersche *et al.*, 1974), but is an inhibitor rather than a stimulator of resorption. Cyclic AMP could be the mediator of both stimulation and inhibition of bone resorption if it acted through pathways that were morphologically and functionally separate.

Once stimulation of bone resorption is established, the bone tissue shows many distinct biochemical features. After PTH treatment, glucose oxidation is enhanced, lactate and citrate production is increased, and citrate oxidation is impaired (Martin *et al.*, 1965). A number of enzymes are released into the medium in organ cultures of bones treated with PTH. These include a collagenase that probably initiates the degradation of matrix, since it can act on insoluble cross-linked collagen to produce large cleavage products (Fig. 4). Collagenase may be activated from a precursor or zymogen form (Woessner, 1973; Vaes, 1972b; Gross, 1974). Further degradation of collagen and of noncollagen glycoproteins and of mucopolysaccharides in bone is probably carried out by a number of acid hydrolases of lysosomal origin (Vaes, 1968). These hydrolases could function to complete the degradation of bone collagen once the initial cleavage by collagenase has occurred, or they could function to break down noncollagenous matrix components. Moreover, there is recent evidence that a lysosomal enzyme, cathepsin B, can degrade insoluble collagen directly (Burleigh *et al.*, 1974). Acid phosphatase activity appears to be associated with both osteoclastic and osteocytic bone resorption by histochemical localization (Wergedal and Baylink, 1969), but its specific role is not known.

Parathyroid hormone-stimulated bone resorption is also characterized by an increase in the synthesis of hexosamine-containing macromolecules (Johnston *et al.*, 1972). Autoradiographic studies show that labeled glucosamine is taken up by osteoclasts and concentrated at their brush borders (Owen and Shetlar, 1968). There is also labeled material on the bone surface adjacent to the osteoclasts. Chemical studies indicate that much of the PTH-stimulated increase in hexosamine labeling is due to increased synthesis and turnover of hyaluronic acid (Luben *et al.*, 1974b). Fibroblastic proliferation, as well as an increase in the number and activity of osteoclasts, occurs in PTH-stimulated bones, and presumably some of these fibroblasts migrate and coalesce to form new osteoclasts. Fibroblasts characteristically produce large amounts of hyaluronic acid, which could be important for their migration (Toole and Gross, 1971). It is also possible that the osteoclasts themselves are responsible for increased hyaluronate synthesis and use the viscoelastic, ion binding, and molecular exclusion properties of this macromolecule to help in their function.

Many of these changes are probably general characteristics of bone resorption regardless of the stimulus, although most studies have been done with PTH. Osteoclastic proliferation, calcium removal, collagenolysis, increased lysosomal enzymes, and increased hexosamine labeling have all been seen in response to other stimulators of resorption.

B. Vitamin D and Bone Resorption

Although the ability of vitamin D to mobilize calcium from bone *in vivo* was demonstrated years ago, *in vitro* studies showed relatively little effect on bone resorption. This discrepancy was due to the requirement for metabolic activation of vitamin D. As noted above, both 25-OHD$_3$ and 1,25-(OH)$_2$D$_3$ can stimulate bone resorption in organ culture (Raisz *et al.*, 1972a), but 1,25-(OH)$_2$D$_3$ is at least 100 times more potent than 25-OHD$_3$ *in vitro* (Fig. 6). Nevertheless, 25-OHD$_3$ could be important in physiological regulation of bone resorption, since it circulates at much higher concentrations than 1,25-(OH)$_2$D$_3$ and at these concentrations can act synergistically with PTH to stimulate bone resorption *in vitro* (Raisz, 1970a). The active vitamin D metabolites, like PTH, increase the activity and number of osteoclasts and are sensitive to inhibitors of RNA and protein synthesis. Moreover, both stimulators cause prolonged resorption after relatively brief exposure. There is evidence that 1,25-(OH)$_2$D$_3$ is concentrated in bone cell nuclei, which could account for its prolonged action (Wong *et al.*, 1972). The synergistic effects of vitamin D metabolites and PTH on bone could explain the marked decrease of PTH responsiveness in animals deficient in vitamin D.

In addition to vitamin D$_3$, other forms of vitamin D probably also require 25-hydroxylation, but some may not require 1-hydroxylation. Dihydrotachysterol is of particular interest because it is considered to have a greater hypercalcemic effect, relative to its effect on intestinal calcium transport. This compound is ineffective in organ culture, but the 25-hydroxy derivative is about as potent as 25-OHD$_3$ in stimulating bone resorption (Trummel *et al.*, 1971).

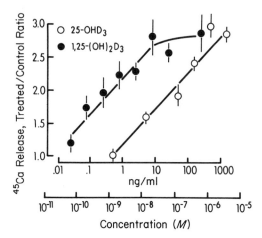

Fig. 6. Dose–response curves for stimulation of bone resorption from fetal rat bones *in vitro* by 1,25-(OH)$_2$D$_3$ and 25-OHD$_3$. Paired bones previously labeled with ^{45}Ca were cultured for 48 hours with or without the indicated doses of vitamin D metabolites and the treated–control radio of release of ^{45}Ca into the medium was measured. The dose–response curves are parallel and have similar maxima, but dihydroxyvitamin D is approximately 100 times as potent as its precursor. (From Raisz *et al.*, 1972a, *Science* **175,** 4023. Copyright 1972 by the American Association for the Advancement of Science).

C. Calcitonin and Bone Resorption

Soon after the discovery of calcitonin, its ability to inhibit the movement of mineral from bone to blood was demonstrated both *in vivo* and *in vitro* (Hirsch and Munson, 1969). This effect has generally been attributed to direct inhibition of calcium removal from bone, but the alternative possibility that the ion primarily affected is phosphate has been suggested (Talmage *et al.*, 1972). The magnitude of the acute hypocalcemia produced by calcitonin appears to depend upon the rate of bone resorption at the time. Young animals with rapid bone turnover, animals in which resorption is stimulated by pharmacological means or by low calcium diets, and patients with diseases characterized by increased resorption show the greatest hypocalcemic effects. The acute effects of calcitonin on mineral transport appear to be mediated, at least in part, by a direct effect on the osteoclast. Calcitonin produces a marked decrease in the amount of active ruffled border in osteoclasts, which can be correlated with inhibition of mineral removal (Holtrop *et al.*, 1974; Kallio *et al.*, 1972). Calcitonin increases the membrane potential of isolated osteoclasts, an effect opposite to that of PTH, which may be related to the change in ruffled borders. When calcitonin is given in organ culture, the effects on mineral and matrix removal are not always parallel. Breakdown of matrix may persist (Brand and Raisz, 1972) in fetal bone cultures, which contain much partially mineralized collagen. The effects on enzyme release are variable (Reynolds, 1968; Vaes, 1972a). When calcitonin is administered *in vivo,* mineral and matrix resorption, as measured by calcium and hydroxyproline excretion, are inhibited in a parallel fashion (Rasmussen and Pechet, 1970), presumably because the bone is fully mineralized and calcium must be removed before lytic enzymes can act on the matrix.

The effects of calcitonin on bone resorption are rapid in onset, dissipate once the hormone is removed, and appear to be independent of RNA and protein synthesis. The speed of recovery from calcitonin depends on removal of the hormone and, as noted earlier, this is quite variable for different species. For example, the greater apparent potency as well as duration of action of salmon calcitonin compared with porcine calcitonin probably results from its longer half-life. Even if administration is continued, the effect of calcitonin may be overcome by increasing the secretion of PTH. Increased PTH levels have been demonstrated after calcitonin administration and are correlated with a disappearance of the initial hypocalcemic effect (Riggs *et al.,* 1971). After prolonged use, foreign calcitonins may show loss of effectiveness because of antibody formation (Singer *et al.,* 1972).

Even when active calcitonin is present continuously and PTH is not increased, inhibition of resorption may not be sustained. *In vitro* this phenomenon has been termed *escape* (Fig. 7). Bones in which osteoclastic resorption is stimulated either by PTH or vitamin D will show marked inhibition of resorption by calcitonin, but with time, resorption increases again despite the continued administration of the inhibitor. This loss of sensitivity appears to depend on the continuous presence of calcitonin. Sensitivity may be restored if the hormone is removed for a day or two (Raisz *et al.,* 1967).

We know little about the action of calcitonin on bone at the molecular level. The rapid effects of calcitonin, its independence from changes in RNA and protein synthesis, the fact that concurrent administration of calcitonin and PTH does not prevent the subsequent induction of resorption by PTH, and the fact that osteoclasts lose their brush borders but show little other morphological change after calcitonin administration all indicate that calcitonin probably acts on transport systems rather than by causing cell modulation. The number of osteoclasts and lytic osteocytes appears to decrease with chronic administration of calcitonin, but it is not known whether this is a direct effect of the hormone.

D. Other Hormones That Affect Bone Resorption

There are many hormones that affect bone resorption but have not yet been proved to be physiological regulators of this process. Bone-resorbing

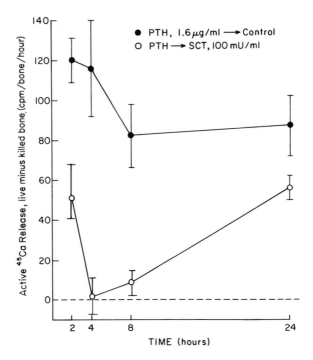

Fig. 7. Effect of calcitonin on bone resorption in organ culture. The points are means and the vertical lines standard errors for 4–12 cultures. When fetal rat long bones labeled with ^{45}Ca were pretreated with PTH for 48 hours and transferred to fresh medium, live bones showed a sustained active ^{45}Ca release compared to killed controls. This release was rapidly inhibited by adding salmon calcitonin (SCT) to the medium, but despite addition of fresh SCT, by 24 hours the SCT-treated bones had begun to resorb again. These changes were accompanied by an initial decrease and a later increase in the proportion of osteoclasts which showed active ruffled borders. (Data from Raisz *et al.,* 1973.)

cells, like bone-forming cells, require thyroxine for normal activity, so that bone resorption is reduced in thyroxine deficiency. With thyroxine excess, both formation and resorption are increased (Krane *et al.,* 1956). There may be a greater effect on resorption, since many hyperthyroid patients develop slight to moderate hypercalcemia and others, particularly older women, show a decrease in bone mass with symptomatic osteoporosis. Direct stimulation of resorption by thyroid hormones was recently demonstrated in tissue culture (Mundy *et al.,* 1976).

Glucocorticoids have different effects on bone resorption, depending upon the model system used for study. The induction of prolonged resorption by brief administration of PTH and vitamin D metabolites can be inhibited by pretreatment with cortisol at concentrations of $10^{-6}M$ or less (Raisz *et al.,* 1972c). Pretreatment with glucocorticoids also diminishes the response to PTH *in vivo* (Magargal *et al.*, 1969). Inhibition is incomplete and can be overcome by high concentrations of PTH or vitamin D given continuously (Raisz *et al.*, 1972c; Stern, 1969). The inhibitory glucocorticoid effect may be due to an inhibition of the transformation of precursor cells to osteoclasts (Jee *et al.*, 1972). *In vivo* glucocorticoid excess can stimulate bone resorption, but this could be an indirect effect. Glucocorticoids inhibit calcium absorption in the gut and increase calcium excretion in the urine, which in turn could lead to increased PTH secretion and hence increased bone resorption (Jee *et al.*, 1972).

In vivo the administration of estrogens or androgens is usually associated with decreased bone resorption, and in organ culture high concentrations of these agents can inhibit resorption (Stern, 1969; Atkins *et al.*, 1972). It is not clear whether sex hormones have a physiological role in controlling resorption.

There are a number of other agents that can affect bone resorption but whose physiological and pathological importance is even less clear. Glucagon can inhibit bone resorption, but only at relatively high concentrations (Stern and Bell, 1970). Prostaglandins stimulate resorption *in vitro* at low concentrations, but even these levels probably do not occur in the circulation under physiological conditions, and prostaglandins do not cause hypercalcemia *in vivo* (Klein and Raisz, 1970). Prostaglandins may be important in pathological bone resorption both in neoplastic disease (Tashjian *et al.*, 1972) and in the inflammatory response associated with humoral immunity (Raisz *et al.*, 1974).

E. Nonhormonal Influences on Bone Resorption

The rate of bone resorption can be greatly affected by the ions in the surrounding medium. These effects can be quite complex. Increasing the amount of calcium available can enhance the initial response to PTH (Raisz *et al.*, 1972a), but once resorption is stimulated, the osteoclasts can function independently of the ambient calcium concentration (Raisz and Niemann, 1969). Phosphate (Raisz and Niemann, 1969), pyrophosphate (Orimo *et al.*, 1969), and diphosphonates (Russell *et al.*, 1970), which are pyrophosphate analogues, have all been shown to inhibit bone resorption, but the results are not uniform under different experimental conditions. It is possible that these ions act by altering mineralization at the resorbing surface and that the prior state of that surface will determine how effective they are. The diphosphonates were thought to act as pyrophosphate analogues that were more effective because they were not hydrolyzed; however, recently high doses of diphosphonate were found to decrease $1,25\text{-}(OH)_2D_3$ formation by the kidney, which could account for its dual inhibitory effects on resorption and mineralization (Hill *et al.*, 1973). Magnesium deficiency is associated with hypocalcemia, and this has been attributed to decreased responsiveness of the skeleton to PTH in man (Estep *et al.,* 1969; Reddy *et al.,* 1973); however, in some animal experiments no change in the response to PTH was observed (Hahn *et al.,* 1972).

Bone resorption, particularly in response to PTH, is generally increased in acidosis and decreased in alkalosis. Carbonic anhydrase inhibitors can block the response to PTH (Minkin and Jennings, 1972). These observations have led to the concept that generation of acid from CO_2 and the formation of organic acids are important for resorption, either because they affect calcium removal from bone or because they activate lysosomal enzymes that break down matrix (Vaes, 1968). Decreased intracellular hydrogen ion concentration in alkalotic or carbonic anhydrase inhibited cells might also increase nonspecific binding of calcium to various constituents of the cell at sites where protons and calcium compete and thus alter calcium transport and other calcium-dependent reactions.

VII. CELLULAR CALCIUM REGULATION

This chapter has emphasized regulation of mineral metabolism at the organ level. Nevertheless, complete understanding of disorders of mineral metabolism will require a better knowledge of the general cellular physiology of calcium and other related ions and the mechanisms by which these ions are transported intracellularly. We know that in those cells in which it can be estimated, particularly muscle and nerve, the ionized calcium concentration is low, probably about 10^{-6} to $10^{-7} M$, compared to an extracellular concentration of $10^{-3} M$ (Borle, 1967). Much of the calcium connected with the cell is not ionized but bound to a number of different sites on the surface of the cell, within the membrane and in various subcellular particles. The binding substances probably include phospholipids (Cotmore *et al.,* 1971), glycoproteins (Sottogasa *et al.,* 1972), and phosphoproteins. The last may be of particular importance for intracellular calcium regulation since there are protein kinases that can alter phosphorylation of intracellular protein, and these enzymes can be controlled by the second messenger for many hormonal actions—cyclic AMP (Rasmussen *et al.,* 1972). Glycoproteins containing sialic acid could be responsible for calcium binding on the outer cell coat, or glycocalyx, where much of the cell calcium is found. This binding, as well as phospholipid binding in the membrane, could control the passive fluxes of calcium in and out of cells by facilitating or impeding diffusion. It is presumed that all cells contain an active calcium extrusion pump that enables them to maintain the lower intracellular ionic concentration and is dependent for its source of energy on a calcium-activated membrane ATPase (Schatzmann and Vincenzi, 1969; Brinkley, 1973).

Mitochondria are known to take up calcium and release it by active processes that can be altered by hormones (Lehninger, 1970). Whether mitochondrial calcium movements are important for metabolic regulation (Borle, 1972) or simply represent a scavenger function when intracellular calcium is high has not been established.

Within the cell, a variety of sites have been identified where calcium movements are important in regulating cellular function. In muscle, initiation of contraction depends on movement of calcium from storage sites to activate an actin–myosin ATPase, and relaxation depends on energy-dependent removal of this calcium to the sarcoplasmic reticulum (Martonosi *et al.,* 1971). Many forms of cellular secretion that involve extrusion of material stored in granules are calcium dependent, and it is possible that calcium binding to the secretory granules is essential for the extrusion process (Rubin, 1970). This role of calcium may explain the stimulatory effects of calcium infusions on gastric and pancreatic secretions—both exocrine and endocrine (Barreras, 1973; Levant *et al.,* 1973; D'Souza and Floch, 1973).

Calcium may also be the mediator for certain humoral effects on cell growth (Perris, 1971). The essential role of extracellular calcium in regulating nerve excitation has long been recognized. There is recent evidence that transport of both calcium and monovalent cations in the nerve membrane is responsible for nerve excitation (Watanabe and Tasaki, 1971).

Although calcium entry across the cell membrane appears to occur largely by passive diffusion, the rate of entry can be markedly altered when cells are activated. This is true not only for neural tissue, but such effects probably also occur in response to PTH and vitamin D; for example, PTH probably increases passive calcium entry into bone and kidney cells and possibly hepatic cells (Chausmer *et al.,* 1972), and vitamin D can alter passive entry of calcium in intestinal cells. These agents probably also act on active calcium transport, but these effects may be more indirect, depending on synthesis of binding proteins or some more complex cell transformation. Calcium exchange also increases when liver cells are activated by other hormones, such as glucagon (Friedmann and Rasmussen, 1970). It is not yet clear whether calcitonin affects passive entry of calcium or acts primarily on active transport.

In view of the importance of calcium in cell function, it is not surprising that disorders of calcium metabolism can produce a wide variety of subtle clinical abnormalities in apparently unrelated systems. In hyperparathyroidism, a long list of abnormalities has been found in a wide variety of organ systems (Raisz, 1971). Among the most recently observed is an abnormality of insulin metabolism (Kim *et al.*, 1971) and of the function of a specific type of motor nerve fiber (Aurbach *et al.*, 1973).

GENERAL REFERENCES

The following general references provide extensive background information and documentation for many of the points made in this chapter.

Aurbach, G., ed. (1976). Volume on calcium regulation and bone metabolism. "Handbook of Physiology, Sect. 7, Vol. VII, Williams & Wilkins, Baltimore, Maryland. Extensive reviews of endocrine regulation of skeletal metabolism.

Bourne, G. H., ed. (1972). "The Biochemistry and Physiology of Bone," 2nd ed. Academic Press, New York. This three-volume, multiauthored text contains detailed chapters of varied quality but provides good surveys of the earlier literature.

Raisz, L. G., Mundy, G. R., Dietrich, J. W., and Canalis, E. M. (1976). Hormonal regulation of mineral metabolism. *In* "International Review of Physiology" (S. M. McCann, ed.), Vol. X. Medical and Technical Publishing Co., Ltd., Lancaster, England. This is a review of the pertinent literature from 1972 to July, 1975.

Talmage, R. V., Owen, M., and Parsons, J. A., eds. (1975). "Calcium Regulating Hormones," Proc. 5th Parathyroid Conf. Experta Med. Found., Amsterdam. With its predecessors, these proceedings review many new developments in this field.

Vaughan, J. (1975). "The Physiology of Bone," 2nd ed. Oxford Univ. Press, London and New York. An excellent introductory volume.

REFERENCES

Adams, E. (1970). *Int. Rev. Connect. Tissue Res.* **5,** 1.

Agus, Z. S., Puschett, J. B., Senesky, D., and Goldberg, M. (1971). *J. Clin. Invest.* **50,** 617.

Agus, Z. S., Gardner, L. B., Beck, L. H., and Goldberg, M. (1973). *Am. J. Physiol.* **224,** 1143.

Albright, F., and Reifenstein, E. (1948). "The Parathyroid Glands and Metabolic Bone Disease." Williams & Wilkins, Baltimore, Maryland.

Alcock, N. W. (1972). *Clin. Orthop. Relat. Res.* **86,** 287.

Ali, S. Y., Sajdera, S. W., and Anderson, H. C. (1970). *Proc. Natl. Acad. Sci. U.S.A.* **67,** 1513.

Anderson, H. C. (1969). *J. Cell Biol.* **41,** 59.

Anderson, H. C., and Reynolds, J. J. (1973). *Dev. Biol.* **34,** 211.

Atkins, D., Zanelli, J. M., Peacock, M., and Nordin, B. E. C. (1972). *J. Endocrinol.* **54,** 107.

Aurbach, G. D., Mallette, L. E., Patten, B. M., Heath, D. A., Doppman, J. L., and Bilezikian, J. P. (1973). *Ann. Intern. Med.* **79,** 566.

Avioli, L. V. (1972). *Arch. Intern. Med.* **129,** 345.

Avioli, L. V. (1974). *In* "Heparin" (R. A. Bradshaw and S. Wessler, eds.), p. 375. Plenum, New York.

Bar, A., and Wasserman, R. H. (1973). *Biochem. Biophys. Res. Commun.* **54,** 191.

Barreras, R. F. (1973). *Gastroenterology* **64**, 1168.

Bassett, C. A. L. (1968). *Calcif. Tissue Res.* **1**, 252.

Baylink, D., and Wergedal, J. (1971). *Am. J. Physiol.* **221**, 669.

Baylink, D., Stauffer, M., Wergedal, J., and Rich, C. (1970). *J. Clin. Invest.* **49**, 1122.

Baylink, D., Wergedal, J., and Stauffer, M. (1971). *J. Clin. Invest.* **50**, 2519.

Baylink, D., Wergedal, J., and Thompson, E. (1972). *J. Histochem. Cytochem.* **20**, 279.

Bélanger, L. F. (1969). *Calcif. Tissue Res.* **4**, 1.

Biddulph, J. M. (1972). *Endocrinology* **90**, 1113.

Bingham, P. J., and Raisz, L. G. (1974). *Calcif. Tissue Res.* **14**, 31.

Bingham, P. J., Brazell, I. A., and Owen, M. (1969). *J. Endocrinol.* **45**, 387.

Bishop, M. C., and Smith, R. (1971). *Clin. Chim. Acta* **33**, 403.

Borle, A. B. (1967). *Clin. Orthop. Relat. Res.* **52**, 267.

Borle, A. B. (1972). *J. Membr. Biol.* **10**, 45.

Brand, J. S., and Raisz, L. G. (1972). *Endocrinology* **90**, 479.

Brinkley, F. J., Jr. (1973). *Fed. Proc., Fed. Am. Soc. Exp. Biol.* **32**, 1735.

Burleigh, M. C., Barrett, A. J., and Lazarus, G. S. (1974). *Biochem. J.* **137**, 387.

Byers, P. H., McKenney, K. H., Lichtenstein, J. R., and Martin, G. R. (1974). *Biochemistry* **13**, 5243.

Byers, P. H., Click, E. M., Harper, E., and Bornstein, P. (1975). *Proc. Natl. Acad. Sci. U.S.A.* **72**, 3009.

Cañas, F., Brand, J. S., Neuman, W. F., and Terepka, A. R. (1969). *Am. J. Physiol.* **216**, 1092.

Charbon, G. A. (1969). *Arch. Int. Pharmacodyn. Ther.* **178**, 296.

Chase, L. R., and Aurbach, G. D. (1970). *J. Biol. Chem.* **245**, 1520.

Chausmer, A. B., Sherman, B. S., and Wallach, S. (1972). *Endocrinology* **90**, 663.

Chen, T. L., and Raisz, L. G. (1974). *Calcif. Tissue Res.* **17**, 113.

Church, R. L., Pfeiffer, S. F., and Tanzer, M. L. (1971). *Proc. Natl. Acad. Sci. U.S.A.* **68**, 3241.

Church, R. L., Yaeger, J. A., and Tanzer, M. L. (1974). *J. Mol. Biol.* **86**, 785.

Clark, I., and Rivera-Cordero, F. (1970). *Endocrinology* **88**, 302.

Cooper, C. W., Schwesinger, W. A., Ontjes, D. A., Mahgoub, A. M., and Munson, P. L. (1972). *Endocrinology* **91**, 1079.

Copp, D. H., Cameron, E. C., Cheney, B. A., Davidson, A. G., and Henze, K. G. (1962). *Endocrinology* **70**, 638.

Cotmore, J. M., Nichols, G., Jr., and Wuthier, R. E. (1971). *Science* **172**, 1339.

Cuervo, L. A., Pita, J. C., and Howell, D. S. (1973). *Calcif. Tissue Res.* **13**, 1.

Daughaday, W. H. (1971). *Am. J. Med.* **50**, 277.

DeLuca, H. F. (1973). *Kidney Int.* **4**, 80.

Diegelmann, R. F., Bernstein, L., and Peterkofsky, B. (1973). *J. Biol. Chem.* **248**, 6514.

Dietrich, J. W., Canalis, E. M., Maina, D., and Raisz, L. G. (1976). *Endocrinology* **98**, 943.

Doty, S. B., and Schofield, B. H. (1972). *In* "Calcium, Parathyroid Hormone and the Calcitonins" (R. V. Talmage and P. L. Munson, eds.), Int. Congr. Ser. No. 243, p. 353. Excerpta Med. Found., Amsterdam.

D'Souza, A., and Floch, M. H. (1973). *Am. J. Clin. Nutr.* **26**, 352.

Ehrlich, H. P., and Bornstein, P. (1972). *Nature (London), New Biol.* **239**, 257.

Emtage, J. S., Lawson, D. E. M., and Kodicek, E. (1973). *Nature (London)* **246**, 100.

Estep, H. S., Shaw, W. A., Watlington, C., Hobe, R., Holland, W., and Tucker, S. (1969). *J. Clin. Endocrinol. Metab.* **29**, 842.

Eyre, D. R., and Glimcher, M. J. (1973). *Biochem. J.* **135**, 393.

Fleisch, H., and Neuman, W. F. (1960). *J. Am. Chem. Soc.* **82**, 3783.

Fleisch, H., and Russell, R. G. G. (1970). *Int. Encycl. Pharmacol. Ther.* Sect. 51, Vol. **1**, p. 61.

Friedenstein, A. J., and Lalykina, K. S. (1972). *Eur. J. Immunol.* **2**, 602.

Friedmann, N., and Rasmussen, H. (1970). *Biochim. Biophys. Acta* **222**, 41.

Frisancho, A. R., Garn, S. M., and Ascoli, W. (1970). *Hum. Biol.* **42**, 639.

Garn, S. M. (1972). *Orthop. Clin. N. Am.* **3**, 503.

Glimcher, M. J., and Krane, S. N. (1968). *Treatise Collagen* **2**, Part B, 68.

Goldhaber, P. (1965). *Science* **147**, 407.

Goldhaber, P., Rabadjija, L., Beyer, W. R., and Kornhauser, A. (1973). *J. Am. Dent. Assoc.* **87**, 1027.

Gray, T. K., Bieberdorf, F. A., and Fordtran, J. S. (1973). *J. Clin. Invest.* **52**, 3084.

Gross, J. (1974). *Harvey Lect.* **68**, 351.

Hahn, T. J., Chase, L. R., and Avioli, L. V. (1972). *J. Clin. Invest.* **51**, 886.

Harris, W. H., and Heaney, R. P. (1969). *N. Engl. J. Med.* **280**, 193, 253, and 303.

Haussler, M. R., Nigode, L., and Rasmussen, H. (1970). *Nature (London)* **228**, 1199.

Heersche, J. N. M., Marcus, R., and Aurbach, G. D. (1974). *Endocrinology* **94**, 241.

Herring, G. M., Andrews, A. T. deB., and Chipperfield, A. R. (1971). *In* "Cellular Mechanisms for Calcium Transfer and Homeostasis" (G. Nichols, Jr. and R. H. Wasserman, eds.), p. 63. Academic Press, New York.

Herrmann-Erlee, M. P. M., and van der Meer, J. M. (1974). *Endocrinology* **94**, 424.

Hill, L. F., Lumb, G. A., Mawer, E. B., and Stanbury, S. W. (1973). *Clin. Sci.* **44**, 335.

Hirsch, P. F., and Munson, P. L. (1969). *Physiol. Rev.* **49**, 548.

Holtrop, M. E., and Weinger, J. M. (1972). *In* "Calcium, Parathyroid Hormone and the Calcitonins" (R. V. Talmage and P. L. Munson, eds.), Int. Congr. Ser. No. 243, p. 365. Excerpta Med. Found., Amsterdam.

Holtrop, M. E., Raisz, L. G., and Simmons, H. (1974). *J. Cell Biol.* **60**, 346.

Horton, J. E., Raisz, L. G., Simmons, H. A., Oppenheim, J. J., and Mergenhagen, S. E. (1972). *Science* **177**, 793.

Howard, J. E., Thomas, W. C., Sr., Barker, L. M., Smith, L. H., and Wadkins, C. L. (1967). *Johns Hopkins Med. J.* **120**, 119.

Howell, D. S. (1971). *J. Bone Joint Surg., Am. Vol.* **53**, 250.

Hulmes, D. J. S., Miller, A., Parry, D. A. D., Piez, K. A., and Woodhead-Galloway, J. (1973). *J. Mol. Biol.* **79**, 137.

Husdan, H., Rapoport, A., and Locke, S. (1973). *Metab., Clin. Exp.* **22**, 787.

Ireland, P., and Fordtran, J. S. (1973). *J. Clin. Invest.* **52**, 2672.

Irwin, M. I., and Kienholz, E. W. (1973). *J. Nutr.* **103**, 1019.

Jee, W. S., and Nolan, P. D. (1963). *Nature (London)* **200**, 225.

Jee, W. S. S., Roberts, W. F., Park, H. Z., Julian, G., and Kramer, M. (1972). *In* "Calcium, Parathyroid Hormone and the Calcitonins" (R. V. Talmage and P. L. Munson, eds.), Int. Congr. Ser. No. 243, p. 430. Excerpta Med. Found., Amsterdam.

Jimenez, S., Harsch, M., and Rosenbloom, J. (1973). *Biochem. Biophys. Res. Commun.* **52**, 106.

Johnston, C. C., Jr., Smith, D. M., and Severson, A. R. (1972). *In* "Calcium, Parathyroid Hormone and the Calcitonins" (R. V. Talmage and P. L. Munson, eds.),. Int. Congr. Ser. No. 243, p. 338. Excerpta Med. Found., Amsterdam.

Jowsey, J., and Raisz, L. G. (1968). *Endocrinology* **82**, 382.

Jung, A., Bisaz, S., Bartholdi, P., and Fleisch, H. (1973). *Calcif. Tissue Res.* **13**, 27.

Kallio, D. M., Garant, P. R., and Minkin, C. (1972). *J. Ultrastruct. Res.* **39**, 205.

Katz, E. P., and Li, S.-T. (1972). *Biochem. Biophys. Res. Commun.* **46**, 1368.

Katz, E. P., and Li, S.-T. (1973). *J. Mol. Biol.* **80**, 1.

Kim, H., Kalkhoff, R. K., Costrini, N. V., Cerletty, J. M., and Jacobson, M. (1971). *J. Clin. Invest.* **50**, 2596.

Kimberg, D. V. (1969). *N. Engl. J. Med.* **280**, 1396.

Kivirikko, K. I. (1970). *Int. Rev. Connect. Tissue Res.* **5**, 93.

Klein, D. C., and Raisz, L. G. (1970). *Endocrinology* **86**, 1436.

Klein, D. C., and Raisz, L. G. (1971). *Endocrinology* **89**, 818.

Krane, S. M., Brownell, G. L., Stanbury, J. B., and Corrigan, H. (1956). *J. Clin. Invest.* **35**, 874.

Krane, S. M., Muñoz, A. J., and Harris, E. D., Jr. (1970). *J. Clin. Invest.* **49**, 716.

Kuttan, R., and Radhakrishnan, A. N. (1973). *Adv. Enzymol.* **37**, 273.

Laflamme, G. H., and Jowsey, J. (1972). *J. Clin. Invest.* **51**, 2834.

Lane, J. M., and Miller, E. J. (1969). *Biochemistry* **8**, 2134.

Lehninger, A. L. (1970). *Biochem. J.* **119**, 129.

LeRoith, D., and Pimstone, B. L. (1973). *Clin. Sci.* **44**, 305.

Levant, J. A., Walsh, J. H., and Isenberg, J. I. (1973). *N. Engl. J. Med.* **289**, 555.

Lichtman, M., and Miller, D. R. (1970). *J. Lab. Clin. Med.* **76**, 267.

Liu, C. C., Baylink, D. J., and Wergedahl, J. (1974). *Endocrinology* **95**, 1011.

Luben, R. A., Goggins, J. F., and Raisz, L. G. (1974a). *Endocrinology* **94**, 737.

Luben, R. A., Mundy, G. R., Trummel, C. L., and Raisz, L. G. (1974b). *J. Clin. Invest.* **53**, 1473.

Lukert, B. P., Stanbury, S. W., and Mawer, E. B. (1973). *Endocrinology* **93**, 718.

Magargal, L. E., Magargal, H., and Reidenberg, M. (1969). *J. Pharmacol. Exp. Ther.* **169**, 138.

Marino, A. A., Becker, R. O., and Soderholm, S. C. (1971). *Calcif. Tissue Res.* **8**, 177.

Marshall, J. H. (1969). *Miner. Metab.* **3**, 2–122.

Martin, G. R., Mecca, C. E., Schiffman, E., and Goldhaber, P. (1965). *In* "The Parathyroid Glands, Ultrastructure, Secretion and Function" (P. J. Gaillard, R. V. Talmage, and A. M. Budy, eds.), p. 261. Univ. of Chicago Press, Chicago, Illinois.

Martonosi, A., Purcell, A. J., and Halpin, R. A. (1971). *In* "Cellular Mechanisms for Calcium Transfer and Homeostasis" (G. Nichols, Jr. and R. H. Wasserman, eds.), p. 175. Academic Press, New York.

Marx, S. J., Fedak, S. D., and Aurbach, G. D. (1972a). *J. Biol. Chem.* **247**, 6913.

Marx, S. J., Woodward, C. J., and Aurbach, G. D. (1972b). *Science* **178**, 999.

Massry, S. G., Friedler, R. M., and Coburn, J. W. (1973). *Arch. Intern. Med.* **131**, 828.

Matthews, J. L., Martin, J. H., Arsenis, C., Eisenstein, R., and Kuettner, K. (1971). *In* "Cellular Mechanisms for Calcium Transfer and Homeostasis" (G. Nichols, Jr. and R. H. Wasserman, eds.), p. 239. Academic Press, New York.

Mears, D. C. (1971). *Endocrinology* **99**, 1021.

Meilman, E., Urivetzky, M. M., and Rapoport, C. M. (1963). *J. Clin. Invest.* **42**, 40.

Miller, E. J. (1971). *Biochemistry* **10**, 1652.

Miller, E. J. (1972). *In* "Developmental Aspects of Oral Biology" (H. C. Slavkin and L. A. Bavetta, eds.), p. 275. Academic Press, New York.

Miller, E. J., and Lunde, L. G. (1973). *Biochemistry* **12**, 3153.

Miller, E. J., Lane, J. M., and Piez, K. A. (1969). *Biochemistry* **8**, 30.

Minkin, C., and Jennings, J. M. (1972). *Science* **176**, 1031.

Mundy, G. R., Luben, R. A., Raisz, L. G., Cooper, R. A., Schechter, G. P., and Salmon, S. E. (1974). *N. Engl. J. Med.* **291**, 1041.

Mundy, G. R., Shapiro, J. L., Bandelin, J. G., Canalis, E. M., and Raisz, L. G. (1976). *J. Clin. Invest.* **58**, 529.

Nagant de Deuxchaisnes, C., and Krane, S. M. (1967). *Am. J. Med.* **43**, 508.

Neuman, W. F. (1972). In "Calcium, Parathyroid Hormone and the Calcitonins" (R. V. Talmage and P. L. Munson, eds.), Int. Congr. Ser. No. 243, p. 389. Excerpta Med. Found., Amsterdam.

Neuman, W. F., and Neuman, M. W. (1958). "The Chemical Dynamics of Bone Mineral." Univ. of Chicago Press, Chicago, Illinois.

Neuman, W. F., and Ramp, W. K. (1971). In "Cellular Mechanisms for Calcium Transfer and Homeostasis" (G. Nichols, Jr. and R. H. Wasserman, eds.), p. 197. Academic Press, New York.

Ney, R. L., Kelly, G., and Bartter, F. C. (1968). Endocrinology 82, 760.

Nigra, T. P., Friedland, M., and Martin, G. R. (1972). J. Invest. Dermatol. 59, 44.

Nusgens, B., and Lapiere, C. M. (1973). Clin. Chim. Acta 48, 203.

Olsen, B. R., Berg, R. A., Kishida, Y., and Prockop, D. J. (1973). Science 182, 825.

Olson, E. B., DeLuca, H. F., and Potts, J. T., Jr. (1972). In "Calcium, Parathyroid Hormone and the Calcitonins" (R. V. Talmage and P. L. Munson, eds.), Int. Congr. Ser. No. 243, p. 240. Excerpta Med. Found., Amsterdam.

Omdahl, J. L., and DeLuca, H. F. (1972). J. Biol. Chem. 247, 5520.

Omdahl, J. L., and DeLuca, H. F. (1973). Physiol. Rev. 53, 327.

Orimo, H., Fujita, T., and Yoshikawa, M. (1969). Endocrinol. Jpn. 16, 415.

Owen, M. (1970). Int. Rev. Cytol. 28, 213.

Owen, M., and Shetlar, M. R. (1968). Nature (London) 220, 1335.

Paillard, F., Ardaillou, R., Malendin, H., Fillastre, J.-P., and Prier, S. (1972). J. Lab. Clin. Med. 80, 200.

Park, E., Church, R. L., and Tanzer, M. L. (1975). Immunology 28, 781.

Parsons, J. A., and Robinson, C. J. (1968). In "Parathyroid Hormone and Thyrocalcitonin (Calcitonin)" (R. V. Talmage and L. F. Bélanger, eds.), Int. Congr. Ser. No. 159, p. 329. Excerpta Med. Found., Amsterdam.

Parsons, J. A., Neer, R. M., and Potts, J. T., Jr. (1971). Endocrinology 89, 735.

Peck, W. A., Messinger, K., and Carpenter, J. (1972). Proc. Int. Congr. Endocrinol., 4th, 1972, Excerpta Med. Found. Int. Congr. Ser. No. 256, abstract 256, p. 93.

Perris, A. D. (1971). In "Cellular Mechanisms for Calcium Transfer and Homeostasis" (G. Nichols, Jr. and R. H. Wasserman, eds.), p. 101. Academic Press, New York.

Phang, J. M., Downing, S. J., and Weiss, I. W. (1970). Biochim. Biophys. Acta 211, 605.

Piez, K. A., Balian, G., Click, E. M., and Bornstein, P. (1972). Biochem. Biophys. Res. Commun. 48, 990.

Pinnell, S. R., Fox, R., and Krane, S. M. (1971). Biochim. Biophys. Acta 229, 119.

Pita, J. C., Cuervo, L. A., Madruga, J. E., Mueller, F. J., and Howell, D. S. (1970). J. Clin. Invest. 49, 2188.

Pope, F. M., Martin, G. R., Lichtenstein, J. R., Penttinen, R., Gerson, B., Rowe, D. V., and McKusick, V. Z. (1975). Proc. Natl. Acad. Sci. U.S.A. 72, 1314.

Posner, A. S. (1973). Fed. Proc., Fed. Am. Soc. Exp. Biol. 32, 1933.

Puschett, J. B., Fernandez, P. C., Boyle, I. T., Gray, R. W., Omdahl, J. L., and DeLuca, H. F. (1972a). Proc. Soc. Exp. Biol. Med. 141, 379.

Puschett, J. B., Moranz, J. B., and Kurnick, W. S. (1972b). J. Clin. Invest. 51, 373.

Raisz, L. G. (1965). Proc. Soc. Exp. Biol. Med. 119, 614.

Raisz, L. G. (1970a). N. Engl. J. Med. 282, 909.

Raisz, L. G. (1970b). Arch. Intern. Med. 126, 887.

Raisz, L. G. (1971). N. Engl. J. Med. 285, 1006.

Raisz, L. G., and Bingham, P. J. (1972). Annu. Rev. Pharmacol. 12, 337.

Raisz, L. G., and Horton, J. E. (1973). In "Clinical Aspects of Metabolic Bone Disease" (B. Frame, A. M. Parfitt, and H. Duncan, eds.), Int. Congr. Ser. No. 270, p. 517. Excerpta Med. Found., Amsterdam.

Raisz, L. G., and Niemann, I. (1969). *Endocrinology* **85**, 446.

Raisz, L. G., Au, W. Y. W., Friedman, J., and Niemann, I. (1967). *Am. J. Med.* **43**, 684.

Raisz, L. G., Trummel, C. L., Holick, M. F., and DeLuca, H. F. (1972a). *Science* **175**, 4023.

Raisz, L. G., Trummel, C. L., and Simmons, H. (1972b). *Endocrinology* **90**, 744.

Raisz, L. G., Trummel, C. L., Wener, J. A., and Simmons, H. A. (1972c). *Endocrinology* **90**, 961.

Raisz, L. G., Holtrop, M., and Simmons, H. A. (1973). *Endocrinology* **93**, 556.

Raisz, L. G., Sandberg, A., Goodson, J. M., Simmons, H. A., and Mergenhagen, S. E. (1974). *Science* **185**, 789.

Rasmussen, H., and Bordier, P. (1973). *N. Engl. J. Med.* **289**, 25.

Rasmussen, H., and Pechet, M. (1970). *Int. Encyl. Pharmacol. Ther.* Sect. 51, Vol. I, p. 237.

Rasmussen, H., Kurokawa, K., Mason, J., and Goodman, D. B. P. (1972). *In* "Calcium, Parathyroid Hormone and the Calcitonins" (R. V. Talmage and P. L. Munson, eds.), Int. Congr. Ser. No. 243, p. 492. Excerpta Med. Found., Amsterdam.

Reddy, C. R., Coburn, J. W., Hartenbower, D. L., Friedler, R. M., Brickman, A. S., Massry, S. G., and Jowsey, J. (1973). *J. Clin. Invest.* **52**, 3000.

Reynolds, J. J. (1968). *Proc. R. Soc. London, Ser. B* **170**, 61.

Riggs, B. L., Arnaud, C. D., Goldsmith, R. S., Taylor, W. F., McCall, J. T., and Sessler, A. D. (1971). *J. Clin. Endocrinol. Metab.* **33**, 115.

Robertson, W. G., Peacock, M., Atkins, D., and Webster, L. A. (1972). *Clin. Sci.* **43**, 715.

Robison, R. (1923). *Biochem. J.* **17**, 286.

Rubin, R. P. (1970). *Pharmacol. Rev.* **22**, 389.

Rushton, M. L., Sammons, H. G., and Robinson, B. H. B. (1971). *Clin. Chim. Acta* **35**, 5.

Russell, R. G. G., Muhlbauer, R. C., Bisaz, S., Williams, D. A., and Fleisch, H. (1970). *Calcif. Tissue Res.* **6**, 183.

Russell, R. G. G., Bisaz, S., Donath, A., Morgan, D. B., and Fleisch, H. (1971). *J. Clin. Invest.* **50**, 961.

Sakamoto, S., Goldhaber, P., and Glimcher, M. J. (1973). *Calcif. Tissue Res.* **12**, 247.

Schatzmann, H. J., and Vincenzi, F. F. (1969). *J. Physiol. (London)* **201**, 369.

Schlesinger, S., MacGillivray, M. H., and Munschauer, R. W. (1973). *J. Pediatr.* **83**, 233.

Scott, B. L. (1967). *J. Cell Biol.* **35**, 115.

Silvis, S. E., and Paragas, P. D., Jr. (1972). *Gastroenterology* **62**, 513.

Singer, F. R., Aldred, J. P., Neer, R. M., Krane, S. M., Potts, J. T., Jr., and Bloch, K. J. (1972). *J. Clin. Invest.* **51**, 2331.

Smith, D. M., Nance, W. E., Kang, K. W., Christian, J. C., and Johnston, C. C., Jr. (1973). *J. Clin. Invest.* **52**, 2800.

Sottocasa, G. S., Panfili, E., deBernard, B., Paulo, G., Vasington, F. D., and Carafoli, E. (1972). *Biochem. Biophys. Res. Commun.* **47**, 808.

Spector, A. R., and Glimcher, M. J. (1972). *Biochim. Biophys. Acta* **263**, 593.

Spielvogel, A. M., Farley, R. O., and Norman, A. W. (1972). *Exp. Cell Res.* **74**, 359.

Stauffer, M., Baylink, D., Wergedal, J., and Rich, C. (1973). *Am. J. Physiol.* **225**, 269.

Stern, B., Golub, L., and Goldhaber, P. (1970). *J. Periodontol. Res.* **5**, 116.

Stern, P. H. (1969). *J. Pharmacol. Exp. Ther.* **168**, 211.

Stern, P. H., and Bell, N. H. (1970). *Endocrinology* **87**, 111.

Talmage, R. V., Anderson, J. J. B., and Cooper, C. W. (1972). *Endocrinology* **90**, 1185.

Tanzer, M. L. (1973). *Science* **180**, 561.

Tashjian, A. H., Jr., Voelkel, E. F., Levine, L., and Goldhaber, P. (1972). *J. Exp. Med.* **136**, 1329.

Thorngren, K.-G., and Hansson, L. I. (1973). *Acta Endocrinol. (Copenhagen)* **74**, 24.

Tonna, E. (1960). *Nature (London)* **185**, 405.

Toole, B. P., and Gross, J. (1971). *Dev. Biol.* **25**, 57.

Triffitt, J. T., and Owen, M. (1973). *Biochem. J.* **136,** 125.

Trummel, C. L., Raisz, L. G., Hallick, R. B., and DeLuca, H. F. (1971). *Biochem. Biophys. Res. Commun.* **44,** 1095.

Urist, M. R. (1970). *In* "Biological Mineralization" (I. Zipkin, ed.), p. 757. Wiley, New York.

Vaes, G. (1968). *J. Cell Biol.* **39,** 676.

Vaes, G. (1972a). *J. Dent. Res.* **51,** 362.

Vaes, G. (1972b). *Biochem. J.* **126,** 275.

Vaughan, J. M. (1973). "The Effect of Irradiation on the Skeleton." Oxford Univ. Press, London and New York.

Wasserman, R. H., and Taylor, A. N. (1973). *J. Nutr.* **103,** 586.

Wasserman, R. H., Corradino, R. A., Taylor, A. N., and Morrissey, R. L. (1971). *In* "Cellular Mechanisms for Calcium Transfer and Homeostasis" (G. Nichols, Jr. and R. H. Wasserman, eds.), p. 293. Academic Press, New York.

Watanabe, A., and Tasaki, I. (1971). *In* "Cellular Mechanisms for Calcium Transfer and Homeostasis" (G. Nichols, Jr. and R. H. Wasserman, eds.), p. 77. Academic Press, New York.

Wergedal, J. E., and Baylink, D. J. (1969). *J. Histochem. Cytochem.* **17,** 799.

Wergedal, J. E., Stauffer, N., Baylink, D., and Rich, C. (1973). *J. Clin. Invest.* **52,** 1052.

Woessner, J. F. (1973). *Clin. Orthop. Relat. Res.* **96,** 310.

Wong, R. G., Adams, T. H., Roberts, P. A., and Norman, A. W. (1970). *Biochim. Biophys. Acta* **219,** 61.

Wong, R. G., Myrtle, J. F., Tsai, H. C., and Norman, A. W. (1972). *J. Biol. Chem.* **247,** 5728.

Wuthier, R. E. (1971). *Calcif. Tissue Res.* **8,** 36.

Yamanishi, Y., Iguchi, M., Ohyama, H., and Matsumura, Y. (1972). *J. Clin. Endocrinol. Metab.* **35,** 55.

2

Kidney Function in Calcium and Phosphate Metabolism

OLAV L. M. BIJVOET

Production of urine is the most conspicuous expression of kidney function but not always the most significant. In 1844 Ludwig first proposed the theory of glomerular filtration and selective tubular reabsorption to explain the formation of urine; according to Cushny's "modern theory" formulated in 1917, some substances are passively filtered in the renal glomeruli and actively reabsorbed through the walls of the renal tubules together with water at a rate required to produce an "optimal" concentration in the fluid reabsorbed into the extracellular fluid. In this manner, optimal concentrations of important solutes are maintained in the blood. The level of concentration in the reabsorbed fluid would then characterize renal function in respect to a given substance. With some modifications, this theory still describes renal handling of calcium and phosphate. It will be shown that variations in renal function will, in the steady state, be reflected in variations in plasma calcium or phosphate concentration, whereas variations in the excretion rate merely reflect corresponding variations in the net input of these substances into the extracellular fluid from sites other than the kidney, for instance, bone or gut. It is clear that the role of the kidney in extracellular calcium and phosphate homeostasis must be considered in relation to the physiology of other organs. But in order to provide a sufficient background for the understanding of the function of the kidney as an organ, the sections on phosphate and calcium will begin with a discussion of the sites and nature of renal tubular transport mechanisms within the kidney and the quantitative relationships between the filtration, reabsorption, and excretion of calcium and phosphate.

Other functions of the kidney related to calcium metabolism but not discussed in this chapter are the inactivation by the kidney of circulating parathyroid hormone, calcitonin, or 25-hydroxycholecalciferol and the formation of metabolically active metabolites from 25-hydroxycholecalciferol.

I. RENAL PHOSPHATE TRANSPORT

A. The Elements of Renal Phosphate Transport

The glomeruli produce an ultrafiltrate of serum. As this ultrafiltrate passes along the renal tubules, its composition is altered because specific substances are subtracted by reabsorption and added by tubular secretion. Three processes, therefore, determine the final composition of urine: ultrafiltration, tubular reabsorption, and tubular secretion.

1. Glomerular Filtration

Micropuncture studies in amphibians and rats, although beset by many technical difficulties, should provide a direct comparison of the simultaneous concentrations of phosphate in serum and in the glomerular filtrate. The results of many such studies seem to indicate that these concentrations do not differ. Walser (1961a) has pointed out that the phosphate concentrations in glomerular filtrate and in serum can only be equal when about 13% of the serum phosphate is not filterable. One reason is that in measuring serum phosphate concentrations, the volume occupied by proteins is not taken into account. In addition, the presence of serum proteins on only one side of the ultrafiltering membrane will induce an electrochemical gradient across the membrane, and, as a result, the distribution of ions along the two sides of the membrane will be unequal (the Donnan equilibrium). He further reviewed existing *in vitro* ultrafiltration studies of serum phosphate and found that many were unreliable because factors, such as pH, pCO_2, or temperature, had not been taken into account. However the best available controlled studies and his own studies in man show that, whatever the absolute value of the serum phosphate concentration, the ultrafiltrates of serum have approximately the same phosphate concentration as the serum itself. On this basis, he reasoned that on the average 13% of the serum phosphate is protein-bound and nonfilterable (Walser, 1961a) (Table I). Therefore, it just so happens that, despite considerable protein binding, the phosphate concentration in glomerular filtrate equals the serum phosphate concentration [PO_4 (w/v)]. This is true for a wide range of serum phosphate concentrations. The filterable fraction of phosphate does apparently not change when phosphate is infused to raise its concentration in the blood to 10 mg per 100 ml. However, rapid and marked elevations of calcium and phosphate levels can result in formation of nonfilterable colloidal complexes of calcium phosphate (McLean and Hinricks, 1938). The filtration rate of phosphate in the kidney (filtered load, L_{PO_4}, weight/time) can, therefore, be calculated as the product of serum phosphate concentration and glomerular filtration rate [G.F.R. (volume/time)] [Eq. (1)]

$$L_{PO_4} = [PO_4] \times G.F.R. \tag{1}$$

TABLE I

Concentrations of Phosphate in Normal Human Plasma[a]

Phosphate	Concentration (mg/100 ml)	% Total
Free $HPO_4{}^{2-}$	1.55	43
Free $H_2PO_4{}^-$	0.34	10
Protein bound	0.43	12
$NaHPO_4{}^-$	1.02	29
$CaHPO_4$	0.12	3
$MgHPO_4$	0.10	3
Total	3.56	100

[a] Reproduced from Walser (1961a).

Henceforth in this chapter the amount filtered per unit time will be designated as filtered load (L_{PO_4}) and defined as [PO$_4$] × G.F.R. Moreover, the serum phosphate concentration [PO$_4$] can be considered as equal to the amount of phosphate filtered per unit volume of glomerular filtrate [Eq. (2)].

$$[PO_4] = L_{PO_4}/G.F.R. \tag{2}$$

2. Tubular Reabsorption and Secretion

Renal tubular handling of phosphate is still not completely understood. In man and in mammals the rate of phosphate excretion [$U_{PO_4}V$ (weight/time)] is always less than the filtration rate. There is, therefore, a net reabsorption of phosphate. The net reabsorption rate [T_{PO_4} (weight/time)] is defined as the difference between filtered load and excretion rate and can only be measured indirectly [Eq. (3)].

$$T_{PO_4} = [PO_4] \times G.F.R. - U_{PO_4}V \tag{3}$$

The occurrence of net phosphate reabsorption does not, however, preclude secretion of phosphate somewhere along the renal tubules, provided the reabsorption rate exceeds the secretion rate. Micropuncture studies in rats and dogs as well as stop-flow studies in dogs suggest a localization of phosphate reabsorption in the first part of the proximal tubules (Strickler et al., 1964; Malvin et al., 1958; Agus et al., 1971, 1973). This is also the site where intravenously administered ^{32}P has been demonstrated by autoradiography in cat tubules (Taugner et al., 1960). The renal sites of action of certain diuretics, such as acetazolamide and furosemide, include the proximal tubules, and these drugs have been shown to produce an acute increase in phosphate excretion. In contrast, diuretics with more distal sites of action do not affect the excretion rate at all. But much of the information regarding sites of action of diuretics has been derived from the premise that phosphate is primarily reabsorbed in the proximal nephron, and there are still many uncertainties regarding the localizations of the actions of diuretics. Moreover, the results of recent combined isotope and micropuncture studies and of modified stop-flow analysis and microperfusions seem explicable only by assuming combined proximal and distal reabsorption (Agus et al., 1973; Amiel et al., 1970; Beck and Goldberg, 1973; Brunette et al., 1973; Davies et al., 1966; LeGrimellec et al., 1974). The quantitative and physiological importance of distal reabsorption process in relation to the better known proximal one has not yet been elucidated.

Proximal phosphate reabsorption has currently been considered as due to a single reabsorption mechanism. However, on the basis of observations made during phosphate infusions in children with vitamin D-resistant rickets, it has been postulated that proximal reabsorption may involve two components: a transport system that can be influenced by parathyroid hormone (PTH) and a second, PTH-insensitive, residual component that permits phosphate flux from lumen to serum but might under exceptional circumstances allow a flux in the opposite direction (Glorieux and Scriver, 1972). This brings the discussion to the problem of phosphate secretion. Phosphorus-32 injected into the renal artery of dogs during stop-flow studies does not appear in the urine, in contrast to other substances like potassium, sodium, and calcium. This argues against the existence of phosphate secretion (Bronner and Thompson, 1961). In nonmammals however, aglomerular fishes (Marshall and Grafflin, 1933), chickens (Levinsky and Davidson, 1957), and alligators (Hernandez and Coulson, 1956), tubular secretion of inorganic phosphate has been demonstrated. There are also reports suggesting phosphate secretion in cats and dogs, but these experiments involved parenteral administration of organic phosphate esters and not inorganic phosphate (Taugner *et al.,* 1953; Schmid *et al.,* 1956). Therefore, the possibility of phosphate influx across the luminal walls of renal tubules is not entirely excluded. This may explain why in recent micropuncture studies in rats the specific activity of ^{32}P marked intraluminal phosphate became reduced (Boudry *et al.,* 1973). In dogs, acute tubular damage was observed to decrease phosphate excretion much more than creatinine excretion. This was interpreted as being due to a combination of proximal back diffusion of proportional amounts of phosphate and creatinine and of distal inhibition of phosphate secretion (Nicholson and Shepherd, 1959). However, differences in diffusion rates between phosphate and creatinine through the damaged tubules may explain the observations just as well (Bartter, 1961).

In summary, phosphate reabsorption occurs early in the proximal tubules and may be effected by more than one transport system. A second site of reabsorption in more distal parts of the nephron has been suggested. The existence of phosphate secretion is a debated subject. Active secretion has not been demonstrated, but phosphate influx or exchange across the tubular wall may exist.

The mechanism by which phosphate is transported across the cells of the renal tubule is uncertain. It seems likely that the movement of phosphate across the luminal border occurs against an electrochemical gradient and that the phosphate transport is an active process (Strickler *et al.,* 1964; Amiel *et al.,* 1970). There is a maximum reabsorption rate (Strickler *et al.,* 1964), indicating saturation kinetics, and there is competition with reabsorption of glucose (Pitts and Alexander, 1944), *p*-aminohippurate (West and Rapaport, 1949) and amino acids (Michael and Drammond, 1967).

Thus far, the term reabsorption was used for cellular transport processes. The term reabsorption rate, however, as applied to measurements *in vivo,* has a derived meaning and is operationally defined as the net difference between filtered load and excretion rate. Reabsorption, thus defined, may be the net result of several different transport processes.

B. Renal Phosphate Transport as a Whole

In this section, the kidney, or rather both kidneys are treated as one single organ, and, here, the term phosphate transport does not designate the mechanism of phosphate transport in individual nephrons, but rather the net difference between filtered load and excretion rate. Both, filtered load and excretion rate can be measured directly; filtered load as $[PO_4] \times$ G.F.R. [see Eq. (1)] and excretion rate as $U_{PO_4}V$. Thus, this section concerns the relation between these two terms when the excretion rate at various levels of filtered load is studied (Pitts and Alexander, 1944; Anderson, 1955; Bijvoet, 1969; Stamp and Stacey, 1970). Since filtered load equals $[PO_4] \times$ G.F.R., it can be varied by two ways: either by altering $[PO_4]$ or by altering G.F.R. First the effect on $U_{PO_4}V$ will be discussed when plasma phosphate concentration is raised by giving a phosphate infusion while G.F.R. remains constant. To bring into prominence the effects of tubular phosphate transport on the relation between $U_{PO_4}V$ and $[PO_4]$ at a constant G.F.R., the data are compared with similar data on inulin, a substance that is likewise filtered at the glomerulus but shows no tubular transport. Figure 1 shows the relationship between the plasma inulin concentration and the excretion rate of inulin during intravenous infusions of inulin in man (Bijvoet, 1969). Because inulin is filtered entirely at the glomerulus and is neither reabsorbed nor secreted in the tubules, any increment in filtered inulin ($[In] \times$ G.F.R.) is excreted entirely. Therefore,

$$[In] \times \text{G.F.R.} = U_{In}V \qquad (4)$$

The slope of the line in Fig. 1 relating the inulin excretion rate ($U_{In}V$) to the plasma inulin concentration [In] is, therefore, numerically equal to the glomerular filtration rate [Eq. (5)].

$$\text{G.F.R.} = U_{In}V/[In] \qquad (5)$$

This ratio between $U_{In}V$ and [In] is the inulin clearance. An infusion of phosphate was given at the same time and in the same manner as the inulin infusion. If no phosphate reabsorption had occurred, the line relating phosphate excretion rate ($U_{PO_4}V$) to plasma phosphate concentration $[PO_4]$ would have been the same as that for inulin, and the phosphate excretion

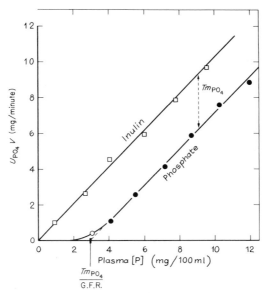

Fig. 1. The relationship between the urinary excretion rate of phosphate $U_{PO_4}V$ in mg/minute and plasma phosphate [P] in mg/100 ml in a healthy individual when fasting (open circle) and during an infusion of phosphate (closed circles). Note that plasma [P] equals the phosphate concentration in the renal glomerular filtrate. The open squares show the relationship between urinary excretion rate and plasma concentration of inulin when inulin was infused simultaneously. (The inulin results are divided by 10.) The slope of the line through the infusion data for phosphate is the same as the slope of the line through the inulin data and is, therefore, the glomerular filtration rate (10^{-2} ml/minute). The vertical distance between the two straight lines, or the negative intercept with the ordinate of the extrapolated straight line through the closed circles, is the maximum rate of tubular reabsorption of phosphate (Tm_{PO_4} in mg/minute). The intercept of the line through the closed circles with the abscissa is the maximum tubular reabsorption of phosphate per 100 ml of glomerular filtrate (Tm_{PO_4}/G.F.R. in mg/100 ml) which has also been called the "theoretical renal phosphate threshold." (From Bijvoet, 1969.)

rate ($U_{PO_4}V$) would have been equal to the filtered phosphate load [PO₄] × G.F.R.) as in Eq. (4). However, during phosphate infusion, at whatever value of [PO₄], phosphate excretion is always less than the filtered load by a value equal to the vertical distance between the inulin line and the phosphate line. This distance is, of course, the net reabsorption rate (T_{PO4}) [Eq. (3)].

$$T_{PO_4} = [PO_4] \times G.F.R. - U_{PO_4}V \qquad (3)$$

Figure 1 shows that when the serum phosphate concentration is increased above its value in the fasting state, indicated by an open circle. The rate of reabsorption (T_{PO_4}) then is initially increased but rapidly reaches a *constant maximum* rate. Any further increment in the filtered load due to an increment of $[PO_4]$ is excreted entirely. It may be convenient at this point to explain some terminology currently used in studies of phosphate reabsorption and originally derived from terms used in similar studies of glucose reabsorption. The *constant maximum* reabsorption rate of phosphate obtained at an artificially high phosphate concentration is designated as the tubular maximum of phosphate $[Tm_{PO_4}$ (weight/time)]. The gradual increase in phosphate reabsorption to this maximum as the serum phosphate $[PO_4]$ is increased (see Fig. 1) is called "phosphate splay." The extrapolated regression line through the phosphate data in Fig. 1 cuts the abscissa at a point which is called the "phosphate threshold." This threshold is a serum phosphate concentration. If phosphate reabsorption would not have splayed at lower serum phosphate values, then phosphate reabsorption would, at this threshold concentration for phosphate $[PO_4]_{thresh}$ have been equal to its constant maximum rate (Tm_{PO_4}) and at the same time equal to the filtered load $[PO_4]_{thresh} \times G.F.R.$ Hence [Eq. (6)].

$$[PO_4]_{thresh} \times G.F.R. = Tm_{PO_4} \tag{6}$$

Therefore, the threshold concentration for phosphate $[PO_4]_{thresh}$ equals $Tm_{PO_4}/G.F.R.$ (weight/volume). The relevance of this threshold concentration for the homeostasis of the serum phosphate is clear from Fig. 1. Below the threshold concentration most of the filtered phosphate is reclaimed by the renal tubules and not much is excreted; above the threshold concentration a substantial part of the filtered phosphate is rejected and excreted into the urine. Furthermore, above the threshold, the concentration at which phosphate is returned to the blood by the tubules is limited to $Tm_{PO_4}/G.F.R.$ (a value equal to the threshold value) because the maximum rate of phosphate reabsorption is Tm_{PO_4} and, since only about one percent of the filtered water reaches the urine, the rate of net water reabsorption approximates G.F.R. The kidney, therefore, tends to maintain plasma phosphate concentration around that value.

The existence of a "phosphate threshold" in man was already postulated in 1925 by Adolph and in 1928 by Brain *et al.* Ellsworth (1932) and Albright *et al.* (1932) suggested in 1932 that the abnormally high or low serum phosphate concentrations occurring in hypoparathyroidism or hyperparathyroidism were due to alterations of the phosphate threshold. Yet the existence of a *Tm* for phosphate was first demonstrated in dogs by Harrison and Harrison only in 1941. Many authors have since confirmed this in dogs, rats, and man. It was, however, noted that even though the value of Tm_{PO_4} did not vary within each set of experiments, there was considerable variation among the various individuals. Much of the individual variation could be accounted for by differences in G.F.R. (Fig. 2). The maximum tubular reabsorption per volume of glomerular filtrate,

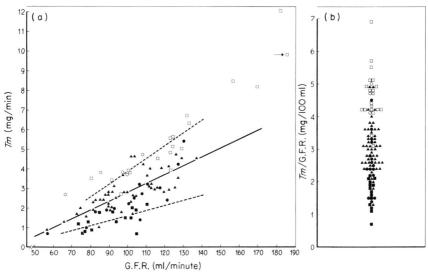

Fig. 2. (a) The relationship between maximum tubular reabsorption rate (*Tm* in mg/minute) and glomerular filtration rate (G.F.R. in liters/minute) in 100 patients. The dashed lines are regression lines calculated for thyreotoxic (open squares) and hypoparathyroid (open circles) patients ($y = 65x - 2.0, r = 0.93, n = 23$) and for hyperparathyroid patients (closed squares) $y = 25x - 0.6, r = 0.64, r = 0.64, n = 14$). The solid line was calculated through the remaining data. ($y = 44x - 1.2, r = 0.77, n = 63$). (b) Distribution of the 100 patients in (a) with respect to *Tm*/G.F.R. mg/100 ml. The symbols refer to the diagnosis: open squares, thyrotoxicosis; open circles, hypoparathyroidism; closed circles, kidney stones or nephrocalcinosis; closed squares, hyperparathyroidism; and closed triangles, other diseases. Note that much of the variation in Tm_{PO_4} is due to variation in G.F.R. and that when the data are plotted according to the Tm_{PO_4}/G.F.R., groups of diseases can be discriminated. (From Bijvoet, 1969).

Tm_{PO_4}/G.F.R. (the phosphate threshold), normally varies much less and characterizes the tubular phosphate reabsorption activity of the kidney (Bijvoet, 1969; Anderson and Parsons, 1963; Hellman *et al.*, 1964); it indicates how the kidney contributes toward the regulation of the serum phosphate concentration.

The maximum tubular reabsorption per volume of glomerular filtrate, Tm_{PO_4}/G.F.R., probably measures a fundamental property of reabsorptive activity. Shannon and Fisher (1938) postulated that *Tm* for glucose corresponds to a maximum rate for a transport process and hence that it is a function of the total amount of enzyme available for transport in the tubules. A maximum reabsorptive rate per unit of G.F.R. (*Tm*/G.F.R.) might then characterize the quantity of transporting carrier available per unit of kidney mass and thus be related to the carrier activity. The existence of splay in phosphate reabsorption may be due to intrinsic properties of the kidney, either anatomical, since all single nephrons do not have an identical G.F.R. or Tm_{PO_4}, or enzymatic in that splay might reflect a limited affinity of the transporting enzyme for the substrate (Bijvoet, 1969).

The relation between tubular reabsorption and glomerular filtration is not only constant between subjects but Tm_{PO_4}/G.F.R. may remain constant when G.F.R. varies within the same individual (Hellman et al., 1964). This is an instance of "glomerulotubular balance," a mechanism as yet insufficiently understood, that maintains balance between glomerular and tubular function (Wesson, 1973). This glomerulotubular balance keeps phosphate reabsorption near its equilibrium value that can be measured as Tm_{PO_4}/G.F.R. or threshold concentration. It had already been surmised by Cushny (1917) and Smith et al. (1943), Smith (1956), and Harrison and Harrison (1941) that the renal threshold concentration, Tm_{PO_4}/G.F.R., not only describes the renal phosphate reabsorption in relation to extracellular fluid homeostasis but actually is a main determinant of serum phosphate concentration. Recently, it has been demonstrated that most of the variation of fasting serum phosphate concentration in man is, in fact, due to variation in Tm_{PO_4}/G.F.R. (Bijvoet, 1969). Clinical assessment of renal phosphate transport should aim at actual measurement of Tm_{PO_4}/G.F.R., that is the renal threshold concentration for phosphate. Measurement of Tm_{PO_4}/G.F.R. is considered in the next section.

C. Measurement of Phosphate Reabsorption

1. Introduction

There are many clinical conditions in which the tubular reabsorption of phosphate has changed; in such cases, measurement of the extent to which phosphate reabsorption is altered may help in diagnosis and in understanding or in assessing the response to treatment. To obtain this information Tm_{PO_4}/G.F.R. can be measured directly by infusing phosphate and plotting the relationship between the phosphate excretion rate ($U_{PO_4}V$) and the serum phosphate concentration [PO_4] for various values of the latter as in Fig. 1 (Stamp and Stacey, 1970). However, this method is time consuming, and it cannot be repeated easily because repeated phosphate infusions disturb the steady state. Recently, it has been demonstrated that Tm_{PO_4}/G.F.R. can be determined directly from simple measurements in a fasting person and without infusions (Bijvoet et al., 1969; Bijvoet and Morgan, 1971; Bijvoet and Van der Sluys Veer, 1972; Bijvoet, 1972). Before this became possible, an alternative and often used approach has been to make some empirical "estimate" of the tubular reabsorption of phosphate. Many such estimates of phosphate reabsorption have been devised (Bijvoet et al., 1969; Bijvoet and Morgan, 1971; Bijvoet, 1972). They are based on relationships between the urinary excretion rate $(U_{PO_4}V)$, serum phosphate concentration [PO$_4$], and glomerular filtration rate (G.F.R.). The last is often taken equal to creatinine clearance ($C_{creat} = U_{creat}V/$[creat]). These estimates will be discussed in the last part of this section. Two particular estimates will be discussed here, the ratio of phosphate clearance ($C_{PO_4} = U_{PO_4}V/$[PO$_4$]) to creatinine clearance, indicated as C_{PO_4}/C_{creat}, and the fractional phosphate reabsorption (T.R.P.) (Bernstein *et al.*, 1965). This is because these parameters are used in the calculation of $Tm_{PO_4}/$G.F.R. (Bijvoet *et al.*, 1969; Bijvoet and Morgan, 1971; Bijvoet and Van der Sluys Veer, 1972; Bijvoet, 1972). T.R.P. and C_{PO_4}/C_{creat} are easily obtained from determinations of phosphate and creatinine concentration in serum ([PO$_4$] and [creat]) and in a simultaneous untimed urine sample (U_{PO_4} and U_{creat}) [Eq. (7)]. All that is needed is simultaneous collection of

$$C_{creat}/C_{PO_4} = \frac{U_{PO_4}V \times [creat]}{[PO_4] \times U_{creat}V} = \frac{U_{PO_4}V \times [creat]}{U_{creat} \times [PO_4]} \tag{7}$$

urine and plasma samples without taking the volume into account. Collections should preferably be made in the morning between 8 and 10 AM. The patient should void at 8 AM. Discard this urine sample and have the patient drink 200 ml distilled water. Take a blood and urine sample at 10 AM for phosphate and creatinine determinations.

The ratio C_{PO_4}/C_{creat} is equal to the excreted fraction of the filtered phosphate load ($U_{PO_4}V/L_{PO_4}$) [Eq. (8)] because $L_{PO_4} = $ [PO$_4$] $\times$ G.F.R. [see Eq. (1)] and $C_{creat} = $ G.F.R.

$$\frac{U_{PO_4}V}{L_{PO_4}} = \frac{U_{PO}V}{[PO_4] \times G.F.R.} = \frac{U_{PO_4} \times [creat]}{[PO_4] \times U_{creat}} = \frac{C_{PO_4}}{C_{creat}} \tag{8}$$

The term T.R.P., the fractional phosphate reabsorption or the reabsorbed fraction of the phosphate load, is nothing but the complement of C_{PO_4}/C_{creat} [Eq. (9)]

$$T.R.P. = \frac{L_{PO_4} - U_{PO_4}V}{L_{PO_4}} = 1 - \frac{U_{PO_4}V}{L_{PO_4}} = 1 - \frac{C_{PO_4}}{C_{creat}} \tag{9}$$

Phosphate clearances or derived measurements should always be made in the fasting state and over short periods because feeding and circadian rhythm affect the results.

2. *Measurement of $Tm_{PO_4}/G.F.R.$ without Phosphate Infusion*

In Fig. 1, at any plasma phosphate concentration, phosphate excretion rate $(U_{PO_4}V)$ is equal to the vertical distance between the phosphate line and the abscissa at that value and phosphate load (L_{PO_4}) to the vertical distance between the inulin line and the abscissa and that value. It is clear

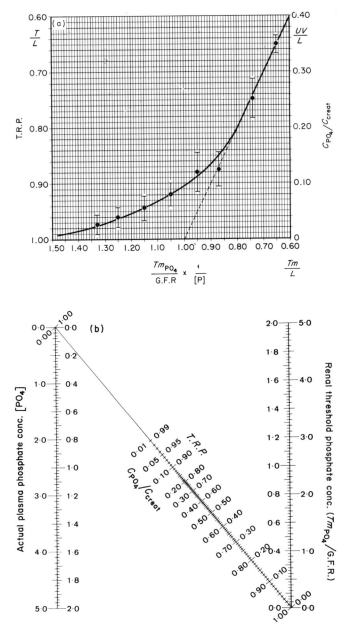

Fig. 3. (a) The relationship between fractional reabsorption of filtered phosphate (T/L = T.R.P.) or fractional excretion of filtered phosphate ($UV/L = C_{PO_4}/C_{creat}$) and the ratio of the renal phosphate threshold to plasma phosphate $[(Tm_{PO_4}/\text{G.F.R.})/[P] = Tm/L]$ in 100 persons when fasting and during an infusion of phosphate. The values are shown for each successive interval of 0.1 of Tm/L. The figure can be used as a nomogram [see (b)] for the estimation of the phosphate reabsorption ($Tm_{PO_4}/\text{G.F.R.}$) for simultaneous measurements of

that the ratio of $U_{PO_4}V$ to L_{PO_4} is high when the threshold concentration $(Tm_{PO_4}/\text{G.F.R.})$ is lower than the actual serum phosphate concentration and low when threshold concentration is higher. That is, the ratio $U_{PO_4}V/L_{PO_4}$ or C_{PO_4}/C_{creat} is inversely related to the ratio of threshold concentration to serum phosphate.

In Fig. 3a C_{PO_4}/C_{creat} and T.R.P. have been compared with the ratio of renal phosphate threshold to plasma phosphate in 100 persons (Bijvoet *et al.*, 1969; Bijvoet and Morgan, 1971; Bijvoet and Van der Sluys Veer, 1972; Bijvoet, 1972). Figure 3a can be used as a nomogram for the calculation of $Tm_{PO_4}/\text{G.F.R.}$ from C_{PO_4}/C_{creat} or T.R.P. within splay when the relation is not linear, that is for values of C_{PO_4}/C_{creat} below 0.20. Simply find for any value of C_{PO_4}/C_{creat} or T.R.P., the corresponding value of $(Tm_{PO_4}/\text{G.F.R.})/[\text{PO}_4]$, and multiply that value by $[\text{PO}_4]$ to obtain $Tm_{PO_4}/\text{G.F.R.}$ For values of C_{PO_4}/C_{creat} above 0.20 (T.R.P. below 0.80) when phosphate reabsorption is above splay, $Tm_{PO_4}/\text{G.F.R.}$ can be directly calculated as T.R.P. $\times [\text{PO}_4]$ since then

$$\text{T.R.P.} \times [\text{PO}_4] = \frac{T_{PO_4} \times [\text{PO}_4]}{L_{PO_4}} = \frac{Tm_{PO_4} \times [\text{PO}_4]}{[\text{PO}_4] \times \text{G.F.R.}} = \frac{Tm_{PO_4}}{\text{G.F.R.}} \quad (10)$$

Note: the curved part of the function in Fig. 3a can be described by an empirical equation that can be solved with a moderately advanced scientific calculator, slide rule, or set of tables. When $C_{PO_4}/C_{creat} < 0.20$

$$\frac{Tm_{PO_4}}{\text{G.F.R.}} = [\text{PO}_4]e^p$$

where

$$p = 10.318 \left(\frac{C_{PO_4}}{C_{creat}}\right)^2 - 5.1848 \left(\frac{C_{PO_4}}{C_{creat}}\right) + 0.4022 \quad (11)$$

T.R.P. (or C_{PO_4}/C_{creat}) and [P]. T.R.P. can be calculated from the concentrations of phosphate and creatinine in plasma ([P] and [creat]) and in urine [(U_{PO_4}) and (U_{creat})]. The rate of flow of urine (V) is not required.

$$\text{T.R.P.} = T/L = 1 - \frac{UV}{L}$$

$$\frac{UV}{L} = \frac{C_{PO_4}}{C_{creat}} = \frac{(P_{PO_4}) \times V}{[P]} \times \frac{[\text{creat}]}{(U_{creat}) \times V} = \frac{(U_{PO_4}) \times [\text{creat}]}{[P] \times (U_{creat})}$$

When $C_{PO_4}/C_{creat} > 0.20$ (T.R.P. < 0.80) then $Tm_{PO_4}/\text{G.F.R.} = \text{T.R.P.} \times [P]$. When $C_{PO_4}/C_{creat} < 0.20$ (T.R.P. > 0.80) then the corresponding value of $(Tm_{PO_4}/\text{G.F.R.})/[P]$ can be obtained using the relationship shown by the continuous line in the figure. $Tm_{PO_4}/\text{G.F.R.}$ is then this value multiplied by [P]. (From Bijvoet and Morgan, 1971; Bijvoet, 1972). (b) Nomogram derived by Walton and Bijvoet (1975) which allows direct derivation of $Tm_{PO_4}/\text{G.F.R.}$

when $C_{PO_4}/C_{creat} > 0.20$

$$\frac{Tm_{PO_4}}{\text{G.F.R.}} = \frac{1 - C_{PO_4}}{C_{creat}} \times [PO_4] \qquad (12)$$

From these data a nomogram has been derived (Walton and Bijvoet, 1975) which allows the direct derivation of $Tm_{PO_4}/\text{G.F.R.}$ (Fig. 3b).

To use the nomogram, the patient is fasted overnight and a urine sample (which need not be accurately timed but which should be collected over a reasonably short period, say 1–2 hours) and a blood sample are obtained. T.R.P. or C_{PO_4}/C_{creat} can then be derived from urine and plasma creatinine and phosphate concentrations as explained in Section I,C,1. The nomogram can then be used to derive $Tm_{PO_4}/\text{G.F.R.}$ A straight line through the appropriate values of $[PO_4]$ and T.R.P. (or C_{PO_4}/C_{creat}) passes through the corresponding value of $Tm_{PO_4}/\text{G.F.R.}$ $Tm_{PO_4}/\text{G.F.R.}$ and $[PO_4]$ are expressed in the same units. The scales and units are arbitrary, but the same should be used for both $[PO_4]$ and $Tm_{PO_4}/\text{G.F.R.}$ Two scales were chosen: The 0.0–2.0 scale is suitable for estimating values of $Tm_{PO_4}/\text{G.F.R.}$ close to the normal range expressed as (0.80–1.35 mmole/liter), and the 0.0–5.0 scale for values close to the normal range expressed as 2.5–4.2 mg per 100 ml. If necessary, the scales for $[PO_4]$ and $Tm_{PO_4}/\text{G.F.R.}$ can be multiplied or divided by any number (provided that the same number is used for both scales).

3. Traditional Indices of Phosphate Reabsorption

The traditional empirical "estimates" of phosphate reabsorption are defined in Table II. The phosphate clearance is the ratio of phosphate excretion to serum phosphate concentration ($U_{PO_4}V/[PO_4]$). Reference to Fig. 1 makes it clear that phosphate clearance will not only vary inversely with $Tm/\text{G.F.R.}$, it will, in addition, vary with glomerular filtration rate and with serum phosphate concentration. It is, therefore, an imprecise index, and its absolute value does not confer unequivocal information. Normal values may vary from 2 to 33 ml/minute (Ollayos and Winkler, 1943) and from 8 to 38 ml/minute per 1.73 m² body surface (Dean and McCance, 1948) or from 4 to 16 ml/minute when measured in the forenoon (Milne, 1951; Kyle et al., 1958) when serum phosphate concentration varies least. Phosphate clearance measurements could be of value in sequential studies provided G.F.R. and serum phosphate concentration remain constant, but in that case simple measurements of $U_{PO_4}V$ should suffice.

The excreted fraction of phosphate, C_{PO_4}/C_{creat} (Crawford et al., 1950) has been mentioned in the first part of this section. The term T.R.P. (reabsorbed fraction of phosphate load) is the complement of C_{PO_4}/C_{creat} (Bern-

TABLE II

The Definition, Symbol, Calculation and Dimensions, and Average and Range for Normal Individuals of the Variables That Influence the Excretion of Phosphate

Variable	Symbol	Calculation	Dimensions	Average	Range
Plasma phosphate	[P]		mass/volume, mg/100 ml	3.2	2.3–4.4
Glomerular filtration rate	G.F.R.		volume/time, ml/minute	100	80–120
Filtered load	L	[P] × G.F.R.	mass/time, mg/minute	3.2	
Urinary excretion rate	UV		mass/time, mg/minute	0.36	0.14–0.57
Tubular reabsorption rate	T	$L - UV$	mass/time, mg/minute	2.84	
Maximum tubular reabsorption rate	Tm	(see Fig. 1)	mass/time, mg/minute	3.2	
Maximum tubular reabsorption rate per 100 ml glomerular filtrate	$\dfrac{Tm}{\text{G.F.R.}}$	(see Figs. 1 and 2)	mass/volume, mg/100 ml	3.2	2.5–4.2
Phosphate clearance	C_{PO_4}	UV/P	vol/time, ml/minute	12	
Phosphate : creatinine clearance	$\dfrac{C_{PO_4}}{C_{creat}}$	UV/L	no dimension	0.12	
Fractional reabsorption of filtered load	T.R.P.	$T/L = 1 - UV/L$	no dimension	0.88	
Phosphate excretion index	P.E.I.	b	dimension?		±0.09
Index of phosphate excretion	I.P.E.	c	mass/volume, mg/100 ml		±0.50

[a] Also included are the various measures and estimates of the tubular reabsorption of phosphate (Bijvoet and Morgan, 1971).

[b] P.E.I. $= C_{PO_4}/C_{creat} - 0.055$ [P] $+ 0.07$; [P] in mg/100 ml. (From Nordin and Fraser, 1960.)

[c] I.P.E. $= UV/\text{G.F.R.} - ([P] - 2.5)/2$; [P] in mg/100 ml. (From Nordin and Bulusu, 1968.)

stein *et al.*, 1965). But some authors use T.R.P. for [PO$_4$] × G.F.R. − $U_{PO_4}V$, which is in fact T_{PO_4} (Crawford *et al.*, 1950; Pronove and Bartter, 1961). Reference to Figs. 1 and 3 makes clear that C_{PO_4}/C_{creat} and T.R.P. do not merely vary with $Tm_{PO_4}/\text{G.F.R.}$ but are also dependent on serum phosphate concentration. Absolute values of C_{PO_4}/C_{creat} and T.R.P. do not, therefore, convey precise information, and normal values for C_{PO_4}/C_{creat} vary widely from 0.6 to 0.22 (Kyle *et al.*, 1958; Chambers *et al.*, 1956). Nordin and Fraser (1960) and Nordin and Bulusu (1968) assumed a linear regression between C_{PO_4}/C_{creat} and serum phosphate concentration (Nordin and Fraser, 1960) or between $U_{PO_4}V/C_{creat}$ and [PO₄], respectively (Nordin and Smith, 1965), at any given setting of renal phosphate transport and based on that regression their P.E.I. (phosphate excretion index) and I.P.E. (index of phosphate excretion). The actual relation between C_{PO_4}/C_{creat} or $U_{PO_4}V/C_{creat}$ and [PO₄] for a series of values of $Tm_{PO_4}/G.F.R.$ is given in Figs. 4 and 5. Since these actual relations are now known (Bijvoet *et al.*, 1969; Bijvoet and Morgan, 1971; Bijvoet and Van der Sluys Veer, 1972; Bijvoet, 1972) and since $Tm_{PO_4}/G.F.R.$ can be directly calculated from the same data (see above), continued use of I.P.E. or P.E.I. is not indicated. Figures 4 and 5 allow combined interpretation of the data reported in literature in terms of $Tm_{PO_4}/G.F.R.$ and without bias.

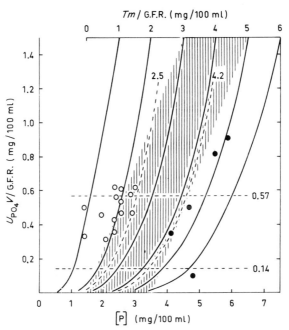

Fig. 4. The relationship between $U_{PO_4}V/G.F.R.$ (mg/100ml) and [PO₄] (mg/100 ml) with respect to $Tm_{PO_4}/G.F.R.$ The lines are drawn at intervals of 1 mg/100 ml in $Tm_{PO_4}/G.F.R.$ The open circles are patients with hyperparathyroidism and the closed circles those with hypoparathyroidism from Fig. 2. The solid lines were calculated from the data of Bijvoet (1969). Note that splay increases as $Tm_{PO_4}/G.F.R.$ increases. The dotted lines repesent the 95% range for $Tm_{PO_4}/G.F.R.$ (2.5–4.2 mg/100 ml) and for $U_{PO_4}V/G.F.R.$ (1.4–5.7 mg/100 ml) in healthy adults (From Anderson 1955; Bijvoet *et al.*, 1964.) The hatched area indicates the normal range of the index of phosphate excretion (I.P.E.) as given by Nordin and Bulusu (1968). (According to Bijvoet *et al.*, 1969.)

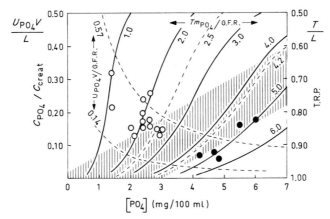

Fig. 5. The relationship between $U_{PO_4}V/L$; (C_{PO_4}/C_{creat}) or T_{PO_4}/L = T.R.P. and serum $[PO_4]$ with respect to $Tm_{PO_4}/G.F.R.$ in the data of Bijvoet (1969). The open circles are patients with hyperparathyroidism and the closed circles the hypoparathyroid patients from Figs. 2 and 3. The solid lines were calculated according to Bijvoet *et al.* (1969) for the average of $Tm_{PO_4}/$ G.F.R. in these groups: The dotted lines represent the 95% range for $Tm_{PO_4}/G.F.R.$ (2.5–4.2 mg/100 ml) and for $U_{PO_4}V/G.F.R.$ (1.4–5.7 mg/100 ml) in healthy adults (Anderson, 1955; Bijvoet *et al.*, 1964). The hatched area indicates the normal range of the phosphate excretion index (P.E.I.) as given by Nordin and Fraser (1960). (According to Bijvoet *et al.*, 1969).

D. The Physiology of Phosphate Excretion

This section deals with renal phosphate handling in relation to phosphate homeostasis of the body. Certain diseases are included in this section on physiology because diseases do not involve new, but only altered, relationships within the organism. These alterations may focus attention upon aspects of the physiological equilibrium that would otherwise be overlooked.

There are two mutually related aspects of phosphate homeostasis: phosphate balance and the steady state of extracellular phosphate concentration. In an ideal steady state, the renal excretion rate of phosphate $U_{PO_4}V$ would be equal to the net input of phosphate into the extracellular fluid at sites other than the kidney. Part of this phosphate input comes of course from dietary phosphate. Food intake and, therefore, phosphate intake is a discontinuous process and will disturb the steady state of the body. One of the characteristics of the observed steady state is the constancy of the extracellular phosphate concentration, reflected in the concentration of serum phosphate $[PO_4]$. It is essential to know how the extrarenal input of phosphate disturbs $[PO_4]$ homeostasis and how the kidney protects the constancy of $[PO_4]$.

1. The Kidney and Serum Phosphate Concentrations

In the preceding section, two factors were mentioned that may influence serum phosphate concentration: (1) the extrarenal phosphate input, mainly phosphate absorbed from the diet that in a steady state would equal excretion rate, $U_{PO_4}V$, and (2) renal phosphate reabsorption that is most characteristically expressed as the renal threshold concentration for phosphate, or $Tm_{PO_4}/G.F.R.$ A third factor the overall efficiency of renal function in relation to the extracellular fluid, depends on the amount of extracellular fluid turned over through glomeruli and tubules per unit time, which is measured as glomerular filtration rate (G.F.R.).

The influence of these three factors, $U_{PO_4}V$, $Tm_{PO_4}/G.F.R.$, and G.F.R. on serum phosphate concentration was studied in 100 persons in whom the absolute values of the factors varied widely (Bijvoet, 1969), but with the following limitation: G.F.R. always exceeded 40 ml/minute because below that filtration rate the daily renal filtered phosphate load at normal serum phosphate concentration would not exceed dietary phosphate intake. Patients were studied after an overnight fast because it was assumed that that was the best approach to a steady state. Table III is a multiple regression analysis relating variations in [PO₄] to variations in $Tm_{PO_4}/G.F.R.$, G.F.R., and $U_{PO_4}V$. The table conclusively shows that nearly 70% of the variance of fasting serum phosphate concentration is determined be the activity of renal phosphate reabsorption, measured as $Tm_{PO_4}/G.F.R.$ Thus, at G.F.R. values above 40 ml/minute and in the fasting state, $Tm_{PO_4}/G.F.R.$ is the major determinant of serum phosphate concentration. Figure 6 illus-

TABLE III

Multiple regression analysis[a,b]

Regression equation for [P]	Residual variance
[P] = +3.3	0.708
[P] = +1.4 + 0.60(Tm/G.F.R.)	0.215
[P] = +1.7 + 0.62(Tm/G.F.R.) − 0.0064(G.F.R.)	0.201
[P] = +1.1 + 0.69(Tm/G.F.R.)[c] − 0.0062(G.F.R.)[d] + 1.5(UV)[c]	0.142

[a] Dependent variable, fasting plasma phosphate concentration ([P]; mg/100 ml); independent variables, tubular phosphate reabsorption (Tm/G.F.R.; mg/100 ml), glomerular filtration rate (G.F.R.; ml/minute), and extrarenal load (UV; mg/minute).
[b] From Bijvoet (1969).
[c] p values = <0.001.
[d] p values = 0.005–0.001

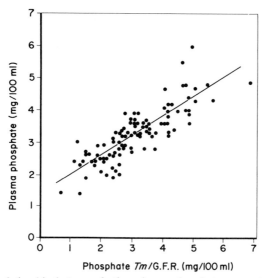

Fig. 6. The relationship between fasting plasma phosphate concentration and $Tm_{PO_4}/$ G.F.R. in 100 experiments. The equation of the regression line is $y = 0.60x + 14, r = 0.84$. (Reproduced from Bijvoet, 1969.)

trates this relation. Table III also shows that at these values of G.F.R. the contribution of glomerular filtration rate to the setting of serum phosphate concentration is small but significant. Figure 7 actually demonstrates this negative partial regression of serum phosphate on G.F.R. at normal

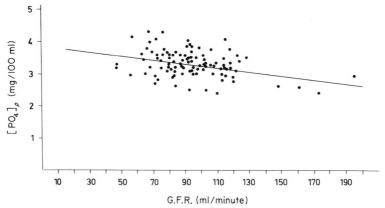

Fig. 7. Negative partial regression of serum phosphate concentration $[PO_4]_p$ on glomerular filtration rate (G.F.R.) at normal or nearly normal values of the latter, in 100 persons. $[PO_4]_p$ was calculated from the data of Bijvoet (1969) using the multiple regression equation for this data. $[PO_4] = 0.69 (Tm_{PO_4}/G.F.R.) - 0.0062 [G.F.R. + 1.5 (U_{PO_4}V)] + 1.15$ and the averages for $Tm_{PO_4}/G.F.R.$ and $U_{PO_4}V$. The level of significance is $0.005 > p > 0.001$.

glomerular filtration rates. Finally, Table III shows that 80% of the variance of serum phosphate is explained when the extrarenal load is also taken into account. The following sections will deal with variations of $U_{PO_4}V$ and $Tm_{PO_4}/G.F.R.$ and with the influence of a low G.F.R. on renal phosphate handling.

2. Physiological Variations of Renal Phosphate Transport

a. Normal Phosphate Excretion Rate. The amount of phosphate excreted per day is equal to the amount of phosphate adsorbed from the diet. The average diet contains about 1500 mg phosphate per day and the average 24-hour renal excretion of phosphate is about 600 mg. Variations in intake and urinary output are closely related (Nordin and Smith, 1965). There are circadian variations in phosphate excretion rate (Wesson, 1964). Phosphate excretion is the lowest in the morning with a minimum at about 11 AM. Thereafter, $U_{PO_4}V$ increases and reaches a maximum value between 6 PM and midnight. It has often been assumed that the rhythm in phosphate excretion is not due to feeding habits, but Albright pointed out that whatever the condition of a patient, phosphate feeding is always followed by an increase in excretion rate (Albright and Reifenstein, 1948). Dossetor *et al.*, (1963) could reverse the rhythm by feeding at night. Feeding seems, therefore, to be an important factor. Yet the phosphate rhythm is not abolished when feeding is distributed equally throughout the day, even though the timing of the rhythm is then changed (Birkenhager *et al.*, 1957). Therefore, other factors may be influential, e.g., muscular activity. Because of the discontinuous nature of phosphate excretion, sequential studies of phosphate excretion should be accompanied by control studies over comparable periods.

The most common cause of a low phosphate excretion rate is a phosphate-poor diet, such as low protein or low calcium diets, or administration of aluminum hydroxyde gels, which bind phosphate in the gut (Chambers *et al.*, 1956; Fauley *et al.*, 1941; Thompson and Hiatt, 1957). Hyperphosphaturia may result from a high phosphate intake or breakdown of bone.

b. The Normal Setting of Phosphate Reabsorption. So far, interest in phosphate reabsorption has mainly concerned the diagnosis of hyperparathyroidism or hypoparathyroidism. However parathyroid hormone (PTH) is not the only factor which influences phosphate reabsorption. Because of its considerable influence on serum phosphate, phosphate reabsorption is the main factor responsible for variations.in serum phosphate with time, age, and disease. The age related variation of $Tm_{PO_4}/G.F.R.$ is considerable. $Tm_{PO_4}/G.F.R.$ is increased in children and adolescents (Corvilain, 1972). The interpretation of $Tm_{PO_4}/G.F.R.$ in childhood requires a separate age-specific normal range (Stalder *et al.*, 1957;

McCrory *et al.*, 1950; Thalassinos *et al.*, 1970). The normal range for healthy adult individuals is between 2.5 and 4.2 mg per 100 ml (Bijvoet *et al.*, 1969; Bijvoet and Morgan, 1971; Bijvoet, 1972). Serum phosphate concentration rises again in women after the menopause, and its concentration was then found to correlate with serum growth hormone concentration (Aitken *et al.*, 1973b), which probably acts on the serum phosphate through increasing Tm_{PO_4}/G.F.R. (Corvilain and Abramov, 1962). It is not known whether there are ciradian variations in Tm_{PO_4}/G.F.R. that might in part be responsible for variations in phosphate excretion rate. However, this is highly probable, since serum phosphate concentration and serum PTH concentration have been shown to vary during the day (Jubiz *et al.*, 1972).

3. The Effect of Parathyroid Hormone on Renal Phosphate Handling

Phosphate reabsorption (Tm_{PO_4}/G.F.R.) is decreased in primary and secondary hyperparathyroidism (see Volume II, Chapters 1, and 2) and increased in hypoparathyroidism (see Volume II, Chapter 3). Parenteral administration of PTH causes an immediate increase in phosphate excretion, and removal of the parathyroids has the opposite effect because of disruption of the steady state. However, it is misleading to characterize as phosphaturic the effects in the kidney of a hormone such as PTH, which merely reduces the level of Tm_{PO_4}/G.F.R. Only a sudden increase in the circulating hormone level can cause a transient increase in phosphate excretion rate. When a steady state is established in hyperparathyroid or hypoparathyroid patients, they cannot be distinguished from healthy persons on the basis of phosphate excretion rate (Chambers *et al.*, 1956). The inhibitory effect of PTH on the renal tubular reabsorption of phosphate was the first action of the hormone to be well documented. It was once considered the most immediate physiological effect of PTH but has as such now been replaced by an increase in cyclic AMP excretion and a transient lowering of the serum calcium concentration. In 1898, Vereecke observed a reduction of phosphate excretion after thyroparathyroidectomy in rabbits. Greenwald (1911) found a dramatic decrease in phosphate excretion after total parathyroidectomy (Collip, 1925). After Collip prepared the first parathyroid extract (see Greenwald, 1911), Greenwald demonstrated that it was "phosphaturic" in rats (Greenwald and Gross, 1925). Albright *et al.* confirmed this effect in healthy persons and in a patient with idiopathic hyperparathyroidism (Albright *et al.*, 1929; Albright and Ellsworth, 1929). Ellsworth (1932) ascribed the effect to the reduction of the renal phosphate threshold. When purified parathyroid extract became available, its inhibiting effect on the renal tubular reabsorption of phosphate was confirmed by unilateral injection in the renal artery of the dog (Pullman *et al.*, 1960).

4. Renal Phosphate Handling and the Diagnosis of Parathyroid Disorders

In the past, a colossal body of literature has accumulated about the possibility of discriminating hyperparathyroid or hypoparathyroid patients from other patients by the use of "phosphate excretion tests." Because it has long been impossible and still difficult to measure serum PTH concentration, the biochemical features used to recognize primary hyperparathyroidism have been hypercalcemia, hypophosphatemia, and a reduced tubular reabsorption of phosphate (see Volume II, Chapter 1). Much of the literature concerned with the feasibility of using measurements of phosphate reabsorption as a diagnostic tool in such patients is controversial. This is mainly due to the indiscriminate use of *phosphate clearance* or the *ratio of phosphate clearance to creatinine clearance* (C_{PO_4}/C_{creat}) or its complement [$1 - (C_{PO_4}/C_{creat})$], called T.R.P., to assess phosphate reabsorption because these measurements were often used empirically without reference to their physiological basis (see Section I,C). The measurement of T.R.P. was introduced in the diagnosis of hyperparathyroidism by Schaaf and Kyle (1954), but others showed that T.R.P. as such was an insufficient discriminant in the diagnosis of hyperparathyroidism (Reynolds *et al.*, 1960). C_{PO_4}/C_{creat}, the ratio of phosphate to creatinine clearance, has been the basis of several indices of phosphate reabsorption. Chambers *et al.* (1956) demonstrated that when patients were deprived of phosphate *(phosphate deprivation test)* there was a greater decrease in C_{PO_4}/C_{creat} in the patients with hyperparathyroidism than in the others. This result can be predicted from Fig. 5. It is explained by the change in the slope of the line relating C_{PO_4}/C_{creat} to [PO_4] with respect to $Tm_{PO_4}/G.F.R.$ Patients with hyperparathyroidism have a lower $Tm_{PO_4}/G.F.R.$ and a steeper slope. A converse procedure has also been used, and its results are explainable in a similar way. It is based on measurement of C_{PO_4}/C_{creat} before and on the fifth day of *administration of inorganic phosphate salts* (2 gm for 3 days and 3 gm for 2 days). C_{PO_4}/C_{creat} rises more in hyperparathyroid patients than in others (Eisenberg, 1968a; Yamahiro and Reynolds, 1962; Massry *et al.*, 1973). Others use the empirically determined relationship between C_{PO_4}/C_{creat} and [PO_4] (Fig. 5) to diagnose hyperparathyroidism (Milne *et al.*, 1952; McGeown, 1961). Nordin and Fraser (1960) devised the *phosphate excretion index* (P.E.I.), which is a linear approximation of the normal relationship between C_{PO_4}/C_{creat} and [PO_4] (Fig. 5 and Table II), but discrimination by means of P.E.I. between normal and abnormal $Tm_{PO_4}/G.F.R.$ fails at low and high levels of

[PO$_4$] (cf. Fig. 5). The index of phosphate excretion (I.P.E.) devised by
Nordin and Bulusu (1968) is a linear approximation of the splay in the
relationship between $U_{PO_4}V$/G.F.R. and [PO$_4$] (Fig. 4 and Table II). It
discriminates between normal and abnormal values of Tm_{PO_4}/G.F.R. over
a wide range of values of [PO$_4$] and can be used as a quick and convenient
"bedside method." However a direct or indirect *assessment of Tm_{PO_4}/*
G.F.R. (Section I,C,2) is the best way to characterize an abnormal phosphate reabsorption in patient. Parathyroid hormone decreases Tm_{PO_4}/
G.F.R. and parathyroidectomy increases it, and Tm_{PO_4}/G.F.R. is characteristically high in hypoparathyroidism and low in hyperparathyroidism
(Fig. 2) (Bijvoet *et al.*, 1964, 1969; Bijvoet and Morgan, 1971; Bijvoet and
Van der Sluys Veer, 1972; Bijvoet, 1972; Hyde *et al.*, 1960). Tm_{PO_4}/G.F.R.
is also depressed in secondary hyperparathyroidism. Examples of secondary hyperparathyroidism are found in rickets, osteomalacia, sprue, and
chronic glomerular failure. A normal Tm_{PO_4}/G.F.R. in hyperparathyroidism is rare and may serve as a warning that other causes of the
hypercalcemia or urolithiasis should be searched for carefully (see Chapter 7). On the other hand, a low Tm_{PO_4}/G.F.R. is not an adequate differentiation between hyperparathyroidism and other causes of urolithiasis
because many patients with "idiopathic hypercalciuria" show a decreased
Tm_{PO_4}/G.F.R., and a lowered Tm_{PO_4}/G.F.R. may occur in tumor-induced
hypercalcemia, possible because hypercalcemia with hypercalciuria
themselves may lower renal tubular phosphate reabsorption (Verbanck
and Toppet, 1961). Another procedure that has been devised to discrimi-
nate hyperparathyroidism from other cases of urolithiasis is the *calcium
infusion test*. It is based on the assumption that autonomous glands in
hyperparathyroid patients will not be able to reduce their hormone production in the presence of hypercalcemia. Many variants exist. According
to the procedure of Kyle *et al.* (1962), C_{PO_4}/C_{creat} is measured between 8
AM and noon on day 1; a calcium infusion providing 10 to 15 mg Ca^{2+} per
kilogram of body weight is given between 8 PM and midnight on the next
day; C_{PO_4}/C_{creat} is again measured between 8 AM and noon and should have
decreased by less than 0.40 in hyperparathyroidism. Since the test is
empirical, it is disturbing that a number of false negative results has been
reported (Pronove and Bartter, 1961; McGeown, 1964). Recently, an alternative procedure was devised (Pak *et al.*, 1972a). The patient receives a
400-mg calcium diet for 3 days. On the third day, a calcium gluconate
infusion is given between 8 AM and noon, providing 15 mg Ca^{2+} per kilogram of body weight. Urine is collected between 8 PM and 8 AM on the day
preceding infusion and on the day of the infusion. $U_{PO_4}V$ should decrease
by less then 25% when the patient is hyperparathyroid.

   In hypoparathyroidism Tm_{PO_4}/G.F.R. is generally raised above 4.2 mg per 100 ml (Fig. 2). Biochemical hypoparathyroidism may be due (1) to accidental damaging of the parathyroid glands, (2) to congenital or acquired inability of the gland to secrete biologically active PTH (idiopathic hypoparathyroidism), or (3) to peripheral hormone resistance (in pseudohypoparathyroidism) (see Volume II, Chapter 3). Albright *et al.* (1942) defined pseudohypoparathyroidism by the failure of the kidney to react to PTH. Chase and Aurbach (1967) found that PTH failed to increase urinary cyclic AMP in patients with pseudohypoparathyroidism. Drezner *et al.* (1973) suggested that two forms of the disease may exist, one form in which PTH fails to decrease Tm_{PO_4}/G.F.R. and to promote cyclic AMP excretion and another form in which cyclic AMP excretion does increase but Tm_{PO_4}/G.F.R.is still insensitive to the hormone. The diagnosis is made with the *Ellsworth–Howard test* (1934). The fasting patient is given 200 units (U.S.P.) parathyroid extract intravenously. The urinary phosphorus content is determined hourly for 3 hours before and for 3–5 hours after injection. Midpoint blood samples are taken over the periods of urine collection. Injection of parathyroid extract should produce a five- to sixfold increase in $U_{PO_4}V$ in healthy persons, a tenfold in hypoparathyroidism, and, at most, a twofold increase in pseudohypoparathyroidism. The decrease of Tm_{PO_4}/G.F.R. is 0.95 ± 0.33 mg per 100 ml in normal subjects, 1.92 ± 0.33 mg per 100 ml in idiopathic hypoparathyroidism, and 0.62 ± 0.32 mg per 100 ml in pseudohypoparathyroidism (Drezner *et al.*, 1973). Cyclic AMP excretion rate should increase at least fourfold.

5. The Effect of Other Hormones on Renal Phosphate Transport

a. Calcitonin. Calcitonin infusions do provoke transient phosphaturia in rat (Robinson *et al.*, 1966) and in man (Bijvoet *et al.*, 1968, 1972; Haas *et al.*, 1971). The effect is not due to secondary stimulation of the parathyroid glands because the action is also seen in thyroparathyroidectomized rats (Raisz, 1972) and in patients with hypoparathyroidism (Bijvoet *et al.*, 1972; Haas *et al.*, 1971). The action is due to lowering of Tm_{PO_4}/G.F.R. (Bijvoet and Froeling, 1973b). In the dog, calcitonin does not affect phosphate excretion, but it does block the increase of phosphate reabsorption due to subsequent administration of 25-hydroxycholecalciferol (Puschett *et al.*, 1974). It is still not clear if calcitonin has a physiological role in man (see Volume II, Chapter 4), but reproducible basal concentrations in the peripheral blood which change appropriately to perturbations of serum calcium have now been described that suggest that this hormone is physiologically important (Silva *et al.*, 1974), and calcitonin may therefore be partially responsible for the phosphaturia that accompanies hypercalcemia (Verbanck and Toppet, 1961) and for the prolonged lowering of Tm_{PO_4}/G.F.R. after 24 hours of infusion of PTH (Froeling and Bijvoet, 1974).

b. *Vitamin D*. Harrison and Harrison (1941) found that phosphate reabsorption in dogs increased after vitamin D administration. However their dogs had intact parathyroid glands, and the rise in phosphate reabsorption may have been due to suppression of the parathyroids. In hypoparathyroidism, treatment with vitamin D has the converse effect in patients, and Tm_{PO_4}/G.F.R. is reduced from elevated to normal values. However, when vitamin D is given to hypoparathyroid patients, its effect on the renal handling of phosphate may be secondary to the elevation of serum calcium, since an increase in serum calcium to normal reduces phosphate reabsorption per se (Lavender and Pullman, 1963; Eisenberg, 1965, 1968b). Micropuncture studies performed in the proximal convolution of normal and parathyroidectomized rats showed that large quantities of cholecalciferol increase tubular reabsorption of phosphate independent of parathyroid function or serum calcium level (Gekle *et al.,* 1971). Cholecalciferol is hydroxylated in the liver to 25-hydroxycholecalciferol (25-OH-D₃), which is again converted in the kidney to 1,25-dihydroxycholecalciferol [1,25-(OH)₂-D₃], the active form of the vitamin that should be considered as a true hormone (see Chapter 5 and Volume II, Chapter 2). Both 25-OH-D₃ and 1,25-(OH)₂-D₃ enhance tubular phosphate reabsorption in the dog and in the rat (Puschett *et al.,* 1972a,b; Popovtzer *et al.,* 1974). These actions, however, are in some manner dependent on PTH, cyclic AMP, or calcitonin. In the dog, all these substances and infusion of calcium, when given before 25-OH-D₃ block the action of 25-OH-D₃ on phosphate transport (Puschett *et al.,* 1972a, 1974). In the rat, 25-OH-D₃ enhances tubular reabsorption of phosphate only when given systemical and not intra-arterial and only in the presence of endogenous or exogenous circulating PTH (Puschett *et al.,* 1972b). In healthy human subjects 1,25-(OH)₂-D₃ given intravenously did not change serum phosphate or renal tubular reabsorption of phosphate, but in patients with X-linked hypophosphatemic rickets intravenous 1,25-(OH)₂-D₃ caused a rapid but transient improvement of tubular reabsorption of phosphate and normalized the response to bovine PTH. When given by mouth it was ineffective (Glorieux *et al.,* 1973). The effect of 1,25-(OH)₂-D₃ in hypophosphatemic rickets is very similar to the effect following calcium infusion in this disease (Glorieux and Scriver, 1972).

The preceding data have not yet been related into one verifiable pattern. All substances mentioned influence the ionic milieu of the cell and given in pharmacological doses may disturb the normal reaction to the hormone. It seems safe, however, to conclude that vitamin D metabolites probably enhance phosphate reabsorption and the reabsorption of calcium and sodium (Puschett *et al.*, 1972a, 1974) in the proximal tubule of the kidney.

 c. Other Hormones. Parathyroid hormone, calcitonin, and vitamin D are not the only hormones that sustain a normal renal phosphate reabsorption and thereby help in maintaining serum phosphate homeostasis. Nor do they or the other hormones affect the phosphate reabsorption which is involved in a direct feedback control of serum phosphate. There is probably no specific hormonal regulation of the serum phosphate.

 Serum phosphate is elevated in the menopause and after oophorectomy (Chapter 6) and decreases again after the administration of estrogens (Donaldson and Nassim, 1954; Aitken *et al.*, 1973a). Estrogens probably decrease phosphate reabsorption (Reifenstein and Albright, 1947; Nassim *et al.*, 1956). However, growth hormone levels may be elevated in postmenopausal women, and it has been suggested that the postmenopausal relative hyperphosphatemia is consistent with an effect on the kidney of increased growth hormone activity (Aitken *et al.*, 1973b). *Growth hormone* excess increases the tubular reabsorption of phosphate in the kidney by a direct effect of the hormone on Tm_{PO_4}/G.F.R. (Corvilain, 1972; Corvilain and Abramov, 1962), and this is the cause of the elevated serum phosphate in patients with active acromegaly (Lambert and Corvilain, 1964; Cattaneo *et al.*, 1964). We have explained earlier in this chapter that excretion rate in a steady state does not reflect tubular handling but rather input of a substance in the extracellular fluid at sites other than the kidney. Tubular handling is reflected in extracellular ion concentration. This point is very well illustrated in *thyrotoxicosis*. In this disease, excess phosphate is excreted into the urine along with calcium (Aub *et al.*, 1929; Robertson, 1942), and this may reflect an increased net bone resorption rate (Adams *et al.*, 1967; Smith *et al.*, 1973). But in thyrotoxicosis the serum phosphate concentration is elevated, and this in turn is due to increased renal tubular reabsorption of phosphate, reflected in an increased renal threshold concentration for phosphate (Tm_{PO_4}/G.F.R.) (Bijvoet *et al.*, 1964; Parsons and Anderson, 1964; Bijvoet and Majoor, 1965). A significant positive correlation was found between Tm_{PO_4}/G.F.R. and the logarithm of serum protein-bound iodine (Bijvoet *et al.*, 1964). It is, therefore, surprising that *triiodothyronine* injections in man and dogs are transiently phosphaturic, indicating that under these conditions thyroid hormone decreases phosphate reabsorption (Beisel *et al.*, 1958, 1960). A probable explanation is that increasing bone resorption by chronic thyroid hormone excess has a slight hypercalcemic effect, which in turn causes reduced production of PTH and relative hypoparathyroidism (Aub *et al.*, 1929; Adams *et al.*, 1967) (Volume II, Chapter 4). *Cortisone* administration decreases the tubular reabsorption of phosphate (Ingbar *et al.*, 1951; Roberts and Pitts, 1953;

Anderson and Foster, 1959). It is not known whether the effect is direct or indirect. Plasma phosphate may be elevated after hypophysectomy or adrenalectomy if replacement therapy is inadequate. An inverse correlation was found between *plasma cortisol* and the fraction of filtered phosphate excreted into the urine (Goldsmith *et al.*, 1965), and a relation between the circadian rhythms of cortisol and serum phosphate has been suggested (Jubiz *et al.*, 1972; Goldsmith *et al.*, 1965).

The hormonal effects on phosphate reabsorption hitherto described can be related to well-known variations of plasma phosphate in disease and therapy. It is not clear what the clinical importance is of the decrease of phosphate reabsorption observed in man after administration of *angiotensin II* (Brodehl and Gellissen, 1966) or in dogs after *vasopressin* administration (Eisinger *et al.*, 1970).

6. Nonhormonal Effects on Renal Phosphate Transport

a. Minerals. A chronic high *phosphate* intake produces a steady state with reduced tubular reabsorption of phosphate (Eisenberg, 1968a; Goldman and Bassett, 1958), reduced calcium excretion, normocalcemia or even slight hypocalcemia, increased immunoreactive parathyroid hormone serum level, and parathyroid hyperplasia (Malm, 1953; Edwards and Hodgkinson, 1965; Reiss *et al.*, 1970; Engfeldt *et al.*, 1954). In dogs, hyperparathyroid changes in bone with net loss of bone were observed (Jowsey and Balambranamiam, 1972). Reducing phosphate intake has the opposite effect (Pronovo *et al.*, 1961; Lotz *et al.*, 1968; Gold *et al.*, 1970). The effects of phosphate feeding on renal tubular phosphate reabsorption are probably mediated by the parathyroid glands, because a slight increase in serum phosphate may cause mild hypocalcemia. It cannot be excluded that slight changes of intracellular phosphate concentration may directly influence the renal reabsorptive process (Foulks, 1955). It is interesting that phosphate depletion is associated with renal bicarbonate wasting, and this phenomenon has been implicated in the hyperchloremic acidosis of hyperparathyroidism (Gold *et al.*, 1973). However, the effect of PTH on bicarbonate reabsorption is probably immediate (Froeling and Bijvoet, 1974) (cf. Section III,A,1,h).

The effect of *calcium infusions* has been discussed earlier (cf. Section I,D,4). One should remember that apart from the parathyroid-mediated stimulation of phosphate reabsorption, infusion of calcium may have an effect *sui generis* on renal transport mechanisms. During calcium infusions, phosphate reabsorption is reduced in hypoparathyroid patients (Verbanck and Toppet, 1961; Eisenberg, 1965), but is increased in X-linked hypophosphatemic rickets (Glorieux and Scriver, 1972). Hypercalcemia also decreases the tubular reabsorption of phosphate, hydrogen, sodium, potassium, and magnesium, and the effect on hydrogen excretion may be operative in the origin of metabolic alkalosis of nonparathyroid hypercalcemia (Verbanck and Toppet, 1961; Amiel, 1964). Hypercalcemia blocks the acute efects of PTH administration on the excretion of phosphate, bicarbonate, and cyclic AMP (Vainsel, 1973; Beck *et al.*, 1974) and blocks the effects of administered 25-hydroxycholecaliferol on the excretion of phosphate, sodium, and calcium (Puschett *et al.*, 1974). Such effects may reflect the importance of intracellular calcium concentration for the proper mediation of hormone actions on cell function (Rasmussen, 1972). An analogous mechanism may be operative in the lowering of phosphate reabsorption by *potassium* depletion (Makler and Stanbury, 1956). Following sudden infusions of *magnesium,* the urinary excretion of phosphate falls despite an increase in serum phosphate. The increase in tubular phosphate reabsorption is due to PTH inhibition, since phosphate excretion is not reduced following an immediate elevation of serum magnesium in dogs without their parathyroid glands (Massry *et al.*, 1970).

Pitts and Alexander (1944) found that sudden alterations in extracellular acid–base balance do not alter Tm_{PO_4} in dogs. But in subsequent studies it was found that sodium bicarbonate infusion induces an acute increase in urinary bicarbonate and phosphate excretion in dogs (Malvin and Lotspeich, 1956; Farlop and Brazeau, 1967) and man (Mostellar and Tuttle, 1964; Puschett and Goldberg, 1969) and reduces $Tm_{PO_4}/$G.F.R. (Malvin and Lotspeich, 1956). Some of this effect may be due not to an alteration of acid–base balance but to an expansion of extracellular volume (Steele, 1970); however, phosphaturia is greater following infusion of sodium bicarbonate than of an equivalent amount of sodium chloride (Puschett and Goldberg, 1969).

Volume expansion due to sodium chloride infusions or hyperoncotic albumin infusion decreases tubular phosphate reabsorption concurrently with a decreased reabsorption of sodium and other electrolytes in the proximal tubule (Steele, 1970; Frick, 1969; Massry *et al.*, 1969; Blythe *et al.*, 1968; Schneider *et al.*, 1973; Knox *et al.*, 1974). Parathyroid hormone may cause all or part of this effect because serum ionized calcium concentration is reduced by the dilutional effect of the infusions (Frick, 1969, 1971; Knox *et al.*, 1974; Spornitz and Frick, 1973). However, in the dog volume loading appears to inhibit tubular reabsorption of phosphate, regardless of the presence or absence of PTH (Hebert *et al.*, 1972) (cf. Section III,A,1,g).

b. Drugs. The $Tm_{PO_4}/$G.F.R. for phosphate may be reduced by infusion of various substances, including *sodium aminohippurate* (West and Rapaport, 1949), certain *amino acids* (Drammond and Michael, 1964; Michael and Drammond, 1967), and *acetoacetate* (Pitts and Alexander,

1944; Cohen *et al.*, 1956). These substances may inhibit the tubular phosphate transport by competing for part of the transport mechanism. *Probenecid*, has an intriguing effect; it has been observed to decrease the tubular reabsorption of phosphate in hypoparathyroid patients or in patients in whom reabsorption of phosphate is increased for unknown reasons (Schneider and Corcoran, 1950; Pascale *et al.*, 1954; Jackson *et al.*, 1956; Schwarz, 1964; Garcia and Yendt, 1970). Schwarz (1964) has observed that probenecid, by inhibiting tubular reabsorption of phosphate, restores the renal response to parathyroid extract in pseudohypoparathyroidism. The Tm_{PO_4}/G.F.R. is increased after prolonged treatment with *heparin* (Bijvoet *et al.*, 1964) and during treatment with disodium ethane-1-hydroxy-1,1-diphosphonate (EHDP) (Recker *et al.*, 1973; Bijvoet *et al.*, 1974). The effect of diuretics on renal tubular reabsorption of phosphate will not be discussed here. The effect of diuretics has generally been studied in relation to the mechanism and localization of phosphate transport, but sustained effects of diuretics on renal phosphate handling are not known (Massry *et al.*, 1973). The reader is further referred to Section II,D,5,c where the effects of diuretics on renal calcium transport are discussed.

c. Diseases. Many of the diseases that influence tubular reabsorption of phosphate have already been mentioned in earlier parts of this section or will be reviewed in Section I,E. In addition, it should be mentioned that the serum phosphate concentration is often elevated in Paget's disease (see Volume II, Chapter 5). The degree of hyperphosphatemia is related to the severity of the disease because a positive correlation was found between the plasma phosphate and the logarithm of hydroxyproline excretion; the hyperphosphatemia is due to increased renal tubular reabsorption of phosphate (Shelling, 1935; Bijvoet and De Vries, 1974). The reason for the elevation of Tm_{PO_4}/G.F.R. is not known. Defective phosphate reabsorption has been found in patients with essential and renovascular hypertension (Heidland *et al.*, 1971). There have been isolated reports in literature on patients with benign bone or soft tissue tumors, associated with vitamin D-resistant rickets or osteomalacia, in whom decreased renal tubular reabsorption of phosphate was a common denominator. The syndrome has recently been considered as a disease entity (Salassa *et al.*, 1970; Dent and Stamp, 1971; Stanbury, 1972a; Mankin, 1974). The first such patient was reported by Prader *et al.* (1959). The hypophosphatemic rickets developed in an 11-year-old girl in association with a "reactive" giant cell tumor or granuloma in one rib. The hypophosphatemia was associated with greatly reduced tubular reabsorption of phosphate without glucosuria or abnormal aminoaciduria. All abnormalities disappeared after resection of the tumor, and the rickets healed completely without any other form of therapy. The tumors include hemangioma of bone, giant cell tumor, nonossifying fibroma of bone, and ossifying mesenchymal tumor of the larynx. These tumor may be quite trivial and only discovered by meticulous inspection of the skin. In all patients, removal of the tumor was promptly followed by normalization of phosphate reabsorption and cure of bone lesions. Salassa *et al.* (1970) suggested that these tumors produce ectopic humoral substances that cause hypophosphatemic osteomalacia.

E. Diseases of the Kidney and Serum Phosphate Homeostasis

It was shown in Section I,D that the role of the kidney in mediating hormonal adjustment of extracellular phosphate homeostasis is mediated through the effect of these hormones on tubular reabsorption of phosphate. The rate of glomerular filtration determines the efficiency of this renal function. Disorders of tubular transport and of glomerular filtration rate each have their specific influence on calcium and phosphate homeostasis (see Volume II, Chapter 2).

1. Disorders of Renal Tubular Phosphate Transport

After the discovery of vitamin D and the elucidation of the role of sunlight in the formation of cholecalciferol in the skin, the syndromes of rickets or osteomalacia, defined by their response to treatment with vitamin D, could be accurately described. This led to increased precision in diagnosis and better differentiation from other syndromes and diseases (Albright *et al.,* 1937; Dent, 1969). In the 1930's a new form of rickets was recognized that was resistant to the usual doses of vitamin D and that now has dissolved itself into a number of diseases due to a spectrum of renal tubular abnormalities (Mankin, 1974; Albright *et al.,* 1937). A common denominator of these diseases is a failure of the proximal tubules to reabsorb phosphate, leading to an abnormally low phosphate concentration in the plasma. The rickets or osteomalacia may be secondary to the hypophosphatemia. The simplest form in which the phosphate reabsorption defect occurs is in isolated form as X-linked hypophosphatemic osteomalacia. The disturbance of phosphate transport may occur in that disease in organs other than the kidney (Short *et al.,* 1973). In other diseases belonging to the same general group, the defect in phosphate reabsorption may be associated with defective reabsorption of glucose, amino acids, bicarbonate, and water and impaired urinary acidification ability. In one of these syndromes anatomical deformities in the tubules have been found (Darmady and Stranack, 1957); in others the abnormalities form part of more general metabolic defects. Some of the syndromes, in particular those associated with renal tubular acidosis, may be acquired and due to toxic damage of the kidney secondary to systemic disorders. This group of diseases is discussed in this volume, Chapter 5.

2. Chronic Renal Failure

Chronic renal failure with decreased glomerular filtration rate is associated with bone disease (Stanbury, 1972b). There are several distinct causes for disturbed calcium metabolism in renal failure: (1) Loss of structural integrity of the kidney leads to loss of function as an endocrine organ and defective formation of 1,25-dihydroxycholecalciferol—the active metabolite of cholecalciferol that is necessary for proper expression of its function (Stanbury, 1972b). This may be responsible for the acquired vitamin D resistance of chronic renal failure. (2) The decrease of glomerular filtration rate leads to less efficient regulation of serum phosphate excretion by the kidney, high serum phosphate, and secondary hyperparathyroidism. (3) Chronic metabolic acidosis due to renal failure may affect bone metabolism. There may be other associated factors, but we will only discuss the mechanism of hyperphosphatemia (see Volume II, Chapter 2).

Goldman et al. (1954) noted that patients with glomerular filtration rates below 30 ml/minute have an elevated serum phosphate concentration. Bricker (1969) argued that any reduction in glomerular filtration rate would tend to produce an increase in serum phosphate and a reciprocal reduction in serum calcium that would be corrected by appropriate elevation of PTH secretion. At slightly decreased glomerular filtration rates, the effect of variations of G.F.R. on serum phosphate are difficult to observe because the effect of variation of phosphate intake and of tubular reabsorption are much greater, but use of the technique of multiple regression analysis has enabled the effect of each of these factors on the serum phosphate [PO$_4$] to be defined separately and has shown a negative correlation between [PO$_4$] and G.F.R. at filtration rates in the normal range (Bijvoet, 1969). This negative partial correlation is illustrated in Fig. 7. The stimulation of parathyroid function by slight hyperphosphatemia has also been experimentally confirmed. Feeding excess phosphate to animals leads to transient elevation of the serum phosphate, parathyroid hyperplasia, and secondary reduction of renal tubular reabsorption of phosphate (Drake et al., 1937; Baumann and Sprinson, 1939; Engfeldt et al., 1954). The phosphate intake in the rat was found to be linearly related to the size of the parathyroid glands (Kaye, 1974). Reiss et al. (1969) could find increased serum concentrations of PTH when glomerular filtration rate was still as high as 70–80 ml/minute and demonstrated a progressive increase in concentrations as renal failure advanced (Reiss and Canterbury, 1971). Finally, Slatopolsky and co-workers (1971) showed in dogs that if the intake of phosphate is reduced in proportion to glomerular filtration rate, secondary hyperparathyroidism is prevented (Slatopolsky et al., 1972; Slatopolsky and Bricker, 1973).

Most of these data are empirical, and some confusion may arise by the indiscriminate use in such studies of T.R.P. or the ratio of phosphate to creatinine clearance, C_{PO_4}/C_{creat}, as an index of renal tubular phosphate reabsorption activity or as an index of the effect of PTH on the kidney. The theoretical basis for the observed effects on the serum phosphate concentration of phosphate feeding and of glomerular filtration rate is relatively simple (Bijvoet, 1969, 1972; Bijvoet et al., 1969; Bijvoet and Morgan, 1971; Morgan, 1973). Excreted phosphate is the nonreabsorbed phosphate. When phosphate reabsorption is maximal, this relation is shown in Eq. (13).

$$U_{PO_4}V = \text{G.F.R.} \times [PO_4] - Tm_{PO_4} \tag{13}$$

Rearrangement gives Eq (14).

$$[PO_4] = \frac{Tm_{PO_4}}{\text{G.F.R.}} + \frac{U_{PO_4}V}{\text{G.F.R.}} \tag{14}$$

It is thus possible to calculate the relation between serum phosphate concentration $[PO_4]$ and glomerular filtration rate for any value of G.F.R., at a set value of $Tm_{PO_4}/\text{G.F.R.}$ The value of T.R.P. can then be derived from Eq. (10).

$$\text{T.R.P.} = \frac{Tm_{PO_4}/\text{G.F.R.}}{[PO_4]} \tag{10}$$

The results are given in Fig. 8. In calculation of Fig. 8 "splay" (see Sections I,B and I,C,2) has been taken into account as derived from earlier studies (Bijvoet, 1969). The predicted relation between $[PO_4]$ and G.F.R. shows a curvilinear increase in $[PO_4]$ as G.F.R. decreases. It explains the sudden rise of $[PO_4]$ at G.F.R. values below 30 ml/minute that has been observed by Goldman et al. (1954), and the predicted relations agree remarkably well with the observed relation between $[PO_4]$ and G.F.R. observed by Kleeman et al. (1970). Consideration of the relation between T.R.P. and G.F.R. shown in Fig. 8b, where they are compared with data of Slatopolsky et al. (1968), is important because it shows that T.R.P. should decrease curvilinearly with G.F.R. when tubular reabsorption ($Tm_{PO_4}/\text{G.F.R.}$) remains unaltered. Thus, in renal failure, a decreased T.R.P. does not primarily reflect secondary hyperparathyroidism. This has also been confirmed experimentally (Popovtzer et al., 1972).

In addition, when G.F.R. is low, T.R.P. becomes very sensitive to small

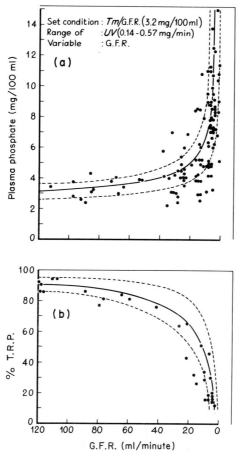

Fig. 8. (a) The relationship between plasma phosphate (mg/100 ml) and G.F.R. (ml/minute) in healthy individuals and patients with chronic renal disease taken from the data of Kleeman *et al.* (1970). The continuous line shows the theoretical relationship when only G.F.R. is varied and Tm_{PO_4}/G.F.R. remains constant at the average normal value. The dashed lines similarly show the ranges of value due to a variation in $U_{PO_4}V$ through the range found in normal subjects. Note that the effect of variations in phosphate load ($U_{PO_4}V$) on [PO$_4$] increases with decreasing G.F.R. (b) The relationship between percent T.R.P. and G.R.F. in healthy individuals and patients with chronic renal failure, taken from the data of Slatopolsky *et al.* (1968). The continuous and dotted lines show the relationships derived under the same conditions as above. (Reproduced from Bijvoet and Morgan, 1971.)

changes in $U_{PO_4}V$ (as may happen with small changes in phosphate intake) independent of any change in the parathyroid-sensitive phosphate reabsorption, thus demonstrating that T.R.P. should not be used as an index of phosphate reabsorption in renal failure. Figure 8 demonstrates that the same variations in phosphate absorption from the gut, which are assumed to be reflected in proportional variations in $U_{PO_4}V$, lead to a much greater increase or decrease of plasma phosphate when glomerular filtration rate is low than when glomerular filtration rate is normal. This agrees with experimental observations (Friis *et al.*, 1968). In renal failure, small changes of G.F.R. and of phosphate intake become more important for the serum phosphate concentration than parathyroid-mediated effects on the renal tubules. The relative effect of extrarenal phosphate input, be it from bone or gut, may actually exceed the importance of renal factors (Kleeman *et al.*, 1970; Slatopolsky *et al.*, 1968). This may explain why with decreasing G.F.R. circadian variations in [PO₄] become excessive and the fasting [PO₄] then no longer relates to the average [PO₄] level over 24 hours. This also explains why serum [PO₄] levels may actually *fall* in uremic patients undergoing parathyroidectomy (Stanbury *et al.*, 1960), when after parathyroidectomy the net rate at which phosphate is transported from bone to blood is reduced. Because of its effect on bone resorption, a high level of PTH may increase the net movement of phosphate to blood and thereby actually cause a *rise* in serum phosphate concentration instead of decreasing the serum [PO₄] by its effect on the kidney. The increased sensitivity of serum phosphate to phosphate input also explains why parenterally administered vitamin D may, as a result of its effect on bone, increase the serum phosphate.

These considerations that make easily intelligible the otherwise paradoxical clinical observations stress again the importance of reducing phosphate intake in uremia. The observation of Slatopolsky and co-workers (1971, 1972) that reduction of phosphate intake in proportion to the decrease of G.F.R. will restore the serum phosphate to normal is also predictable (Fig. 9), since at, for instance, half the G.F.R. phosphate output is halved when [PO₄] and Tm_{PO_4}/G.F.R. remain constant and thus only half the input is needed to maintain the same [PO₄]. This will help to alleviate the stress on the parathyroid glands. However, as shown, the parathyroid glands need not play a role in that reduction of phosphate concentration. Normalization of T.R.P. is in those circumstances mainly a mathematical result because of Eq. (9).

$$\text{T.R.P.} = 1 - \frac{U_{PO_4}V}{[PO_4] \times \text{G.F.R.}} \tag{9}$$

T.R.P. should remain normal when [PO₄] is normal and the ratio of $U_{PO_4}V$ to G.F.R. is normal.

It remains to be seen if values of Tm_{PO_4}/G.F.R. as measured in renal failure may be compared with normal values in persons of the same age

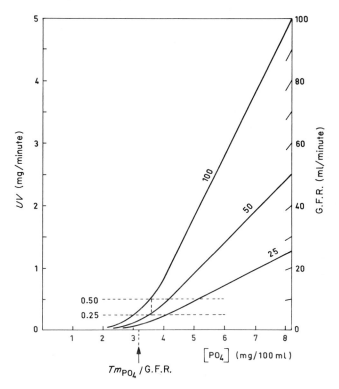

Fig. 9. The relationship between the urinary excretion rate of phosphate ($U_{PO_4}V$, mg/minute) and the plasma phosphate ([PO$_4$], mg/100 ml) with respect to G.F.R. (ml/minute). In a steady state $U_{PO_4}V$ equals the phosphate absorbed from the diet. Note that a proportional reduction of G.F.R. and of phosphate absorbed from the diet will leave the plasma [PO$_4$] unaffected and that the increase in plasma [PO$_4$] due to a given increase in phosphate intake (UV) is inversely proportional to G.F.R. Data from the observation that $d(U_{PO_4}V)/d[PO_4]$ equals G.F.R. even at very low rates of G.F.R. (Arner, 1964); splay was calculated according to Bijvoet (1969).

and sex. Splay may change in renal failure (Bricker *et al.*, 1965), but serum phosphate concentration is generally so high that reabsorption rate will be maximal anyway and can be calculated as shown in Eq. (10).

$$\frac{Tm_{PO_4}}{\text{G.F.R.}} = \text{T.R.P.} \times [PO_4] \tag{10}$$

However, the balance between glomerular and tubular function may be markedly disturbed in uremia (Seldin *et al.*, 1971) so that an ''abnormal'' Tm/G.F.R. ratio may be indicative of anatomical as well as of functional disturbances.

II. RENAL CALCIUM TRANSPORT

A. The Elements of Renal Calcium Transport

Studies of the renal transport of calcium are less open to interpretation than studies of phosphate transport and are still largely empirical. There are several reasons for this. First, the concentration of calcium in the glomerular filtrate is less than the serum calcium concentration and is, therefore, less easily assessed. Second, calcium reabsorption in the renal tubules occurs at various sites, each with different sensitivity to factors affecting tubular reabsorption. Third, not all of the calcium in the renal tubular fluid is ionized, and not all forms are reabsorbed equally well. Unlike changes in serum phosphate due to altered renal phosphate transport, changes in serum calcium [Ca] are quickly sensed by and corrected through the parathyroids; therefore, hormonal or mineral actions on renal calcium transport that would otherwise affect serum calcium concentration are not always easily recognized.

1. Glomerular Filtration

Calcium is present in the serum in various forms (Table IV). Somewhat less than 50% of plasma calcium is ionized, and 46% of total calcium is bound to protein, the remainder forming complexes with phosphate, citrate, and other organic anions (Walser, 1961a, 1969). Not all serum calcium is filterable through the glomeruli. The filtered load of calcium (L_{Ca}, weight/time) is therefore equal to the product of the glomerular filtration rate (G.F.R., volume/time) and the fraction (f) of serum calcium ([Ca], w/v) which passes through the glomerular membrane.

$$L_{Ca} = \text{G.F.R.} \times f \times [\text{Ca}] \tag{15}$$

A precise value for f, the ultrafilterable fraction of serum calcium, is difficult to obtain. From the few direct micropuncture studies that have been

TABLE IV

Concentrations of Calcium in Normal Human Plasma[a]

Calcium	Concentration (mg/100 ml)	% total
Free calcium ions	4.72	47.5
Protein bound	4.56	46.0
$CaHPO_4$	0.16	1.6
Calcium citrate	0.16	1.7
Unidentified	0.32	3.2
Total	9.92	100

[a] Reproduced from Walser (1961a).

carried out in rodents, it was concluded that the calcium concentration in the glomerular filtrate was equal to the ultrafilterable calcium (Lassiter *et al.*, 1963). Direct measurements of ultrafilterable calcium are complicated and not used routinely. Ultrafiltration methods are very sensitive to pH and pCO$_2$, and there may be differences between the permeability of the membranes and the glomeruli. The composition of serum calcium may vary for different calcium concentrations or for different diseases. It is, therefore, not possible to give anything but an approximate value for the ultrafilterable fraction, which normally lies between 58 and 65% (Walser, 1969). In a healthy person, the filtered load, the product of glomerular filtration rate (120 ml/minute) and ultrafilterable fraction (0.60) of serum calcium (10 mg/100 ml), is about 10,000 mg/day. In the remainder of this chapter, the amount of calcium filtered per unit time (L_{Ca}) will be defined as $f \times$ [Ca] $\times$ G.F.R. The amount of calcium filtered per unit volume glomerular filtrate equals [Eqs. (15) and (16)]:

$$L_{Ca}/\text{G.F.R.} = f \times [\text{Ca}] \tag{16}$$

2. Tubular Reabsorption and Secretion

In man, the calcium excretion rate is on the average less than 400 mg/day. Since in that time about 10,000 mg of calcium is filtered at the glomeruli, more than 96% is reabsorbed, and less than 4% of the filtered calcium is excreted. Direct studies of renal tubular reabsorption in dogs using micropuncture and stop-flow techniques and in rodents using micropuncture or microperfusion have revealed at least two sites of active calcium reabsorption (Lassiter *et al.*, 1963; Beck and Goldberg, 1973; Agus *et al.*, 1973; Howard *et al.*, 1959; Wesson and Lauler, 1959; Duarte and Watson, 1967; Widrow and Levinsky, 1962; Frick *et al.*, 1965). In rodents about two-thirds of the calcium reabsorption occurs in the proximal tubules, 20 to 25% in the ascending limb of Henle and 10% in the distal convoluted tubules (Lassiter *et al.*, 1963). Several properties characterize calcium reabsorption in the proximal tubules: It is linked with sodium reabsorption (Agus *et al.*, 1973; Howard *et al.*, 1959; Duarte and Watson, 1967; Frick *et al.*, 1965); it is insensitive to PTH (Frick *et al.*, 1965). Recently it has been suggested that parathyroid inhibits proximal calcium reabsorption, but this action may be secondary to an effect on proximal Na reabsorption (Agus *et al.*, 1973); and, finally, the rate of proximal calcium reabsorption appears to vary directly with the intraluminal calcium concentration and is not limited by a maximal rate or *Tm* (Frick *et al.*, 1965). The second calcium reabsorption process was localized in the rat in the ascending limb of Henle's loop proximal to sodium reabsorption (Lassiter *et al.*, 1963). Stop-flow studies in dogs and micropuncture studies in rodents localized the effect of PTH in distal parts of the nephron (Lassiter *et al.*, 1963; Howard *et al.*, 1959; Wesson and Lauler, 1959; Widrow and Levinsky, 1962). There is evidence that at least one component of the tubular reabsorption of calcium is rate *(Tm)* limited (see Section II,B). By inference it seems likely that this must be the distal process. There is evidence for the existence of calcium influx through the tubular walls into the tubular lumen. In dogs, radioactive calcium injected into the renal artery during stop-flow experiments appears earlier than marked creatinine administered simultaneously (Bronner and Thompson, 1961). Net influx into the proximal tubules has also been demonstrated in rats during microperfusion with calcium-free solutions (Frick *et al.*, 1965). There are indications that medullary recycling exists between the ascending and descending limbs of the loop of Henle for calcium and magnesium with sodium, potassium, and chloride but not with phosphate (De Rouffignac *et al.*, 1973). The calcium transport in the distal nephron must be accomplished by a very active calcium pump, since both micropuncture and stop-flow studies revealed tubular fluid to ultrafilterable plasma ratios of calcium well below unity (Lassiter *et al.*, 1963; Howard *et al.*, 1959; Wesson and Lauler, 1959; Grollman *et al.*, 1963) despite an electrical potential difference across the tubule that should lead to the appearance of tubular fluid to ultrafilterable plasma ratios above 1.0.

B. Renal Calcium Transport as a Whole

In clinical studies the net calcium reabsorption [T_{Ca} (mass/time)] is defined as shown in Eq. (17).

$$T_{Ca} = f \times [Ca] \times G.F.R. - U_{Ca}V \tag{17}$$

Net calcium reabsorption is simply the net result of several transport processes along the nephron. Tubular reabsorption per unit volume of glomerular filtrate (T_{Ca}/G.F.R., mass/volume) would be about equal to the concentration of calcium in the fluid reabsorbed by the tubules (see Section I,B) and is defined as shown in Eq. (18).

$$T_{Ca}/G.F.R. = f \times [Ca] - U_{Ca}V/G.F.R. \tag{18}$$

There is some justification for expressing reabsorption in terms of glomerular filtration rate. Studies of Massry and co-workers indicate a glomerulotubular balance (cf. Section I,B) for calcium (Massry *et al.*, 1967; Massry and Kleeman, 1972). For practical purposes T_{Ca}/G.F.R. indicates the net calcium concentration in the fluid reabsorbed by the kidney into the blood.

Calcium reabsorption can, therefore, be studied by comparing $f \times [Ca]$ with $U_{Ca}V$/G.F.R. during calcium infusion. In dogs, no evidence of a maximum limiting rate of the tubular reabsorption *(Tm)* of calcium was found; reabsorption continued to rise as the glomerular filtration of calcium was steadily increased by means of calcium infusion (Chen and Neuman, 1955; Poulos, 1957). In man, Copp (1960) reported data showing a *Tm* for calcium. His experiments have never been confirmed. Kleeman *et al.* (1961) noted that fractional calcium excretion (C_{Ca}/C_{creat}) increased with increasing serum [Ca]; and later Peacock and co-workers (1969) found that when plasma calcium is steadily increased, a constant proportion of any increase in filtered load above a given value is excreted (Peacock and Nordin, 1968a; Peacock *et al.*, 1969). This is illustrated in Fig. 10 adapted from the work of Peacock *et al.* (1969; Bijvoet and Van der Sluys Veer, 1972). In their studies it was tactily assumed that patients show variations in the rate of calcium reabsorption that are due to and proportional to variations in G.F.R. as has already been demonstrated for phosphate (see Section I,B). To eliminate variations in reabsorption due to variations in G.F.R., the reabsorption rate was studied in terms of $f \times$ [Ca] as well as $U_{Ca}V$/G.F.R. [see Eq. (18)]. $U_{Ca}V$/G.F.R. can simply be calculated from the ratio of calcium to creatinine concentration in the urine multiplied by serum creatinine concentration (cf. Section I,C). Another simplification was introduced since in their studies ultrafilterable calcium was always a constant fraction, 0.58, of the total calcium, all data on the abscissa should be multiplied by 0.58. It is clear from Fig. 10 that during calcium infusion a linear relationship between $U_{Ca}V$/G.F.R. and serum [Ca] was obtained. The relationship resembles that for phosphate (Fig. 4); however, unlike phosphate excretion, not all of the increase in filtered load per unit G.F.R. is excreted. The slope relating $U_{Ca}V$/G.F.R. to $f \times$ [Ca] is not equal to unity but to 0.51. In terms of total calcium, the slope equals 0.30. Peacock and Nordin (1968a) called the intercept of the line relating all observations with the abscissa the calcium threshold. Any increase in [Ca] above this threshold increases $U_{Ca}V$/G.F.R. by 0.30 of that increase. Note that splay for calcium excretion is much less than that for phosphate.

Calcium reabsorption probably occurs at two or more different sites in the tubules (see Section II,A). One site of reabsorption is proximal. Micropuncture studies suggest a concentration-dependent reabsorption rate. With such a mechanism, a constant fraction of filtered calcium would be excreted (Fig. 11). If the distal reabsorption rate is assumed to be *Tm*-limited this would cause excretion at all values of [Ca] to be less than that by a constant value equal to Tm_{Ca}/G.F.R., thereby shifting the line downward by that value. This would cause the regression line relating $U_{Ca}V$/G.F.R. to [Ca] to intersect the abscissa at the point called the "calcium threshold." Note in Fig. 11 that if proximal reabsorption is a fraction *(t)* of

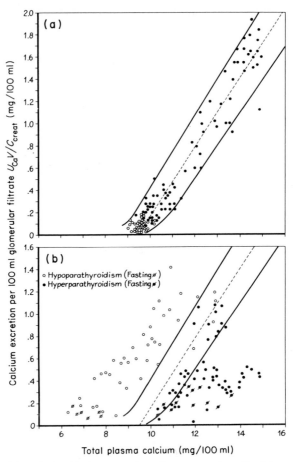

Fig. 10. (a) The relationship between the urinary excretion of calcium per 100 ml of glomerular filtrate ($U_{Ca}V/C_{creat}$) and the total serum calcium in healthy adults when fasting (open circles) and during calcium loading (closed circles); the dashed line represents a regression line through the closed circles. The continuous lines are drawn to indicate a "normal range." (b) The relationship between calcium excretion over 100 ml of G.F.R. and serum calcium in patients with hypoparathyroidism (open circles) and hyperparathyroidism (closed circles) when fasting (dash through the symbol) and when loaded with calcium. Normal limits as in (a). (According to Peacock *et al.*, 1969.)

filtered calcium, the slope of $U_{Ca}V$/G.F.R. with respect to [Ca] is equal to $f \times (1 - t)$. Thus Tm_{Ca}/G.F.R. equals $f \times (1 - t) \times$ threshold. The relationship between filtered fraction *(f)*, proximal reabsorbed fraction *(t)*, distal reabsorption Tm_{Ca}/G.F.R. and renal threshold concentration for calcium [Ca]$_{thresh}$ therefore becomes

$$[Ca]_{thresh} = \frac{Tm_{Ca}/G.F.R.}{f(1-t)} \tag{19}$$

Peacock and Nordin (1968a) found a mean renal threshold concentration for calcium of 9.5 mg per 100 ml in healthy adults. They found a slope of $U_{Ca}V/G.F.R.$ with respect to [Ca] of 0.30. From these data, it can be calculated that the fractional proximal calcium reabsorption *(t)* is about

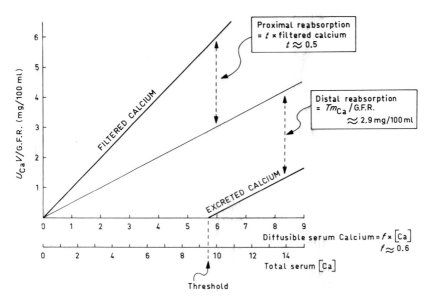

Fig. 11. Theoretical relationship between the urinary excretion of calcium per 100 ml of glomerular filtrate ($U_{Ca}V/G.F.R.$) and the total [Ca] and the diffusible serum calcium concentration (f × [Ca], $f = 0.60$). The uppermost line labeled filtered calcium represents $U_{Ca}V/$ G.F.R. when there is no tubular calcium reabsorption. The middle line represents $U_{Ca}V/$ G.F.R. when a constant fraction *(t)* of filtered calcium (t × f × [Ca], t = 0.5, t × f = 0.3) is reabsorbed in the proximal tubules. Note that excreted calcium would then be equal to

$$U_{Ca}V/G.F.R. = (1 - t) \times f \times [Ca] = 0.3 \times [Ca]$$

The lower line labeled excreted calcium represents $U_{Ca}V/G.F.R.$ when calcium is also reabsorbed in more distal regions of the nephron at a constant maximum rate per unit G.F.R. ($Tm_{Ca}/G.F.R. = 2.9$ mg/100 ml). Note that excreted calcium would then be equal to

$$U_{Ca}V/G.F.R. = (1 - t) \times f \times [Ca] - Tm_{Ca}/G.F.R.$$

and that when $U_{Ca}V/G.F.R.$ equals zero, [Ca] equals threshold and $Tm_{Ca}/G.F.R.$ equals $(1 - t) \times f \times$ threshold. From this it follows that $U_{Ca}V/G.F.R. = (1 - t) \times f \times [Ca] -$ threshold), or $U_{Ca}V/G.F.R. = 0.3$ ([Ca] − 9.5), which is the relationship described by Peacock and Nordin (1968a) and Peacock *et al.* (1969) that is shown in Fig. 10.

50% and the rate of distal reabsorption 2.9 mg per 100 ml. Two direct consequences of Eq. (19) are that the apparent threshold concentration for calcium varies directly with Tm_{Ca}/G.F.R. and inversely with $(1 - t)$. A 50% decrease of t from 0.5 to 0.25 would lower the threshold concentration to $(1 - 0.5)/(1 - 0.25) = 0.66$ of its original value, that is from 9.5 to 6.3 mg per 100 ml without changing distal Tm_{Ca}/G.F.R. The same analysis has been used by Mioni *et al.* (1971) to differentiate between proximal and distal disturbances of calcium reabsorption in renal disease. The renal threshold concentration for calcium is considered to determine the average around which serum [Ca] varies (Mioni *et al.*, 1971). When [Ca] increases above that level, the excretion rate increases rapidly; when [Ca] decreases, the excretion rate will fall to very low values. The relationship between kidney function and the level of serum [Ca] will be discussed later in more detail (see Section II,D,1).

C. Measurement of Calcium Reabsorption

In comparison with the great variety of indices for phosphate excretion, the measurement of calcium reabsorption seems neglected. The terms hypercalciuria or hypocalciuria refer to steady states with increased or decreased excretion rates of calcium and as such indicate increased or decreased extrarenal input of calcium into the extracellular fluid and not an altered calcium reabsorption. Some information about variations in renal calcium reabsorption can be gained by comparing $U_{Ca}V$, G.F.R. and serum [Ca] using Fig. 10 as basis of comparison (Peacock and Nordin, 1973). $U_{Ca}V$/G.F.R. is calculated as the ratio of urine calcium to creatinine concentrations multiplied by the serum creatinine concentration. Any value lying below the lines indicating a normal relationship between $U_{Ca}V$/G.F.R. and [Ca] would indicate increased net calcium reabsorption; the converse would apply to values lying above. Any $U_{Ca}V$/G.F.R. value above normal but within the normal range for the relationship between $U_{Ca}V$/G.F.R. and [Ca] would indicate an elevated [Ca] due to either increased calcium input into the extracellular fluid or low G.F.R. (numerator or denominator of the term $U_{Ca}V$/G.F.R.) with normal net tubular reabsorption. Figure 10 should, however, not be used indiscriminately, for any value outside the normal relation between $U_{Ca}V$/G.F.R. and [Ca] could be related to any of the following disturbances: (a) an abnormal filtered fraction of calcium due to altered protein bound or complexed calcium as for instance in cirrhosis or myeloma; (b) an altered proximal reabsorption, as may occur in renal failure or when proximal sodium chloride reabsorption is altered (see below); (c) an altered distal reabsorption; or (d) a combination of these factors [cf. Eq. (19)]. One should also remember that in constructing Fig. 10 from infusion data the possible effect of an increasing serum [Ca] on parathyroid-mediated calcium reabsorption (see Section II,D,1) and of acute hypercalcemia on renal reabsorption of calcium (Verbanck and Toppet, 1961; Massry *et al.*, 1968a) has not been considered.

Yet the use of Fig. 10 as a basis of comparison offers some advantage over the use of calcium clearance or the ratio of calcium to creatinine clearance because the exact relationship between calcium clearances and the tubular reabsorption of calcium is even less well defined and the absolute values of these clearances have no meaning. In acute studies, conclusions about qualitative changes in calcium transport can, of course, be derived from transient calciuric or hypocalciuric effects, provided no concomitant changes in serum [Ca] occur in the same direction. In comparing groups of studies, changes in or differences between excretion rates offer information about tubular calcium transport only when there are no corresponding differences in serum [Ca] or G.F.R. However, in this case one needs sensitive measurements of serum calcium concentration, because Fig. 10 suggests that an increase in [Ca] of 0.1 mg per 100 ml could well be responsible for an increase in calcium excretion rate of about 60 mg Ca per 24 hours, when there are no compensatory changes in tubular calcium transport.

D. The Physiology of Calcium Excretion

In this section, renal calcium handling will be discussed in relation to extracellular calcium homeostasis and calcium balance. The preceding discussion of renal phosphate handling emphasized the importance of the kidney for serum phosphate homeostasis. Phosphate transport in other organs is probably of less importance in that respect, and there is no endocrine organ that senses extracellular phosphate concentration and regulates renal tubular phosphate reabsorption in relation to this. Therefore, serum phosphate concentration is primarily controlled, or rather fixed, by the kidney. On the contrary, serum calcium concentration is not controlled by the kidney but by the parathyroid glands. These glands achieve constancy of extracellular calcium concentration through modulation by PTH of the rates of ion transport in three target organs: kidney, bone, and possibly gut. Accordingly, the importance and the nature of the action of PTH on calcium reabsorption in the kidney will be discussed first and then the relative roles of kidney and bone in mediating the effects of PTH on serum calcium.

1. The Effect of Parathyroid Hormone on Renal Calcium Handling

Albright and Reifenstein (1948) stated already that there were two trains of thought with regard to the effect of PTH on serum calcium. One school believed that the hormone acts directly on bone tissue causing its dissolution and that serum calcium changes are secondary to the bone changes. Albright himself adhered to the second view that the hormone acts on the electrolyte equilibria of the body through its effect on the kidney and that the bone changes are secondary to the chemical changes. He postulated that PTH modulates serum [PO$_4$] through its effect on the kidney. A high serum phosphate might then inhibit dissolution of calcium phosphate from bone, and a low phosphate might enhance it. These effects then mediate the influence of PTH secretion on serum calcium concentration. However, the work of Barnicot (1948) and of Gaillard (1961) showed that PTH itself can mobilize calcium from bone. Talmage *et al.* (1953) then demonstrated that the parathyroids could maintain calcium homeostasis in nephrectomized rats and could, therefore, do this by a direct action on bone. The emphasis then shifted to the extrarenal effects of the parathyroids in calcium homeostasis. However, the first evidence that the kidneys might also be directly involved in calcium homeostasis also came from Talmage and co-workers (1955; Talmage and Kraintz, 1954; Talmage, 1956–1957). They showed that in rats PTH injections transiently decreased calcium excretion and thus increased tubular reabsorption of calcium, leading to a rise in serum [Ca]. When, however, PTH administration was continued and sufficient time had elapsed, a steady state developed, where the effect on the excretion rate was reversed. The excretion rate was now increased because, in the steady state, the excretion rate reflected PTH-induced bone resorption. These authors also explained that although the absolute rate of excretion of calcium was increased, the calcium excretion rate was low in relation to the elevated serum [Ca]. Thus, an untreated rat would have excreted more calcium at the same serum calcium level. Hence, tubular reabsorption of calcium remained increased. Talmage and co-workers (1955) interpreted their data as meaning that the parathyroids maintain serum calcium concentration by action on both bone and kidneys and that PTH increases the renal calcium threshold (Talmage and Kraintz, 1954; Talmage *et al.*, 1955; Talmage, 1956–1957)

There are now three types of evidence to show that PTH increases the tubular reabsorption of calcium. One type is based on transient changes in calcium excretion rate when the steady state is disrupted by parathyroidectomy or PTH administration. The second type of evidence is based on the effect of PTH administration on the intraluminal calcium content of the renal tubules in micropuncture or stop-flow studies. The third type is based on the relation between calcium excretion rate and serum calcium concentration in hyperparathyroid or hypoparathyroid states.

a. Disruption of the Steady State. In rats, dogs, and frogs, there is a rise in urinary calcium excretion rate coinciding with a drop in serum calcium concentration following parathyroidectomy (Talmage and Kraintz, 1954; Talmage *et al.*, 1955; Talmage, 1956–1957; Berthaux *et al.*, 1960; Kleeman *et al.*, 1960; Cortelyou *et al.*, 1960). This has also been observed in patients with parathyroid adenoma subjected to parathyroidectomy (Kleeman *et al.*, 1961; Canary and Kyle, 1959). The increment lasts only for a short time until the serum calcium concentration has decreased to the point where the excretion rate returns to normal. However, in dogs (Buchanan, 1961) and man (Lafferty and Pearson, 1963), the phenomenon does not occur invariably. A transient decrease in calcium excretion following PTH administration has been found in rats (Talmage and Kraintz, 1954; Talmage *et al.*, 1955). In normal men or dogs, such changes have been more difficult to demonstrate and even opposite effects have been found (Massry *et al.*, 1973; Walser, 1969). There are several possible explanations for these difficulties: (1) The effect may be masked by concurrent increase of net bone resorption (Talmage and Kraintz, 1954; Talmage *et al.*, 1955; Talmage, 1956–1957). (2) PTH may have a dual action in the kidney consisting of a transient inhibition of proximal calcium and sodium reabsorption and a continued acceleration of distal calcium reabsorption rate, the initial total effect being no change but the final effect being a net increase of reabsorption (Agus *et al.*, 1971, 1973) (cf. Sections II,D,5,b and III,A,1,i). (3) There may be a delay before the effect of PTH on calcium reabsorption becomes fully expressed (Froeling and Bijvoet, 1974; LeGrimellec *et al.*, 1974). However, in hypoparathyroid patients with a normal serum calcium concentration maintained by calcium infusion, PTH was observed to acutely reduce calcium excretion (Eisenberg, 1965).

b. Micropuncture and Stop-Flow Studies. With these techniques, it was shown that PTH accelerates tubular reabsorption of calcium in distal parts of the nephron (Lassiter *et al.*, 1963, Agus *et al.*, 1971, 1973; Howard *et al.*, 1959; Wesson and Lauler, 1959; Widrow and Levinsky, 1962; Frick *et al.*, 1965). The first clear demonstration of a distal site of action was given by Widrow and Levinsky (1962) in the dog with a stop-flow technique. They found a distal tubular site at which intraluminal calcium concentration in normal dogs is low. This distal dip is almost abolished by parathyroidectomy and is restored by parathyroid extract. Purified PTH also has this effect (MacIntrye *et al.*, 1963). Earlier micropuncture studies in rats showed that PTH has no effect on proximal calcium reabsorption (Frick *et al.*, 1965), but more recently micropunctures in dogs have produced evidence suggesting that PTH reduces proximal tubular reabsorption of calcium (with sodium) but increased distal reabsorption to a greater extent, the net effect being increased reabsorption (Agus *et al.*, 1971, 1973).

c. The Relation between Calcium Excretion and Serum Calcium in Hyper-

parathyroidism and Hypoparathyroidism. When patients with hyperparathyroidism or hypoparathyroidism are in a steady state, that is have stable serum calcium concentrations, albeit high or low, the excretion rate of calcium is equal to the net input of calcium into the extracellular fluid from bone or gut and does not reflect normality or abnormality of renal tubular calcium reabsorption. However it follows from Eq. (17)

$$U_{Ca}V = f \times [Ca] \times G.F.R. - T_{ca} \qquad (17)$$

that increased reabsorption will be reflected in a lower than normal calcium excretion rate at a given serum calcium concentration. Kleeman *et al.* (1961) and Gordan *et al.* (1962) showed that normal subjects given calcium infusions have higher calcium excretion rates relative to serum calcium (calcium clearance) than hyperparathyroid patients with comparable hypercalcemia. Even if such patients do exhibit hypercalciuria (Albright and Reifenstein, 1948; Canary and Kyle, 1959), this is due to increased resorption of bone or increased calcium absorption in the gut, and healthy persons would excrete much more calcium in the urine at comparable calcium concentrations. The relation between calcium excretion rate and serum calcium concentration in healthy subjects and persons with hyperparathyroidism or hypoparathyroidism during calcium infusion or increased oral calcium intake has been worked out by Peacock *et al.* (1969; Peacock and Nordin, 1968a). (Fig. 10). These authors interpreted their observations to mean that the line in Fig. 10a relating calcium excretion to serum calcium concentration shifts downward (rate-limited distal calcium reabsorption, Tm_{Ca}, increases by a constant amount at any [Ca], cf. Fig. 11) in hyperparathyroidism and upward in hypoparathyroidism, thus causing a higher renal threshold concentration for calcium in hyperparathyroidism and a low threshold in hypoparathyroidism. Their observations confirm anyway that overall renal reabsorption is increased in the hyperparathyroid state and reduced in the hypoparathyroid state. From such data it can be concluded that the action of PTH on the kidney is to increase overall calcium reabsorption and that this will be instrumental in maintaining a high serum calcium concentration.

In the foregoing sections, it was suggested that calcium reabsorption consists of two different mechanisms: one is concentration dependent, localized in the proximal tubules, and controls with G.F.R. the slope of the line relating $U_{Ca}V$ to serum [Ca] (Fig. 11). The other mechanism, localized distally, could be the *Tm*-limited one. This Tm_{Ca} would then be increased by enhanced and decreased by reduced PTH secretion with proportional changes of the renal threshold concentration for calcium and serum [Ca] [cf. Eq. (19)].

2. Kidney, Bone, Hormone, and Serum Calcium

Talmage and co-workers 1953, (1955; Talmage and Kraintz, 1954; Talmage, 1956–1957) showed that both kidney and bone may mediate the effect of PTH on serum calcium. Peacock and co-workers maintain that the kidney is the main mediator (Peacock *et al.*, 1969; Peacock and Nordin, 1968a, 1973; Nordin and Peacock, 1969; Nordin *et al.*, 1972). Based on the correlations found by them between changes in calcium excretion per 100 ml of glomerular filtrate and serum calcium levels (Fig. 10), their proposal is that the fall in blood calcium levels following the removal of a parathyroid adenoma is due to a decreased renal threshold concentration for calcium, and the hypercalcemia of hyperparathyroidism is attributed to the raised threshold. They conclude that the maintenance of a stable serum calcium concentration in healthy persons is solely mediated by the kidney. Although their proposal seems straightforward at first sight, it is overstated and should be qualified (Bijvoet and Van der Sluys Veer, 1972; Bijvoet, 1973). In discussing the relative roles of kidney and bone in the homeostasis of blood calcium, it is important to distinguish between (a) the mean level of the blood calcium concentration in an approximately steady state and (b) the damping of transient variations in the calcium concentration around that level. At normal glomerular filtration rate, when kidney function is normally efficient, the kidney probably determines the mean level of the blood calcium concentration by excreting calcium when serum [Ca] rises above the threshold concentration for calcium and reclaiming all filtered calcium when serum [Ca] decreases below it (Fig. 10). However, the role of the kidney in correcting transient disturbances of the steady state can not be derived from Fig. 10. According to the relationship in Fig. 10, an increase in absorbed calcium of 100 mg/day would increase serum [Ca] by 0.2 mg per 100 ml before the kidney could excrete calcium at the same increased rate. One would expect this to affect PTH secretion and thereby not only calcium excretion but also net bone resorption. Conversely, when the calcium concentration becomes depressed, the kidney cannot generate calcium to increase it, i.e., it cannot reabsorb more calcium from the tubules than is filtered at the glomeruli. The body can, however, counteract challanges to calcium homeostasis by modulating the relative rates of calcium uptake and release in bone. Phang *et al.* (1969) found that prolonged changes in the rate of calcium absorption in the gut produced in humans by altering the calcium content of the diet were only partly balanced by changes in the renal excretion rate; they were further compensated for by relative changes between the rates of gain and loss of calcium in the skeleton. This may explain why at normal levels of calcium intake, the correlation between intake and renal excretion is poor (Nordin and Smith, 1965; Davis *et al.,* 1970). When this mechanism fails, as for instance in myxedematous children with low turnover rates of bone calcium, blood calcium may vary with the calcium intake (Lowe *et al.,* 1962; Klotz and Kanovitz, 1966). Parathyroidectomy (Kleeman *et al.,* 1961) or suppression of the parathyroid glands by hypermagnesemia (Massry *et al.,* 1970) is followed by a far greater decrease in serum calcium than can be accounted for by the urinary losses during the time of observations. Probably, the combined parathyroid effects on bone and kidney maintain serum calcium homeostasis.

Figure 12 shows the effect in man of continuous intravenous infusion for 24 hours of parathyroid extract or hormone at ten times the endogenous production rate, on serum [Ca], $U_{Ca}V$, cumulative calcium loss (that is the cumulative loss of calcium above normal $U_{Ca}V$), and hydroxyproline excretion (Bijvoet and Froeling, 1973b; Froeling and Bijvoet, 1974). The change in the excretion rate of hydroxyproline reflects an action on bone (Avioli and Prockop, 1967). The slowness of the change in the excretion rate at the start or termination of the infusion is not due to extracellular dilution, since in man a sudden decrease in bone turnover due to calcitonin administration has been shown to result in a steep decline of the hydroxyproline excretion rate (Bijvoet *et al.,* 1972). The increase in plasma calcium induced by PTH was clearly due to an action of the hormone in bone, since the excretion rate was unchanged and it occurred in parallel with the increased hydroxyproline production. However, the increased load would have been excreted, as was the case with hydroxyproline, if tubular reabsorption had not been set at a higher level. It is, therefore, concluded that the higher setting of serum calcium concentration was due to action in the kidney, but that the actual rise of serum calcium to that higher concentration was due to a dual action in the kidney and in bone (Bijvoet and Froeling, 1973b; Froeling and Bijvoet, 1974). The two organs probably each have a specific function in the homeostasis of serum calcium by PTH. It should be noted that the PTH-induced rise in serum calcium is slow; the increase in bone resorption and the increase in renal tubular calcium reabsorption develop slowly. The slowness of reaction of the renal tubules has already been discussed in the preceding section. It could be possible that the parathyroid-dependent homeostasis of serum calcium mainly pertains to prolonged disturbances of calcium balance and that minute-to-minute homeostasis is due to other mechanisms, such as calcium buffering in bone (Neuman and Neuman, 1957) and variations in the production rate of calcitonin, a hormone with a much more rapid effect on calcium transport in the kidney and the bone (Bijvoet *et al.,* 1972; Copp *et al.,* 1962) than PTH.

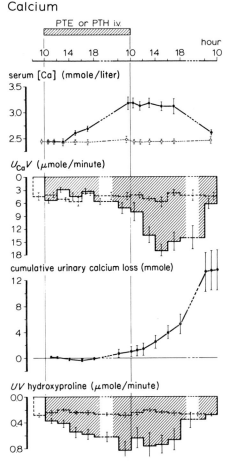

Fig. 12. Effect in man of continuous intravenous infusion for 24 hours of parathyroid extract (PTE), or hormone (PTH), at a rate of 2 U.S.P. units per kilogram body weight per hour, on serum calcium concentration, urinary calcium excretion rate, cumulative calcium loss (differences between control and experimental period), and hydroxyproline excretion. Solid lines and hatched areas represent observations during infusion and postinfusion day. Dashed lines are observations during the 24 hours preceding infusion. (According to Froeling and Bijvoet, 1974.)

3. Physiological Variations of Renal Calcium Transport

a. Normal Calcium Excretion Rate. When the extracellular calcium concentration remains constant, the calcium excretion rate will necessarily reflect the net input of calcium into the extracellular fluid if measured over sufficiently long periods, for instance, several days. This input is the calcium absorbed from the diet plus or minus the net rate of calcium removal from or uptake into the bone. For a group of normal individuals, there is much less correlation between dietary intake and urinary excretion of calcium than that of phosphate; moreover, there is no significant correlation when both are compared between the limits of a normal calcium intake (Davis *et al.*, 1970). This means that either the efficiency of calcium absorption from the diet varies greatly among individuals or that there may be considerable variation in the net removal or gain of calcium in bone. For a single individual, changing calcium intake and thereby absorbed calcium does produce corresponding changes in bone resorption, and only part of the change in input is reflected in calcium excretion (Phang *et al.*, 1969).

The normal rate of calcium excretion is not easy to define. There are even different values for various regions in the world: therefore, not all data apply everywhere. Because of a great relative variation in $U_{Ca}V$ among healthy individuals, a large number of accurate 24-hour urine collections from a representative group is necessary to obtain sufficient information (see Volume II, Chapter 7). Ninety-five percent of the healthy women probably excrete less than 300 mg/day; this upper limit is about 400 mg/day in men (Davis *et al.*, 1970; Nordin *et al.*, 1972a; Robertson and Morgan, 1972). For both sexes, there is a lower limit of the order of 75 mg/day below which calcium excretion does not normally fall (Robertson and Morgan, 1972). A lower excretion rate means that the possibility of malabsorption of calcium in the gut should be investigated. The urinary calcium excretion rate diminishes significantly after 50 years of age in women and 60 years of age in man. This happens despite an unchanged intake. There is a steady loss of bone with aging, and this loss could contribute an extra 30–40 mg calcium to the urine. This indicated that the efficiency of calcium absorption diminishes with age (Davis *et al.*, 1970). Premenopausal women show adaptation to an overnight fast by a reduced calcium excretion rate in the early morning; this is less likely to occur in postmenopausal women (Gallagher and Nordin, 1973; Nordin *et al.*, 1970). When it is assumed that excretion after an overnight fast reflects net bone resorption, the lack of response to an overnight fast may reflect the increased loss of bone that occurs in women after the menopause (Chapter 6).

There is a diurnal variation in calcium excretion rate with a peak in the forenoon (Wesson, 1964; Walser, 1969; Campbell and Webster, 1921; Briscoe and Ragan, 1966), correlating with the peak in sodium excretion (Birkenhager *et al.*, 1959; Robinson *et al.*, 1962). The reason for this diurnal variation is not well known. It may in part be related to variations in intake of calcium, sodium, and nutrients during the day (see Section II,D,5,b)

(Edwards and Hodgkinson, 1965; Heaton and Hodgkinson, 1963). Not all authors find the peak in calcium excretion rate in the same period of the day, and not all authors find similar shifts of the peak in calcium excretion rate when food is given at regular intervals throughout the 24 hours and activity is restricted (Walser, 1969). Although there is considerable variation in calcium excretion rate among individuals, the variation observed for one person may be much less (Morgan *et al.*, 1972). There may, however, be seasonal variations, urinary calcium being maximal in July and August and minimal in February and March (Morgan *et al.*, 1972; McCance and Widdowson, 1942).

b. The Definition of an Abnormal Calcium Excretion Rate. The term hypercalciuria means an abnormally high calcium excretion rate. This term is used for two different things (Robertson and Morgan, 1972). When comparing an individual with the population of healthy adults, the term hypercalciuria means that this individual excretes per 24 hours more calcium than 95% of the healthy adults. However, when we compare two groups, for instance, a group of patients with recurrent stones and a group of healthy subjects, the mean calcium excretion rate of the patients with stones will almost certainly be higher than that of the healthy individuals; however, the two groups may overlap considerably so that the excretion rate of most of the hypercalciuric group will be below the 95% upper limit of normal (Fig. 13).

In the steady state, the calcium excretion rate reflects the net input of calcium into the extracellular fluid from sites other than the kidney. The organs that contribute the most to shifts in net input over long periods of time are the bone and the gut. In the bone, there may be a disequilibrium

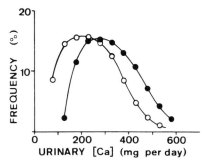

Fig. 13. The frequency distributions (expressed in percent) of the 24-hour excretion of urinary calcium in male patients with idiopathic stones (closed circles) and their age, weight, and sex-matched controls (open circles). Note that similarity of the two curves and that all individual points in the frequency distribution curve of controls exceed the corresponding points for normals by 75 mg/day. Reproduced from Robertson and Morgan (1972).

between calcium uptake and the removal rate. In the gut, dietary calcium as well as the efficiency of calcium absorption from the diet may vary. Therefore, in a steady state, hypercalciuria or hypocalciuria indicate abnormalities in either bone or gut. Nordin *et al*. (1972a) proposed designating the two types of hypercalciuria, that due to gut and that due to bone, as absorptive and resorptive hypercalciuria, respectively. Absorptive hypercalciuria is the most common type (Chapter 7) and can be diagnosed when measurement of the urinary calcium excretion rate at two levels of calcium intake (low and normal) reveals that $U_{Ca}V$ is normal at a low intake but high at a normal intake (Fig. 14). This type of hypercalciuria is apparent in 24-hour or daytime urine but not in fasting urine. If net bone resorption (i.e., the difference between rate of removal of calcium from bone and deposition rate) is sufficiently high, it may produce absolute hypercalciuria. This type of hypercalciuria will not be influenced by diet. It will persist with a low calcium diet and will be also reflected in a high excretion rate in the fasting state (Fig. 14). Thus, in a steady state, an abnormal calcium excretion rate reflects abnormal net calcium transport from the bone, abnormal calcium absorption from the gut, or both.

The serum calcium concentration is normally kept constant between narrow limits; hypercalciuria at a normal serum [Ca] indicates decreased renal calcium reabsorption, and hypocalciuria, increased tubular reabsorption of calcium. However, even if interpretation in terms of increased or decreased renal tubular reabsorption of calcium seems straightforward, the explanation of such a phenomenon is not. For instance, the explanation of an increased calcium excretion rate combined with normocalcemia and

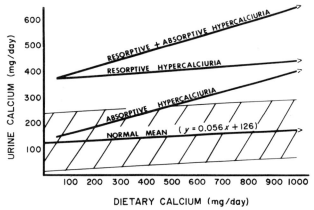

Fig. 14. The normal relationship between the urine calcium (mean ± 2 S.D.) and dietary calcium, and the relationship in various types of hypercalciuria. Reproduced from Nordin *et al*. (1972a).

hence decreased tubular calcium reabsorption rate in thyrotoxicosis is quite different from the explanation of hypercalciuria induced in patients with osteoporosis by infusing calcitonin infusion for several weeks. In the case of thyrotoxicosis, the first event is probably an increase in bone resorption rate with respect to bone formation due to the increased thyroid hormone level (Adams *et al.*, 1967; Smith *et al.*, 1973). This causes an increased input of calcium into the extracellular fluid, and, when tubular reabsorption is unaltered, this extra load of calcium can only be excreted when the filtered load has become elevated by the increase of extracellular and serum calcium concentrations. Any increase in input, resulting in an increase in $U_{Ca}V$ of 100 mg/day, will need an increase in serum [Ca] of about 0.2 mg per 100 ml at a normal G.F.R., and more at reduced G.F.R., (cf. Fig. 10). Consequently the PTH level is probably reduced and the tubular reabsorption decreased; thus the kidney can excrete the extra load at a normal serum [Ca] (Adams *et al.*, 1967; Smith *et al.*, 1973). In the case of a continuous calcitonin infusion, however, the primary event is a decrease in tubular reabsorption of calcium (Copp *et al.*, 1962). Therefore, a larger rate of input of calcium into the extracellular fluid is needed to maintain a normal serum [Ca]. However, calcitonin decreased the bone resorption rate, and thus serum [Ca] and the filtered load tend to drop. This, of course, stimulates the parathyroid glands, and the serum level of PTH is increased with a dual effect on kidney and on bone. In the kidney PTH will increase calcium reabsorption to some degree; however meanwhile in bone, the resorption rate will be increased relative to the bone formation rate, and a steady state develops with normocalcemia and hypercalciuria. Thus, the normocalcemic hypercalciuria may be associated with secondary hypoparathyroidism, as in thyrotoxicosis, or with secondary hyperparathyroidism, as during continuous calcitonin infusion.

These two examples illustrate that the interpretation of a normocalcemic steady state with an altered calcium excretion rate need not always be straightforward. The state of primary hypercalciuria often occurring in patients with recurrent stones might well be comparable to the situation caused by infusion of calcitonin, and might therefore be accompanied by secondary (or tertiary) hyperparathyroidism (see Section II,D,5,d).

c. The Normal Tubular Calcium Reabsorption. Calcium reabsorption cannot be measured directly (see Section II,C). The normal relation between excretion rate, glomerular filtration rate, and serum calcium concentration was defined by Peacock and Nordin (1973) (Fig. 10). Nothing is known about circadian, or day-to-day, variations of renal tubular calcium transport or about variations with age and sex.

4. The Effect of Other Hormones on Renal Calcium Transport

a. *Calcitonin*. It has been shown that in man single intravenous injections of calcitonin cause a transient increase in calcium excretion (Bijvoet and Froeling, 1973b; Bijvoet et al., 1968, 1972; Ardaillou et al., 1967; Singer et al., 1969; Haas et al., 1971). This is followed by a reduction of calcium excretion to below control levels when the serum [Ca] was lowered by the calcitonin injection as in patients with Paget's disease (Bijvoet and Froeling, 1973b; Bijvoet et al., 1968). This reduction of calcium excretion is clearly due to a reduced filtered load, and despite lowering of serum [Ca] and $U_{Ca}V$, the ratio of $U_{Ca}V$ to [Ca] remains elevated above control levels (Bijvoet and Froeling, 1973a). When osteoporotic patients received continuous *intravenous* calcitonin infusions over periods of 1 to 2 months, hypercalciuria developed with a normal serum [Ca], indicating a lowered renal tubular reabsorption of calcium (Bijvoet et al., 1972). In these patients with osteoporosis, serum calcium homeostasis was maintained in spite of reduced renal tubular calcium reabsorption by increased net bone resorption (see Chapter 6). This is another instance when bone plays a role in serum calcium homeostasis. One intramuscular porcine calcitonin injection per day produces no measurable effect on calcium reabsorption when 24-hour urine samples are studied because calcitonin has a half-life time which is measured in minutes, and unlike the effect on bone the effect on the kidney does not outlast the presence of calcitonin in the serum (Bijvoet et al., 1972). Thus, in chronic treatment with calcitonin, spaced intramuscular injections of calcitonin with a short half-life are to be preferred above a form with prolonged half-life or continuous administration because a sustained side effect on tubular reabsorption may provoke secondary hyperparathyroidism and a negative bone balance. Nothing is known about the site of action of calcitonin in the kidney. It has been suggested that the calciuric effect is localized in the proximal tubules (Bijvoet et al., 1971; Paillard et al., 1972). In dogs, calcitonin does not inhibit the reabsorption of calcium, phosphate, and sodium, but it blocks the promotion of reabsorption of these substances by 25-hydroxycholecalciferol (Puschett et al., 1974).

b. *Vitamin D*. Rather little information is available about the effect of vitamin D on renal calcium transport. The physiologically active metabolites of cholecalciferol have only recently become available for study. Clearance studies in dogs, treated with cholecalciferol and 25-hydroxycholecalciferol indicate that these substances may increase proximal renal tubular reabsorption of calcium, phosphate, and sodium (Puschett *et al.*, 1972a; Omdahl and DeLuca, 1973), and 1,25-dihydroxycholecalciferol appears to have the same effect (Puschett *et al.*, 1972b). The action of 25-hydroxycholecalciferol can be blocked by prior administration of calcitonin (Puschett *et al.*, 1974). Earlier studies in rachitic dogs already strongly suggested that vitamin D can increase the tubular reabsorption of calcium, since urine calcium fell when vitamin D was given (Gran, 1960; Ney *et al.*, 1968). Calcium excretion was found to fall during the first 2 to 25 hours after vitamin D administration to rachitic dogs, while serum calcium was unaltered. After 6 days serum calcium levels were higher and urinary calcium increased (Ney *et al.*, 1968). At that point, actions of vitamin D on sites outside the kidney had apparently become manifest. Prolonged vitamin D administration causes calcium excretion rate to rise (Edwards and Hodgkinson, 1965; Gough *et al.*, 1933; Hanna *et al.*, 1963), presumably by promoting input of calcium in the extracellular fluid from gut and bone. For opposite reasons, renal excretion of calcium may be small in rickets and osteomalacia, although the plasma calcium concentration is not necessarily low, and when vitamin D is withdrawn from the diet, the urinary excretion of calcium may almost cease (Chu *et al.*, 1940). The serum [Ca] can be maintained at normal or near normal levels in vitamin D deficiency, in spite of the hypocalciuria that indicates decreased calcium absorption from the gut. The renal tubular reabsorption is, therefore, increased, and this is presumably due to secondary hyperparathyroidism (Erdheim, 1907; Wilder *et al.*, 1934) (see also Section I,D,5,b).

c. Other Hormones. The hypercalciuria of *thyrotoxicosis* has been known for a long time and may reflect an increased net bone resorption rate (Aub *et al.*, 1929; Robertson, 1942; Adams *et al.*, 1967; Smith *et al.*, 1973). The hypercalciuria occurs despite a normal serum [Ca]. Tubular reabsorption of calcium is therefore reduced. This and the accompanying increased renal tubular reabsorption of phosphate may be explained by assuming that the parathyroids counteract the effect of increased net bone resorption on serum [Ca] by reducing the endogenous production rate of PTH (cf. Section I,D,5,c).

Glucocorticoid administration usually tends to augment urinary calcium excretion in human subjects (Edwards and Hodgkinson, 1965; Pechet *et al.*, 1959; Laake, 1960). Urinary calcium excretion is often, although not always, high in Cushing's syndrome and always decreases after treatment (Molinatti *et al.*, 1960; Jowsey and Riggs, 1970). This is probably not due to altered calcium reabsorption from the diet; the data on the effect of corticoids on calcium absorption are conflicting, but net bone resorption is often increased. Usually bone formation is found to be inhibited (Jowsey and Riggs, 1970), although it sometimes is increased (Van der Sluys Veer *et al.*, 1967), and bone resorption may be enhanced (Jowsey and Riggs, 1970), but generally this is insufficiently compensated for by bone formation so that the bone balance is negative (Van der Sluys Veer *et al.*, 1967).

This negative bone balance will account for the sustained hypercalciuria. The hypercalciuria of Cushing's syndrome is normocalcemic, but it is not known whether the reduced tubular reabsorption of calcium is a direct effect of the glucocorticoids or not. In patients with *sarcoidosis* in whom hypercalciuria is due to increased calcium absorption from the gut (Henneman *et al.*, 1954, 1956; Anderson *et al.*, 1954), cortisone decreases the increased urinary calcium excretion as well as the increased calcium absorption from the gut, which causes the hypercalciuria (Henneman *et al.*, 1956; Anderson *et al.*, 1954; Canary *et al.*, 1964). In *Addison's disease*, hypercalciuria and occasionally hypercalcemia may be found. Metabolic acidosis in Addison's disease may be responsible for both (Jowsey and Simons, 1968) but hyperproteinemia may in part explain the elevated total serum [Ca] (Myers *et al.*, 1964).

Patients with *acromegaly* exhibit hypercalciuria without hypercalcemia (Bauer and Aub, 1941; Hanna *et al.*, 1961). The excess calcium excreted is derived from the excess calcium absorbed in the gut (Nunziata *et al.*, 1971; Sjöberg, 1969). In acromegaly, there is excessive bone turnover, but probably no net loss of calcium from the bone (Roelfsema *et al.*, 1970) (see Chapter 6). The normocalcemic hypercalciuria suggests a decreased tubular reabsorption of calcium, but the mechanism responsible for this is obscure. *Growth hormone* may anatognize the effect of PTH on calcium reabsorption in the kidney (Pechet, 1966).

Gallagher and Nordin (1973) reported a significant rise in fasting plasma and urine calcium after removal of the ovaries. *Estrogens* have long been known to reduce the excretion of calcium, especially after continued administration (Shorr, 1945; Anderson, 1950; Ackerman *et al.*, 1954). Gallagher and Nordin (1973) postulated on the basis of *in vitro* tissue culture studies that estrogens inhibit the effect of PTH on bone. The postmenopausal hypercalciuria that is especially manifest in the fasting urine would be the result of increased bone resorption due to an uninhibited PTH action in bone. Earlier, Muller (1969) reported that there is a marked increase in the occurrence of manifest hyperparathyroidism in postmenopausal women (see Chapter 6).

The urinary excretion of calcium and sodium is increased during the administration of *glucagon* (Charbon *et al.*, 1963; Dewonck *et al.*, 1963; Pullman *et al.*, 1967). *Angiotensin* also increased renal excretion of sodium, calcium, and magnesium (Gantt and Carter, 1964). *Catecholamines* were found to increase calcium excretion in rats (Morey and Kenney, 1964).

5. Nonhormonal Effects on Renal Calcium Transport

a. Immobility. It is well known that bed rest and inactivity increase the urinary calcium excretion rate; this has sometimes been associated with small increases in serum [Ca], particularly in paraplegics (Cuthbertson, 1929; Deitrick *et al.,* 1948; Lutwak *et al.,* 1969; Whedon and Shorr, 1957). Hypercalciuria has also been found during weightlessness in space flight (Dunning and Plum, 1957), and it also occurs after a fracture and may then be accompanied by an increase in serum [PO₄] (Bijvoet and Van der Sluys Veer, 1968). The cause of the hypercalciuria is probably an increase in the net bone resorption rate resulting from the absence of weight-bearing, especially on long bones, and the disuse of muscles involved in weight-bearing (Issekutz *et al.,* 1966; Rodahl *et al.,* 1966). The elevated serum [PO₄] may reflect the effect of a secondary decrease in PTH secretion on phosphate transport in the kidney. The supine position of bed rest may also be significant. It is known that passive tilting leads to reductions in sodium and calcium excretion and that the response to an expansion of the extracellular volume is a diminished fractional reabsorption of sodium and water and probably also calcium in the proximal renal tubules. There is a close relationship between the excretion of sodium and calcium in man (Walser, 1969) (cf. next section).

b. Minerals and Nutrients. In man and dogs, there is a close association between the excretion rates of calcium and *sodium* and between calcium and sodium clearances (Walser, 1961b; Robinson *et al.,* 1962). Alterations in dietary sodium while dietary calcium remains constant or *saline* infusions lead to changes in calcium excretion that parallel the resulting changes in sodium excretion (Kleeman *et al.,* 1964). Conversely, sodium excretion increases after an infusion of calcium (Wills *et al.,* 1969). These phenomena may all be ascribed to the association of sodium chloride with calcium transport in the proximal tubules (Lassiter *et al.,* 1963; Agus *et al.,* 1973; Frick *et al.,* 1965; Dirks *et al.,* 1965). There is not always an association between calcium and sodium excretion, particularly when changes in sodium or calcium reabsorption may be ascribed to changes of transport in the distal tubules or of transport of sodium bicarbonate. Treatment with sodium-retaining steroids causes a transient reduction of sodium but not of calcium excretion (Lemann *et al.,* 1970). Administration of PTH leads to a transient increase in sodium bicarbonate excretion with unchanged or reduced calcium excretion (Bijvoet and Froeling, 1973a,b; Froeling and Bijvoet, 1974). Metabolic acidosis induces natriuresis. In acidosis there is a strong correlation between calcium excretion and the ammonium but not the sodium excretion (Lemann *et al.,* 1967). Walser (1969) pointed out that since ammonium ion is added to the urine as a consequence of the sodium for hydrogen exchange, a strong correlation between calcium and sodium plus ammonium excretion may exist. This implies, however, that the sodium for hydrogen exchange is not associated with a change in calcium excretion. A possible explanation is that the gradient type of calcium reabsorption in the proximal tubules is closely linked to the proximal reabsorption of sodium chloride and water, i.e., to volume regulation. Within the proximal tubules, changes in sodium reabsorption correlate positively with those in calcium reabsorption. Micropuncture studies in rodents and dogs show a close relationship between fractional calcium and sodium reabsorption along the proximal tubules (Lassiter *et al.*, 1963; Agus *et al.*, 1973). Perfusion studies of the proximal tubules of the rat using varying concentrations of calcium and sodium strongly suggest that there is a common transport mechanism for calcium and sodium (Frick *et al.*, 1965). There may also be a site of linked reabsorption of sodium and calcium in the ascending limb of the loop of Henle which is related to a sodium and a calcium gradient between the renal papillae and the medulla in the rat and which can be inhibited by furosemide (Thwaites and Trounce, 1972). Distal sodium reabsorption and sodium for hydrogen or potassium exchange may be unrelated to calcium reabsorption. These points will be discussed further in Section III. An argument for this hypothesis is that mineralocorticoids that promote sodium reabsorption at distal sites in the nephron initially leave calcium reabsorption unchanged, but after prolonged administration, increased calcium excretion occurs, probably due to a proximal effect mediated by extracellular fluid volume expansion (Massry *et al.*, 1968b; Rastegas *et al.*, 1972).

It has long been known that experimental *acidosis* induces hypercalciuria and a negative calcium balance in healthy adults (Farquharson *et al.*, 1931; Lemann *et al.*, 1966). Interpretations of this have varied. Albright and Reifenstein (1948) assumed that the calcium losses were derived from bone salts and that the buffering action of the skeleton was the primary event. Prolonged ammonium chloride acidosis indeed leads to the development of osteoporosis in experimental animals (Barzel and Jowsey, 1969; Barzel, 1970). Walser (1961b) has proposed that since metabolic acidosis induces natriuresis, and since natriuresis is usually associated with calciuresis, acidosis primarily augments calcium clearance by virtue of its effect on sodium clearance. Others suggested primary action of acidosis in bone, mediated by the parathyroid glands in response to extracellular pH (Bernstein *et al.*, 1970; Wills, 1970a). It has, however, now been established that the parathyroids are not necessary for the stimulation of bone resorption in metabolic acidosis (Delling and Donath, 1973). Lemann and Lennon (1972) have made it clear that bone is a base reservoir in man. Growing infants are in negative acid balance, presumably due to deposition of base in bone and new body water (Kildeberg *et al.*, 1969). Continuous positive acid balances are induced by healthy individuals during periods of chronic stable ammonium chloride acidosis (Lemann *et al.*, 1966). The possible mechanism by which acidosis induces parathyroid-independent bone loss is unknown. Increased osteoclastic bone resorption has been noted; furthermore, the rate of removal of bone mineral has been found to exceed the resorption of organic components of bone around osteocytes (Barzel and Jowsey, 1969; Delling and Donath, 1973). The hypercalciuria that accompanies acidosis is, therefore, due to an increased net input of bone calcium into the extracellular fluid. Hypercalciuria is associated with a normal serum [Ca]. Lemann *et al.* (1967) even found an increase in ultrafilterable calcium upon administration of ammonium chloride to healthy or hypoparathyroid subjects. Therefore, it is possible that the PTH level is reduced in these patients. In sheep, the serum PTH levels have been found to fall during acute acidosis and to rise during acute alkalosis (Kaplan *et al.*, 1971, 1972). Such a response would be very adequate, since an increased renal tubular reabsorption of bicarbonate would ensue (see Section III). In respiratory acidosis, due to prolonged exposure to an atmosphere of 0.7% CO_2 in air, serum ionized calcium became slightly elevated and calcium excretion rate decreased (Gray *et al.*, 1973).

The influence of *phosphate* feeding and depletion has been reviewed before (Section I,D,6,a). It has also been mentioned that *hypercalcemia* by itself may reduce renal tubular calcium reabsorption, independent of parathyroid function (Verbanck and Toppet, 1961; Massry *et al.*, 1968).

The ingestion of the *nutrients,* glucose, fructose, galactose, or ethanol, or the infusion of glucose or insulin results in an increase in urinary calcium excretion (Edwards and Hodgkinson, 1965; Laake, 1960; Heggeness, 1959; Hodgkinson and Heaton, 1965; Lindeman *et al.*, 1967; Lemann *et al.*, 1969). Carbohydrate-induced calciuria is greater in patients with stones than in healthy subjects (Lemann *et al.*, 1969). When one kidney is removed, the carbohydrate-induced hypercalciuria of the remaining kidney becomes greater than it was before (Bones *et al.*, 1973). The mechanism as well as the significance is as yet not clear. Interestingly, hexoses that are themselves actively transported in the intestine specifically inhibit calcium influx in the luminal mucosa (Patrick and Stirling, 1973).

c. Diuretics. The calcium excretion rate can be considerably modified by administration of diuretics, a fact of considerable importance in clinical medicine. This means that it is possible to use benzothiadiazines to reduce calcium excretion in healthy individuals and in patients with idiopathic hypercalciuria and to use combined furosemide and sodium chloride infusions to increase calcium excretion and combat hypercalcemia.

Benzothiadiazines: Lamberg and Kuhlbach (1959) noted that when they gave chlorothiazide and hydrochlorothiazide to patients with congestive heart failure, the urinary excretion rate of calcium decreased (Lamberg and Kuhlbach, 1959). Many authors confirmed that when these drugs are given for longer periods of time, urinary calcium falls below control levels (Walser and Trounce, 1961; Higgins *et al.*, 1964; Nassim and Higgins, 1965; Yendt *et al.*, 1966; Parfitt, 1972; Brickman *et al.*, 1972). The drug was introduced in the treatment of hypercalciuria in patients with recurrent renal stones (Nassim and Higgins, 1965; Yendt *et al.*, 1966). The exact mechanism by which thiazides diminish $U_{Ca}V$ is unknown (Parfitt, 1972; Brickman *et al.*, 1972). It has been suggested that the diuretic-induced volume depletion may increase proximal tubular reabsorption of sodium and calcium because of the interdependence of proximal sodium chloride and calcium resorption (Suki *et al.*, 1967; Epstein, 1968) (see preceding section). It was indeed noted that reexpansion of the extracellular space due to dietary salt caused the calcium clearance to return to normal during a continuous thiazide dosage (Brickman *et al.*, 1972; Suki *et al.*, 1967). Indeed, micropuncture studies in dogs showed that chlorothiazide, apart from an inhibition of proximal sodium and calcium reabsorption (Fernandez and Puschett, 1973), does reduce sodium reabsorption in the distal nephron without affecting calcium reabsorption (Edwards *et al.*, 1973) and that intravenous administration of chlorothiazide is followed by increased reabsorption of sodium in the proximal tubules when urinary losses are not replaced (Dirks *et al.*, 1966).

However, the sustained decrease in $U_{Ca}V$ during continued thiazide treatment cannot be explained by a renal action alone. If the sole action of thiazide were a direct or indirect increase in the tubular reabsorption of calcium, $U_{Ca}V$ would only be transiently reduced until a steady state at a higher serum [Ca] concentration set in, whereby $U_{Ca}V$ would again equal the rate of net bone resorption plus calcium absorption from the gut. It would be logical to attribute the absence of hypercalcemia to an adaptive decrease of the production rate of PTH. This is followed by reduction of distal tubular reabsorption effecting normalization of serum calcium and by reduction of bone resorption and calcium absorption in the gut effecting a decrease of calcium excretion rate. There is experimental data supporting this thesis, but there is also data that remain unexplained. The parathyroids are certainly involved in the mechanism of action of the thiazides. In dogs treated with thiazides, the parathyroid glands become enlarged (Pickleman *et al.*, 1969). From this, however, was concluded that the thiazides caused parathyroid stimulation. However, no evidence of increased amino acid turnover was found in the glands (Pickleman *et al.*, 1969), and the possibility that the morphological changes were due to accumulation of unexcreted material has to be considered. Recently, it was found that in hypercalciuric patients the serum level of immunoreactive PTH were consistently reduced when they had previously been elevated; this was considered to be related to the decrease in calcium excretion (Coe *et al.*, 1971). Indications have been presented that a reduction of the serum PTH level may also occur in healthy persons (Stote *et al.*, 1972). The evidence for an action of thiazides on calcium absorption from the gut is most controversial; decreased (Nassim and Higgins, 1965; Ehrig *et al.*, 1974) as well as unchanged (Harrison and Rose, 1968) or even increased (Jørgensen and Transbøl, 1974) calcium absorption has been found. However, hydroxyproline excretion has been found to decrease in rats (Jørgensen and Nielsen, 1972) and in man (Pak *et al.*, 1972) indicating a reduction of bone turnover. The implication of the parathyroid glands in the mechanism of action of the thiazides is also evident from studies in hypoparathyroid and hyperparathyroid patients (Parfitt, 1972; Brickman *et al.*, 1972; Van der Sluys Veer *et al.*, 1966). In these patients, one would expect that PTH production cannot be reduced, and, therefore, these patients have no mechanism to counteract elevation of serum calcium, nor should calcium excretion rate be reduced. Indeed, in hypoparathyroid patients, serum calcium does increase and calcium excretion is unchanged (Parfitt, 1972). In hyperparathyroidism, serum calcium concentration increases also, yet the calcium excretion rate does decrease (Brickman *et al.*, 1972). Another unexplained observation is that sodium depletion induces hypocalciuria (Kleeman *et al.*, 1964), yet the reduction of calcium excretion rate in, for instance, furosemide-induced volume depletion, after discontinuation of furosemide is less than the reduction of calcium excretion during thiazide treatment (Brickman *et al.*, 1972). One has, therefore, to assume that the benzothiadiazine diuretics have an additional PTH-independent action on bone resorption.

A property of the thiazides which has been neglected in this context is their effect on acid–base balance. Thiazides cause extracellular alkalosis, and an ammonium chloride load causes less metabolic acidosis with thiazides than without (Garcia and Yendt, 1970; Talso and Carballo, 1960). Patients with hyperparathyroidism are known to have hyperchloremic acidosis (Wills, 1971) (see Section III,A,1,h), which may facilitate the net removal of calcium from bone by PTH (Adams *et al.*, 1970; Lemann *et al.*, 1966). It is, therefore, possible that thiazides counteract the metabolic acidosis in hyperparathyroidism and so reduce bone resorption and calcium excretion. In hypoparathyroidism, on the other hand, there is already a tendency toward metabolic alkalosis (Barzel, 1969), and this tendency explains why this parathyroid-independent mechanism is not operative in hypoparathyroidism. In normoparathyroid patients, both the effect on

PTH, mediated by volume depletion, and the effect on acid–base balance may play a role.

The hypercalcemia induced by thiazides or chlorthalidone, which has a similar action, forms the basis for another *diagnostic procedure in hyperparathyroidism* (Van der Sluys Veer *et al.*, 1966; Adams *et al.*, 1970; Chalmers *et al.*, 1972). It is based on the development of hypercalcemia during administration of thiazides (Van der Sluys Veer *et al.*, 1966), sometimes given in combination with a phosphate-poor diet and aluminum hydroxyde gel (Adams *et al.*, 1970; Chalmers *et al.*, 1972). The test is used in normocalcemic persons suspected of having "normocalcemic hyperparathyroidism" (see Volume II, Chapter 1). A diet, containing 160 mg of calcium and 700 mg of phosphate is given for 12 days, aluminum hydroxide gel four times daily, 60 ml/day, is added from the fifth day and 1 gm chlorothiazide twice daily from the tenth day. Morning blood samples are taken on day 12 and 13, and calcium values are corrected from changes in plasma protein concentration. Failure to maintain normocalcemia is considered indicative of hyperparathyroidism.

Furosemide: Tambyah and Lim (1969) found a significant increase in the urinary excretion of calcium throughout an 8-hour interval after oral administration of a single dose of 80 mg of furosemide. They suggested that the drug may be of value in the treatment of hypercalcemia. This has been confirmed (Suki *et al.*, 1970). The sulfonamide diuretic furosemide probably acts by inhibiting sodium reabsorption in the proximal tubule and in the ascending limb of the loop of Henle (Suki *et al.*, 1965; Knox *et al.*, 1969; Birke *et al.*, 1972; Thwaites and Trounce, 1972; Seldin *et al.*, 1966). The calciuric effect can be explained by an association between the sodium and calcium transport at the site of action (Edwards *et al.*, 1973; Thwaites and Trounce, 1972). The method of *treatment of hypercalcemia with furosemide* has been detailed by Suki *et al.* (1970). Close medical supervision and adequate replacement of deficit of sodium, potassium, magnesium, and water are essential. Prior to administration of the diuretic and when central venous pressure is not elevated, extracellular volume deficit should be corrected with 1 to 3 liters of 0.9% NaCl. Diuresis is induced by the intravenous injection of 80 to 100 mg of furosemide and sustained by the injection of the same dose at intervals of 1 to 2 hours. The urinary excretion rate of water, sodium, potassium, and magnesium should be measured hourly to guide replacement therapy, and serum electrolytes should be measured at intervals of 2 to 4 hours. A solution of 0.9% NaCl and 5% dextrose in water, administered in a ratio of 3 : 1 or 4 : 1 with 20 to 40 mEq of potassium chloride and 10 to 20 mg of magnesium ion per liter of infusate is usually adequate to replenish electrolyte losses (Massry *et al.*, 1973).

Other diuretics: The site of action of other diuretics on the renal tubule is still insufficiently understood in terms of calcium metabolism. *Organic mercurials* cause transient calciuric responses (Wesson, 1962; Parfitt, 1969). The calciuric response is probably related to a natriuric response, and the site of action of these drugs includes the proximal tubules (Sakai and Enomoto, 1964). The carbonic anhydrase inhibitor *acetazolamide* augments cyclic AMP and phosphate excretion and mimics the proximal tubular effects of PTH (Rodriguez *et al.*, 1974). Its effects on calcium excretion are not clear. It may cause proximal calcium loss compensated for by increased tubular reabsorption in more distal sites of the nephron (Beck and Goldberg, 1973). *Ethacrinic* acid produces chloruresis and natriuresis without a change in bicarbonate excretion. It does not inhibit carbonic anhydrase and may inhibit sodium and chloride reabsorption in the proximal tubule and in the ascending limb of the loop of Henle (Goldberg *et al.*, 1964; Clapp *et al.*, 1971; Eknoyan *et al.*, 1970); these are also sites of calcium reabsorption. Ethacrinic acid also causes nearly proportional increments in the calcium and sodium clearance (Eknoyan *et al.*, 1970; Demartini *et al.*, 1967). The aldosterone antagonists, *spironolactone* and *triamterene*, act in more distal sites of the renal tubules. Spironolactone has an acute calciuric and natriuric effect, but calcium and sodium clearances do not change parallel (Ben-Ishay *et al.*, 1972). Triamterene increases the excretion of sodium and chloride in approximately equal amounts. It does not affect calcium excretion (Walker *et al.*, 1972).

d. Diseases. It would be trivial to list here names of diseases associated with increased or decreased calcium excretion or with hypercalcemia or hypocalcemia and associated with abnormal renal handling of calcium. The aim of this chapter is rather to present a background for interpretation of disorders of calcium metabolism in terms of renal function. Besides, many such disorders are mentioned in passing. However, a disorder of considerable clinical importance that has been insufficiently discussed is *idiopathic hypercalciuria.*

Patients with idiopathic recurrent calcium oxalate stones excrete more calcium in the urine than age, weight, and sex-matched controls (Robertson and Morgan, 1972). The association between elevated urinary calcium and recurrent idiopathic urolithiasis has been known for a long time (Flocks, 1939; Liberman *et al.*, 1968). Hodgkinson and Pyrah (1958) found hypercalciuria in 35% of the male patients and 25% of the female patients with recurrent stones and in only 10% of the male and 6% of the female controls. In patients with calcium oxalate stones, 43% were hypercalciuric. Robertson and Morgan (1972) applied probit analysis to data on calcium excretion in patients with stones and controls which were matched for sex and age. They found that the 2 distributions had the same form and could be superimposed when the urinary calcium excretion of every patient with stones was reduced by 75 mg/day. Both distributions were non-Gaussian with significant positive coefficients of skewness (Fig. 13). This asymmetry, however, was not due to an excess of high values at the upper end of the curve but to a distortion at the lower end limiting the frequency with which a low calcium excretion may occur. This means that many patients with urolithiasis may have a "normal" absolute calcium excretion, but that calcium excretion in these patients is still higher than would be expected had they belonged to a normal population. The hypercalciuria of patients with stones is called idiopathic because in these patients no evident causes of increased calcium excretion exist, such as primary hyperparathyroidism, sarcoidosis, thyrotoxicosis, Cushing's syndrome, active acromegaly, idiopathic osteoporosis, vitamin D intoxication, Fanconi syndrome, myeloma, malignancy, or immobility.

The term "idiopathic hypercalciuria" was first used by Albright *et al.* (1955). The idiopathic hypercalciuria is normocalcemic and must, therefore, be associated with a reduced rate of renal tubular calcium reabsorption. As discussed earlier, a sustained increased excretion rate of calcium at a stable serum calcium level can only occur when the net input of calcium into the extracellular fluid is increased. It has now been demonstrated repeatedly that fractional absorption of calcium from the gut is increased in idiopathic hypercalciuria (Liberman *et al.*, 1968; Nordin *et al.*, 1972a; Peacock and Nordin, 1968b; Lichtwitz *et al.*, 1963). The patients absorb more calcium from a normal diet than healthy subjects. When, however, dietary calcium is reduced to very low levels, the difference between the calcium excretion rate in idiopathic hypercalciuria and that of the controls is not as great. Calcium excretion in hypercalciuria should, therefore, be examined at two distinct levels of calcium intake (cf. Section II,D,3,b and Fig. 14). Other disturbances have been found in these patients. With combined balance and calcium isotope studies, Liberman *et al.* (1968) found that they have an enlarged miscible calcium pool and an increased turnover of calcium through the bone. Several authors noted a tendency toward hypophosphatemia (Albright *et al.*, 1955; Lichtwitz *et al.*, 1963), which has been questioned (Edwards and Hodgkinson, 1965); however, in a recent study of patients with recurrent oxalate lithiasis hypophosphatemia, a reduced renal tubular reabsorption of phosphate (Tm_{PO_4}/G.F.R.) and some impairment of the maximum acidification of the urine were found (Fig. 15) (P. G. A. M. Froeling and O. L. M. Bijvoet, unpublished observations). In most individual patients, these fall within the normal range, but the group as a whole has values that are significantly different from normal.

Albright *et al.* (1955) and Henneman *et al.* (1958) have suggested that

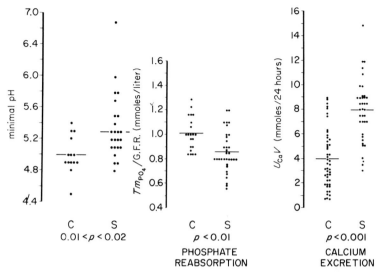

Fig. 15. Calcium excretion rate ($U_{Ca}V$, mmoles/24 hours), phosphate reabsorption activity (Tm_{PO_4}/G.F.R., mmoles/liter), and minimal urinary pH obtained after an oral ammonium chloride load in patients with idiopathic stones (S) and healthy adults (C). After P. G. A. M. Froeling and O. L. M. Bijvoet (unpublished observations).

the primary event in this disease was a reduced renal tubular reabsorption of calcium, caused by kidney damage, presumably by chronic pyelonephritis. The reduced renal calcium reabsorption would lead to reduced serum calcium, compensatory parathyroid hyperplasia, and so to increased calcium absorption from the gut; this sequence would also explain the increased calcium turnover, reduced Tm_{PO_4}/G.F.R., and impairment of urine acidification mentioned above. However, pyelonephritis has not been demonstrated (Edwards and Hodgkinson, 1965; Harrison, 1959). The hypothesis that a disturbance of renal calcium reabsorption is the first step in the sequence of events leading to idiopathic hypercalciuria has often been disputed. With calcium infusion studies, Peacock and Nordin (1968a) found a normal "calcium threshold" (cf. Fig. 10) in hypercalciuric patients. However, it can be assumed that a primary abnormality of renal tubular calcium reabsorption in patients with stones would be partially corrected by secondary hyperparathyroidism (Albright et al., 1955; Henneman et al., 1958), Pak et al. (1972b) considered secondary hyperparathyroidism in idiopathic hypercalciuria as improbable because of the normal reaction to calcium infusions, the normal urine cyclic AMP, and the normal levels of immunoreactive PTH but the data reviewed above show that there is considerable overlap between measurements in patients with stones and healthy controls. Pak et al. (1972b) first removed from the study group those that had abnormal values for their various criteria of hyperparathyroidism and diagnosed them as "normocalcemic hyperparathyroidism," and found hyperparathyroidism in the majority of them. The remaining patients, with normal tests, therefore, belonged to a selected group. Since the increased calcium absorption and the resulting steady state hypercalciuria might be due to the secondary hyperparathyroidism, it is not unexpected that in their surgical patients hypercalciuria was not noticed in the postoperative state. Finn *et al.* (1970) studied a man who received a kidney from his father, who had idiopathic hypercalciuria. The son did not develop hypercalciuria. This was considered an argument against the primary renal nature of the abnormality. However, it actually is not an argument against a possible renal calcium reabsorption defect as the initial cause of the syndrome, since such a defect might be unilateral. The "good" kidney may have been transplanted. In fact, the hypercalciuria in the father became worse after the operation. In patients with unilateral lithiasis, urine samples were collected separately from each kidney; the kidney adjacent to the stone was found to excrete significantly more calcium than the contralateral organ (Sotornik *et al.*, 1972). So far, the hypothesis that reduced tubular calcium reabsorption is the primary event in the disease. In an alternative hypothesis, the primary defect in idiopathic hypercalciuria is believed to be gastrointestinal hyperabsorption of calcium. It is difficult to reconcile such an hypothesis with the increased bone turnover rate found in these patients, which indicates a more general abnormality of the calcium metabolism (Liberman *et al.*, 1968).

The calcium excretion rate can be reduced in idiopathic hypercalciuria by the administration of thiazide diuretics. Theories about the action of these diuretics have been discussed in Section II,D,5,c. Part of their effect on $U_{Ca}V$ is probably due to a stimulation of proximal sodium and calcium reabsorption in the kidney caused by volume depletion (Suki *et al.*, 1967). Coe *et al.* (1971) studied the effect of giving thiazide to patients with idiopathic hypercalciuria. In two-thirds of their patients serum PTH levels exceeded the 95% upper limit of normal. These levels normalized during thiazide treatment. On the basis of the data presented above, the hypothesis that there is secondary hyperparathyroidism in idiopathic hypercalciuria becomes increasingly attractive. The so-called normocalcemic hyperparathyroidism, observed in idiopathic hypercalciuria, may be a secondary rather than a primary disease, and some of the results of thiazide treatment may be due to the abatement of secondary hyperparathyroidism. It is quite possible that the secondary hyperparathyroidism in idiopathic hypercalciuria may become autonomous in some patients. With long-term stimulation, transition from hyperplasia to parathyroid adenoma may well occur, as in some cases of renal failure (Reiss and Canterbury, 1971). The possibility of transition from secondary to primary hyperparathyroidism has been suggested before (Davies *et al.,* 1956; Jowsey, 1968).

In summary, the etiology of idiopathic hypercalciuria has not yet been solved. On the basis of all the available evidence, it is conceivable that idiopathic hypercalciuria, normocalcemic hyperparathyroidism, and "primary" hyperparathyroidism in urolithiasis are different forms of the same disease. The nature of the primary defect in renal calcium reabsorption is still a riddle. There are two ways in which this defect may have originated: The defect may be a renal lesion specifically affecting calcium reabsorption, as originally suggested, or it may be secondary to primary disturbances in other systems, as for instance in the balance between proximal and distal renal reabsorption of sodium.

E. Diseases of the Kidney and Calcium Excretion

1. Diseases of the Kidney Tubules

In Section I,E,1 disorders of tubular transport were mentioned with emphasis on reduction of the renal tubular reabsorption of phosphate. There is another group of tubular disorders, summarized under the name of *renal tubular acidosis*. This is a clinical syndrome of disordered renal acidification characterized biochemically by minimal or no azotemia, hyperchloremic acidosis, inappropriately high urinary pH, bicarbonaturia and reduced urinary excretion of titratable acid and of ammonium (McSherry *et al.,* 1972). It was first identified by Lightwood (1935) and subsequently recognized by Albright *et al.* (1946) as renal tubular in origin. There is an infantile type (Butler *et al.,* 1936; Lightwood *et al.,* 1953) and an adult type (Baines *et al.,* 1945). In adults, there is a less complete form that can only be recognized by studying urine pH under a maximal acid load (Wrong and Davies, 1959). Recently, the syndrome has been classified into a proximal form (type 2) and a distal form (type 1), either of which may be primary or secondary (McSherry *et al.,* 1972; Rodriguez-Soriano and Edelman, 1969; Morris, 1969; Nash *et al.,* 1972). The proximal form of the disorder is characterized by a low renal threshold for bicarbonate, excessive bicarbonate excretion, and alkalinization of urine occurs when this threshold is surpassed. At subthreshold levels of serum bicarbonate, such patients may acidify their urine below pH 5.0. The distal form has a normal bicarbonate threshold but constant slight to moderate bicarbonaturia and inadequate acidification. Urine pH remains elevated above 6.0 regardless of the degree of acidification. The proximal form is often associated with other primary tubular defects described in Section I,E,1. However, in some of these patients and in many with acidosis of the distal type, the disorder is acquired and is a consequence of altered serum globulins, abnormalities of carbohydrate or metal metabolism, endocrinopathies, pyelonephritis, or drug toxicity (Mankin, 1974). Many of the patients belonging to either of the two forms have impaired tubular reabsorption of sodium, potassium, phosphate, and water. They may have hypophosphatemic rickets, and the acidosis may produce net resorption of bone with hypercalciuria (Farquharson et al., 1931; Lemann et al., 1966) (cf. Section II,D,5,b).

Over 70% of the patients have nephrocalcinosis (Baines et al., 1945; Cooke and Kleeman, 1950; Huth et al., 1960). This may partly be caused by the hypercalciuria, but the elevated urine pH and the low citrate content found in the urine of these patients may play an important role in the genesis of the renal parenchymal calcification (Morrissey et al., 1963). A full discussion of the syndrome will be found in Chapter 7.

2. Glomerular Disorders

Two types of glomerular disease, each associated with a decreased net calcium excretion rate, are discussed: the nephrotic syndrome and renal glomerular failure.

a. The Nephrotic Syndrome. It has long been known that patients with the nephrotic syndrome excrete remarkably little calcium into the urine. Jones et al. (1967) have investigated this in detail. They found that hypocalciuria was characteristic. After remission, the urinary calcium rose rapidly. They also remarked that net tubular reabsorption of calcium must be increased in these patients because ultrafilterable serum calcium was significantly increased. The cause of the low $U_{Ca}V$ was decreased calcium absorption from the gut, which Jones et al. believed to be secondary to the renal abnormality. No relationship between disorders of sodium and calcium reabsorption could be demonstrated to explain the increased reabsorption rate. An attractive hypothesis is that hydroxylation of 25-hydroxycholecalciferol in the proximal tubules may be impaired in the nephrotic syndrome, but no evidence of osteomalacia has been detected in these patients, and there are no signs of secondary hyperparathyroidism.

b. Renal Glomerular Failure. Hypocalciuria is a well known characteristic of renal failure. It is due to malabsorption of calcium from the gut and is, therefore, one of the symptoms of the apparent vitamin D insensitivity of the patients (Stanbury, 1972b) (see Volume II, Chapter 2). The hypocalciuria is often accompanied by a low serum calcium and a high serum phosphate concentration (see Section I,E,2). The fractional excretion of calcium is found to be low in early renal failure (Popovtzer *et al.*, 1970), but in advanced renal failure the percentage excretion becomes high (Mioni *et al.*, 1971; Cochran and Nordin, 1971). This means that in the early stages of renal failure tubular reabsorption of calcium is increased and that it decreases below normal when the kidney damage becomes severe. The increased tubular reabsorption of calcium that is found when there is still relatively small reduction of glomerular filtration rate may be another symptom of the secondary hyperparathyroidism in those patients. Mioni *et al.* (1971) gave calcium infusions to such patients and found that the slope of the regression line relating calcium excretion per 100 ml of G.F.R. to serum calcium was unchanged (see Fig. 11) but that the intercept increased. This indicates an increased distal tubular reabsorption, as could be expected when the increase is due to increased serum PTH.

The decrease of calcium reabsorption in later stages is more difficult to explain. It could be due to a decrease of proximal volume reabsorption from the remaining nephrons. A 50% decrease would theoretically lead to a reduction of the renal threshold concentration for calcium from 9.5 to 6.3 mg per 100 ml (cf. Section II,B). When renal failure is advanced, the fractional excretion of calcium is in fact closely correlated with that of sodium (Popovtzer *et al.*, 1969), and the relationship is almost identical to that observed in normal dogs undergoing volume expansion with saline infusion (Massry *et al.*, 1967, 1973; Blythe *et al.*, 1968). The fractional excretion of any increase in filtered load should then increase (slope in Fig. 11). However Mioni *et al.* (1971) found that this fraction remained unchanged and that those patients had a low maximum of distal tubular calcium reabsorption relative to glomerular filtration rate (Tm_{Ca}/G.F.R.). It is possible that the decreased calcium reabsorption relative to glomerular filtration rate is due to anatomical disturbance of the balance between glomerular and tubular functions (Seldin *et al.*, 1971) so that the ratio Tm_{Ca}/G.F.R. is reduced.

Considering the very low efficiency of the kidney in mediating electrolyte homeostasis when G.F.R. is very low (cf. Section I,E,2), it is improbable that the low tubular reabsorption rate for calcium contributes much to the lowering of serum calcium concentration seen in uremic patients.

III. RENAL PHYSIOLOGY AND THE EFFECTS OF PARATHYROID HORMONE AND CALCITONIN ON ELECTROLYTE HOMEOSTASIS

A constant extracellular fluid composition is achieved by adapted and coordinated modulation of the rates of ion transport in specialized target organs, such as kidney, gut, and bone. A description of the actions of PTH and calcitonin in the kidney should not only include the influence of the hormone on the rate of transport of individual ions but also the relationship between these actions and their combined impact on the regulation of extracellular ion balance and homeostasis (Froeling and Bijvoet, 1974). The various renal effects of parathyroid hormone and calcitonin, the quantitative relationship between these effects, and their integration in the control of extracellular ion composition are described here.

A. Parathyroid Hormone

The nature of and the connection between the diverse effects of PTH will mainly be illustrated with data from a study in which bovine PTH was infused at ten times the normal endogenous production rate. Infusions were given to five healthy persons at a rate of 2 U.S.P. units per hour per kilogram of body weight (Bijvoet and Froeling, 1973a,b; Froeling and Bijvoet, 1974). The normal endogenous production rate has been estimated at 300 to 600 U.S.P. units per day (Buckle, 1969; Kleeman et al., 1971). The effects of the infusion on serum electrolytes, electrolyte excretion rate, and cumulative electrolyte losses are illustrated in Figs. 12 and 16–18. These effects may be divided into two categories. One category consists of immediate responses. To these belong changes in the excretion rate of cyclic AMP (Fig. 16) and sodium, potassium, and hydrogen ion (Fig. 17) that reflect actions of the hormone on ion transport in the kidney. A second category consisting of a much slower response is illustrated by the change in the excretion rate of hydroxyproline (Fig. 16). This reflects an action on bone.

1. The Renal Effects of Parathyroid Hormone

a. Cyclic AMP. The effect of PTH on cyclic AMP is maximal right from the start of infusion, while maximum sodium excretion and minimal Tm_{PO_4}/G.F.R. occur later (Froeling and Bijvoet, 1974). Chase and Aurbach (1967) found that PTH activates adenyl cyclase in the renal cortex, increases the concentration of adenyl cyclase in the renal tubules, and causes a rise in urine cyclic AMP (Chase and Aurbach, 1967; Aurbach and Chase, 1970; Melson et al., 1970). Parathyroid hormone does also activate adenyl cyclase in skeletal tissue; however, the increase in urinary cyclic AMP is of renal origin (Kaminski et al., 1970). The urinary cyclic AMP becomes elevated within minutes after PTH administration and precedes its effect on phosphate excretion, and it is therefore assumed that the inhibition of tubular phosphate reabsorption is due to adenyl cyclase activation (Aurbach et al., 1970). This hypothesis is supported by the rise in

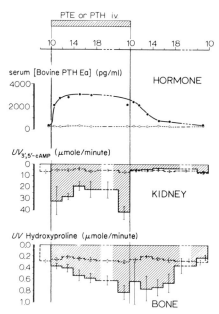

Fig. 16. Effect in man of continuous intravenous infusion for 24 hours of parathyroid extract (PTE), or hormone (PTH), at a rate of 2 U.S.P. units/kg/hour on immunoassayable PTH in serum and on urinary excretion rates of cyclic AMP (*UV* of 3'5'-AMP) and hydroxyproline. Continuous lines and hatched areas represent observations during day of infusion and postinfusion day. Dashed lines are observations during the 24 hours preceding infusion. (From P. G. A. M. Froeling and O. L. M. Bijvoet, 1974.)

phosphate excretion observed in thyroparathyroidectomized rats after infusion of dibutyryl cyclic AMP (Agus *et al.*, 1971). Cyclic AMP also promotes excretion of sodium and potassium, but does not affect tubular reabsorption of calcium (Puschett *et al.*, 1974). There is no effect of PTH in pseudohypoparathyroidism, a syndrome in which the kidney is refractory to the "phosphaturic" effect of the hormone (Aurbach *et al.*, 1970) (cf. Section I,D,4) (see Volume II, Chapter 2). The sustained elevation of cyclic AMP excretion with prolonged infusion (Froeling and Bijvoet, 1974) explains why measurement of urinary cyclic AMP might be useful in the diagnosis of hyperparathyroidism (Dohan *et al.*, 1971; Murad and Pak, 1972). Normal excretion rate ranges from 2.0 to 3.0 μmoles per gram of urinary creatinine (Dohan *et al.*, 1971; Murad and Pak, 1972).

b. Hydroxyproline. The increase in urinary hydroxyproline excretion expresses the action of PTH on collagen metabolism in the bone (Avioli and Prockop, 1967; Benoit *et al.*, 1963). The slowness of change in the excretion rate at the start or termination of the infusion (Fig. 16) is not due to extracellular dilution, since in man a sudden decrease in bone turnover

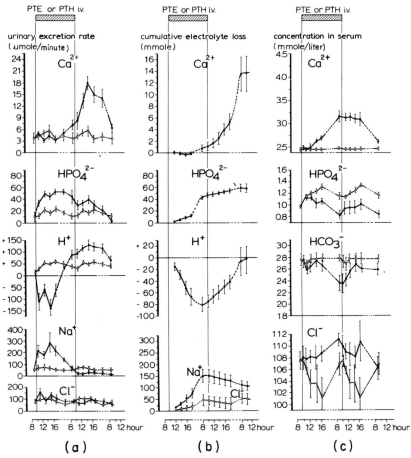

Fig. 17. Effect of continuous intravenous infusion for 24 hours of parathyroid extract (PTE), or hormone (PTH), at a rate of 2 U.S.P. units/kg of body weight/hour; (a) or urinary excretion rate of calcium (Ca), phosphate (PO₄), hydrogen (H), sodium (Na), and chloride (Cl); (b) cumulative loss of these electrolytes, calculated from differences between control and experimental period; and (c) the effect on serum calcium, phosphate, bicarbonate (HCO₃), and chloride. Averages ± S.E. of observations in five persons. Closed circles are sequential observations on the infusion and postinfusion days, and open circles, on the day preceding infusion. (Reproduced from P. G. A. M. Froeling and O. L. M. Bijvoet, 1974.)

due to calcitonin administration results in a steep decline of the hydroxy-proline excretion rate (Bijvoet *et al.*, 1972). The effect of PTH on bone turnover, therefore, develops slowly and outlasts the presence of active hormone in the circulation. This conclusion is in agreement with Rasmussen's observations in rats (Rasmussen *et al.*, 1964) and those of Raisz *et al.* (1972) in tissue culture.

  c. Calcium and Phosphate. The effects of PTH on renal phosphate and calcium transport have already been discussed in Sections I,D,3 and II,D,1. Figure 17 summarizes these effects. Parathyroid hormone mobilizes calcium and phosphate from the bone. By increasing tubular calcium reabsorption, the calcium is retained and serum calcium increases. The mobilized calcium is only excreted after serum calcium has reached a higher level or after the infusion is terminated. In contrast, the mobilized phosphate is excreted immediately because tubular phosphate reabsorption is decreased. In spite of an increased phosphate input into the blood, the net effect is a lowering of serum phosphate.

    d. Magnesium. Data on the effect of PTH on magnesium reabsorption are conflicting. After i.v. injections PTH may reduce magnesium clearance parallel to the calcium clearance (Gill *et al.*, 1967; Paunier *et al.*, 1969–1970). However, hyperparathyroidism is usually associated with increased magnesium loss, even with hypomagnesiemia (MacIntyre, 1963). The early response to parathyroid ablation in rats is an increase in magnesium excretion (Heaton, 1965). There is also similarity between the stop-flow patterns of calcium and magnesium in dogs (Murdaugh and Robinson, 1960). In general, the excretion rate of magnesium seems to vary with the calcium excretion rate, regardless of the concentrations in

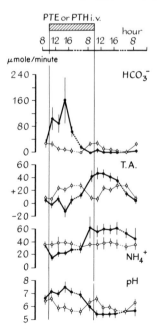

Fig. 18. Effect of continuous intravenous infusion for 24 hours of parathyroid extract (PTE), or hormone (PTH) on urinary excretion rate of bicarbonate (HCO₃⁻), titrable acid (T.A.), and NH₄, and on urine pH (cf. Fig. 17). Reproduced from Bijvoet and Froeling, 1973b).

serum of calcium or magnesium (Froeling and Bijvoet, 1974; Bijvoet *et al.*, 1972; Hornum and Transbøl, 1973).

e. Glucose. Halver (1967) has reviewed the literature on the relationship between the parathyroids and glucose excretion (Halver, 1968; Halver *et al.*, 1968). He has shown that the tubular reabsorptive capacity for glucose was affected by parathyroid function. In primary hyperparathyroidism, Tm/G.F.R. for glucose was found to be increased, and in hypoparathyroidism, this ratio was found to be decreased. The author suggests that PTH has a direct and specific effect on glucose transport across the tubular membrane.

f. Amino Acids. The decreased renal tubular reabsorption of phosphate in rickets is considered to be due to secondary hyperparathyroidism. It is still questionable whether hyperaminoaciduria in rickets is also due to hyperparathyroidism. The degree of hyperaminoaciduria has been found to be correlated with the severity of the rickets; yet, in clinical studies, it has been difficult to find a correlation between aminoaciduria and the degree of disturbance of the phosphate reabsorption (Brodehl *et al.*, 1971). However, in PTH-treated intact rats an almost generalized hyperaminoaciduria has been found (Gekle, 1971).

g. Sodium. Soon after parathyroid extracts became available, it was noted that administration of these extracts to experimental animals and to man was followed by a transient increase in urinary volume and excretion rate of sodium (Shelling, 1935; McCann, 1928; Charbon and Hoekstra, 1963; Hellman *et al.*, 1965). The sodium loss was accompanied by increased potassium diuresis. Micropuncture studies in dogs have shown that in these animals PTH administration caused a 30 to 40% inhibition of sodium reabsorption that was not due to a rise in glomerular filtration rate (Agus *et al.*, 1971). The inhibition of sodium reabsorption was of the same order of magnitude as inhibition of phosphate reabsorption, and both phenomena were also obtained by administration of dibutyryl cyclic AMP (Agus *et al.*, 1971). Since saline loading has comparable effects on sodium and phosphate excretion, it was suggested that the phosphaturic effect of PTH might be secondary to its effect on sodium excretion (Agus *et al.*, 1971). However, saline loading is followed by sodium chloride and calcium diureses, and, in recent studies (Fig. 17), it was found that the excess sodium excreted during PTH administration is accompanied by bicarbonate rather than by chloride (Bijvoet and Froeling, 1973a,b; Froeling and Bijvoet, 1974). It, therefore, seems improbable that the phosphaturic effect of PTH and the phosphaturic effect of volume expansion are due to alteration of the same mechanism of sodium transport. The phosphaturic effect of PTH may instead be due to a change in intracellular pH.

h. Bicarbonate, Hydrogen Ion, and Potassium. Ellsworth and Howard (1934) and Robbins (1937) showed that after injection of parathyroid extract the urinary pH rose; the excretion of water, sodium, and phosphate increased; and no significant change in urine chloride was reported (Ellsworth and Howard, 1934; Robbins, 1937; Ellsworth and Nicholson, 1935). A number of authors noted an increased excretion of bicarbonate (Barzel, 1971; Kleeman and Cooke, 1951; Nordin, 1960). Hellman *et al.* (1965) suggested that the action of PTH in the kidney is associated with inhibition of sodium for hydrogen exchange.

In addition, it has been noted that patients with hyperparathyroidism have elevated serum chloride and lowered serum bicarbonate concentrations (Wills, 1970, 1971; Wills and McGowan, 1963; Palmer *et al.*, 1974). This is due to reduced proximal bicarbonate reabsorption, and parathyroidectomy is followed by elevation of bicarbonate *Tm* (Muldowney *et al.*, 1971). Decreased bicarbonate *Tm* has also been described in malabsorption and uremia (Muldowney *et al.*, 1968, 1972).

The relation between the acute effects of PTH on sodium bicarbonate excretion and the hyperchloremic acidosis found in hyperparathyroidism is apparent from the results of long-term infusions of the hormone illustrated in Figs. 17 and 18. In those studies (Froeling and Bijvoet, 1974), infusion of 2 U.S.P. units of PTH per kilogram body weight per hour caused a loss of sodium amounting to 150 mmoles after 24 hours. The increase in sodium excretion was immediate but transient, and there was sodium retention during the post-infusion day. The natriuresis was not accompanied by significant loss of chloride but was accompanied by considerable retention of hydrogen, mainly due to bicarbonate diuresis (Fig. 18). Any influence on titratable acid and NH₄ excretion can be considered secondary to the bicarbonate loss. Consequently, chloride reabsorption exceeded sodium reabsorption, in contrast to control reabsorption rates, and hyperchloremic acidosis developed. Urine pH initially increased to maximum values, but with development of acidosis and before discontinuation of the infusion, it dropped again. Parathyroid hormone-induced acidosis was therefore of the proximal type. These data actually demonstrate the relationship between the hyperchloremic acidosis in hyperparathyroidism and the altered proximal tubular handling of sodium and bicarbonate induced by PTH in relation to chloride.

In hypercalcemia due to other causes than hyperparathyroidism, metabolic alkalosis has been found. This may not only be due to secondary hypoparathyroidism but also to an inhibitory effect of hypercalcemia on the renal tubular reabsorption of bicarbonate (Verbanck and Toppet, 1961; Amiel, 1964; Vainsel, 1973; Fülgraff and Heidenreich, 1973).

Also associated with the sodium loss is a considerable potassium loss

(Froeling and Bijvoet, 1974), which could partly be connected with the impaired excretion of hydrogen ions but may in addition reflect the effect of an increased distal sodium load.

i. Calcium–Sodium Interdependence. There is a close association between proximal sodium and calcium loss (cf. Section II,D,5,b). Parathyroid hormone appears exceptional because it causes sodium loss without the associated calcium loss. However, as discussed earlier (see Section II,D,5,b), proximal calcium reabsorption is probably associated with sodium chloride reabsorption rather than the sodium for hydrogen exchange. The surprising behavior of PTH may thus be explained. However, recent micropuncture studies show inhibition of proximal calcium reabsorption by PTH in association with increased distal reabsorption (cf. Section II,D,1,b). Even if the overall result of PTH on the kidney is a net increase in reabsorption, this effect may, in fact, only be the final result of a complex relationship between inhibition and stimulation of reabsorption in different parts of the kidney (Agus *et al.,* 1973).

2. Parathyroid Hormone and Serum Ion Homeostasis

The data in the preceding section demonstrate a direct relationship between an excess of PTH and hypercalcemia, hypophosphatemia, and hyperchloremic acidosis. All of these changes in plasma electrolyte concentrations can be shown to be due to specific actions of PTH in the kidney. It has been suggested on the basis of such observations that homeostasis of acid–base equilibrium and calcium metabolism are closely associated and may have been so throughout the history of evolution (Ellsworth and Nicholson, 1935; Wills, 1970a; Wilbur, 1973; Robertson, 1972). The serum PTH levels have indeed been found to fall during acute acidosis in sheep and to rise during alkalosis (Kaplan *et al.,* 1971, 1972). However, the latter observations may simply be related to concurrent changes in ionized calcium. As an alternative possibility, it can be suggested that on a more physiological level the renal effects of PTH are keyed to its actions in bone. With respect to extracellular fluid, bone contains an excess of fixed cation. Net resorption of bone, therefore, not only produces a calcium and phosphate load but also causes a base excess in the extracellular fluid (Lemann and Lennon, 1972). The actions of PTH in the kidney seem ideally adapted for excretion of the excess phosphate and base and retention of the calcium removed from bone and vice versa. From the point of view of the maintenance of extracellular ion homeostasis, the various actions of the hormone in these two organ systems may, therefore, be complementary.

The effect of PTH on hydrogen metabolism may also occur in organs other than the kidney. A high pH in tissue culture reduces PTH-induced bone resorption, and the PTH-induced mineral release will elevate the ambient pH (Raisz, 1965). There are observations that suggest the presence of a functional carbonic anhydrase system in bone linked to the mechanism of bone resorption (Warte, 1972; Minkin and Jennings, 1972). Parathyroid hormone may act on the hydrogen gradient along the functional blood–bone barrier—the barrier concept was recently revived by Neuman and Ramp (1971)—and thus keep the hydrogen ion concentration in bone interstitial fluid high enough for the resorption of minerals induced by the hormone.

B. Calcitonin

1. The Renal Effects of Calcitonin

a. Calcium and Phosphate. In Sections I,D,5,a and II,D,4,a, it was shown that calcitonin decreases renal tubular reabsorption of calcium and phosphate (Bijvoet *et al.,* 1968, 1972; Haas *et al.,* 1971; Bijvoet and Froeling, 1973a; Massry *et al.,* 1968; Ardaillou *et al.,* 1967; Singer *et al.,* 1969). The effects are specific to calcitonin and not due to secondary elevation of PTH because they also occur in hypoparathyroid patients.

b. Cyclic AMP. *In vitro* studies show that calcitonin is capable of stimulating adenylate cyclase from both bone and kidney as well as increasing the accumulation of cyclic AMP in these tissues, although to a much lesser degree than PTH (Murad *et al.,* 1970; Heersche *et al.,* 1974). Administration of calcitonin to hypoparathyroid and normal persons is followed by no increase in cyclic AMP excretion or a very small increase in relation to the 10- to 100-fold rise after PTH administration (Froeling and Bijvoet, 1974; Murad and Pak, 1972; Buchanan, 1961).

c. Hydroxyproline. Acute intravenous administration of calcitonin to patients with Paget's disease and to healthy persons is followed by a transient reduction of hydroxyproline excretion that may reflect a decrease in osteoclast activity. In the healthy person, the absolute decrease is much less, but the relative decrease of hydroxyproline excretion is the same (Chase and Aurbach, 1967; Bijvoet *et al.,* 1970); the decrease is due to a reduction of secretion of hydroxyproline into the plasma rather than altered renal handling (Bijvoet *et al.,* 1968). Long-term calcitonin administration in patients with Paget's disease is assoicated with reduction of the elevated hydroxyproline excretion rate, presumably due to a depression of bone turnover caused by the hormone (Woodhouse, 1972).

d. Sodium. As soon as calcitonin was available for animal and human studies, it became apparent that calcitonin, like PTH, has a significant natriuretic effect and also promotes the excretion of potassium (Bijvoet *et al.,* 1968; Ardaillou *et al.,* 1967). At first it seemed hard to explain why these hormones have opposite effects on the renal tubular reabsorption of calcium, while both promote the excretion of sodium, potassium, and phosphate. However, in later studies it became clear that while PTH affects the sodium for hydrogen exchange in the kidney and has no significant effect on chloride excretion, calcitonin causes nearly equimolar increases in sodium and chloride excretion (Bijvoet and Froeling, 1973a,b; Bijvoet *et al.,* 1971). Bicarbonate excretion may be affected slightly by calcitonin, but not more than can be explained by the overall inhibiting effect on volume reabsorption in the proximal tubule (Bijvoet and Froeling, 1973a,b; Bijvoet *et al.,* 1971).

e. Potassium. Calcitonin also causes a small increase in potassium excretion (Bijvoet and Froeling, 1973a,b). Whereas PTH-induced potassium loss is on the same order as sodium loss, the potassium loss with calcitonin is about 10–20% of the sodium loss and may well be explained by a distal sodium for potassium exchange secondary to the increased escape of sodium from the proximal tubules.

f. Magnesium. Magnesium excretion also changes with calcitonin. In acute and chronic studies, the pattern of magnesium excretion nearly doubles that of calcium excretion, regardless of the serum magnesium concentration (Bijvoet and Froeling, 1973a,b). This suggests again that there is no specific transport system for magnesium (see Section III,A,1,d).

g. Amino Acids. Calcitonin administration is followed by a rise in the excretion rate of α-amino acids, which is mainly due to excretion of glycine, alanine, and histidine (Bijvoet *et al.,* 1971).

2. Calcitonin and Serum Ion Homeostasis

As discussed in this section, any apparent hormonal effect on a mineral transport system should ultimately be reflected in an altered homeostasis in which a steady state is established incorporating the altered hormone level. When calcitonin infusions in man are continued over longer periods, there is a transient renal loss of sodium chloride and water with a decrease in body weight. Afterward a steady state sets in with the lowered body weight, the same sodium excretion rate, and higher than control aldosterone secretion rate and plasma renin activity (Fig. 19). After the calcitonin infusions are terminated, sodium retention occurs and the body weight returns to control values (Bijvoet *et al.,* 1970, 1971). These observations suggest that the inhibition of sodium chloride reabsorption caused by calcitonin may, with prolonged administration, place considerable strain on the other mechanisms responsible for volume homeostasis. It is of interest that the response to an expansion of the extracellular

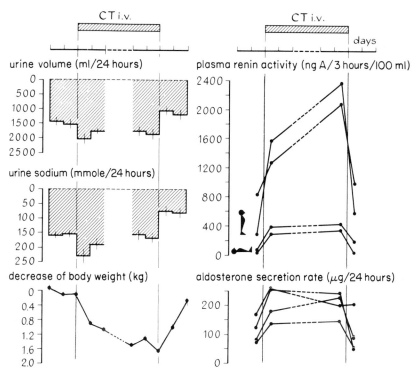

Fig. 19. Composite graph showing the effect (± S.E.) in eight patients of continuous porcine calcitonin (CT) infusions (63 MRCU/24 hours) on daily excretion of water and sodium and on body weight, and the effects in some of these patients on aldosterone secretion rate and plasma renin activity, the latter with patients supine and standing. [Reprinted by permission from O. L. M. Bijvoet *et al.*, *The New England Journal of Medicine* **284**, 681 (1971).]

volume is a diminished reabsorption of sodium, water, calcium, and phosphate in the proximal tubules. These changes in proximal tubular function are identical to the changes produced by calcitonin, and it is, therefore, entirely possible that all renal effects of calcitonin are linked with its effect on sodium chloride transport. In dogs these actions are not apparent, but in these animals calcitonin blocks the effect of 25-hydroxycholecalciferol on reabsorption of electrolytes (Puschett *et al.*, 1974). Calcitonin may alter the ionic composition of the proximal tubular cells necessary for proper expression of their function.

The physiological role of calcitonin in man is still uncertain. A definite observation is that serum calcitonin concentrations are considerably increased in medullary carcinoma (Tashian and Melvin, 1968). Recently, the sensitivity of the radioimmunoassay of calcitonin has been sufficiently increased to enable its measurement in healthy persons as well as increases by induced hypercalcemia and decreases by hypocalcemia following EDTA infusions (Heynen and Franchimont, 1974; Silva *et al.,* 1974).

The question remains: Why do calcitonin and PTH have opposite effects on calcium transport and different effects on bone metabolism but similar effects on sodium transport? The question is probably an artificial one, since the effects of calcitonin and of PTH on tubular sodium transport are of quite different nature. Calcitonin inhibits reabsorption of sodium chloride and causes volume depletion; PTH inhibits sodium bicarbonate reabsorption and causes hyperchloremic acidosis. These two modes of sodium transport may have separate mechanisms and localizations (Whittembury and Proverbio, 1969). In *in vitro* cell systems calcitonin and PTH have opposite effects on intracellular calcium. Parathyroid hormone causes calcium influx; calcitonin causes calcium efflux (Rasmussen, 1972). Although these effects are opposite, the mechanisms of action need not be of opposite nature, but they may well be different. It still remains to be ascertained whether PTH-induced calcium influx is not associated with changes of cellular pH and whether calcitonin-induced calcium efflux may not be linked with a sodium chloride pump. The quite different nature of the effects of these two hormones on electrolyte homeostasis may stem from different roles of these hormones in the earlier stages of evolution. Parathyroid hormone may have been involved in the regulation of acid–base status (Barzel, 1971; Wills, 1970a; Robertson, 1972), and calcitonin may have been involved in volume regulation or osmoregulation (Bijvoet *et al.,* 1971; Pang, 1971, 1973).

ACKNOWLEDGMENTS

The author wishes to thank Françoise Bijvoet-Dessain and Anita, Kathinka, Dominique, Patrick and Danielle Bijvoet for their patience and understanding and Cora Reitsma-La Brujeere who, good humoredly, gave continuous secretarial help.

REFERENCES

Ackerman, P. G., Toro, D. G., Kountz, W. B., and Kheim, T. (1954). *J. Gerontol.* **9,** 450.
Adams, P. H., Jowsey, J., Kelly, P. J., Riggs, B. L., Kinney, V. R., and Jones, J. D. (1967). *Q. J. Med.* **36,** 1.
Adams, P. H., Chalmers, T. M., Hill, L. F., and Truscott, B. (1970). *Brit. Med. J.* **4,** 582.
Adolph, E. F. (1925). *Am. J. Physiol.* **74,** 93.
Agus, Z. S., Puschett, J. B., Senesky, D., and Goldberg, M. (1971). *J. Clin. Invest.* **50,** 617.
Agus, Z. S., Gardner, L. B., Beck, L. H., Goldman, M. (1973). *Am. J. Physiol.* **224,** 1143.

Aitken, J. M., Hart, D. M., Anderson, J. B. J., Lindsay, R., Smith, D. A., and Speirs, C. F. (1973a). *Br. Med. J.* **2**, 325.

Aitken, J. M., Gallagher, M. D. J., Hart, D. M., Newton, D. A. G., and Craig, A. (1973b). *J. Endocrinol.* **59**, 593.

Albright, F., and Ellsworth, R. (1929). *J. Clin. Invest.* **7**, 183.

Albright, F., and Reifenstein, E. C. (1948). "The Parathyroid Glands and Metabolic Bone Disease." Williams & Wilkins, Baltimore, Maryland.

Albright, F., Bauer, W., Ropes, M., and Aub, J. C. (1929). *J. Clin. Invest.* **7**, 139.

Albright, F., Bauer, W., Claflin, D., and Cockrill, J. R. (1932). *J. Clin. Invest.* **11**, 411.

Albright, F., Butler, A. M., and Bloomberg, E. (1937). *Am. J. Dis. Child.* **54**, 529.

Albright, F., Burnett, C. H., Smith, P. H., and Parson, W. (1942). *Endocrinology* **30**, 922.

Albright, F., Burnett, C. H., Parson, W., Reifenstein, E. C., Jr., and Roos, A. (1946). *Medicine (Baltimore)* **25**, 399.

Albright, F., Henneman, P. H., Benedict, P. H., and Forbes, A. P. (1955). *Proc. R. Soc. Med.* **46**, 1077.

Amiel, C. (1964). *Soc. Med. Hop. Paris* **115**, 321.

Amiel, C., Kuntziger, H., and Richet, G. (1970). *Pfluegers Arch.* **317**, 93.

Anderson, I. A. (1950). *Q. J. Med.* **19**, 67.

Anderson, J. (1955). *J. Physiol (London)* **130**, 268.

Anderson, J., and Foster, J. B. (1959). *Clin. Sci.* **18**, 437.

Anderson, J., and Parsons, V. (1963). *Clin. Sci.* **25**, 431.

Anderson, J., Dent, C. E., Harper, C., and Philpot, G. R. (1954). *Lancet* **2**, 720.

Ardaillou, R., Milhaud, G., Rousselet, F., Vuagnat, P., and Ricket, G. (1967). *C.R. Acad. Sci.* **264**, 3037.

Arner, B. (1964). *Acta Med. Scand.* **176**, Suppl. 415.

Aub, J. C., Bauer, W., Heath, C., and Ropes, M. (1929). *J. Clin. Invest.* **7**, 97.

Aurbach, G. D., and Chase, L. R. (1970). *Fed. Proc., Fed. Am. Soc. Exp. Biol.* **29**, 1179.

Aurbach, G. D., Marcus, R., Winickoff, R. W., Epstein, E. J., and Nigra, T. P. (1970). *Metab., Clin. Exp.* **19**, 799.

Avioli, L. V., and Prockop, D. J. (1967). *J. Clin. Invest.* **46**, 217.

Baines, G. H., Barclay, J. A., and Cooke, W. T. (1945). *Q. J. Med.* **14**, 113.

Barnicot, N. A. (1948). *J. Anat.* **82**, 233.

Bartter, F. C. (1961). *In* "The Parathyroids" (R. O. Greep and R. V. Talmage, eds.), p. 388. Thomas, Springfield, Illinois.

Barzel, U. S. (1969). *J. Clin. Endocrinol. Metab.* **29**, 917.

Barzel, U. S. (1970). *In* "Osteoporosis" (U. S. Barzel, ed.), p. 199. Grune & Stratton, New York.

Barzel, U. S. (1971). *Lancet* **1**, 1329.

Barzel, U. S., and Jowsey, J. (1969). *Clin. Sci.* **36**, 517.

Bauer, W., and Aub, J. C. (1941). *J. Clin. Invest.* **20**, 295.

Baumann, E. J., and Sprinson, D. S. (1939). *Am. J. Physiol.* **125**, 741.

Beck, L. H., and Goldberg, M. (1973). *Am. J. Physiol.* **224**, 1136.

Beck, N., Singh, H., Reed, S. W., and Davis, B. B. (1974). *J. Clin. Invest.* **53**, 717.

Beisel, W. R., Zernan, C. J., Jr., Rubini, M. E., and Blythe, W. B. (1958). *Am. J. Physiol.* **195**, 357.

Beisel, W. R., Austen, K. F., and Rubini, M. E. (1960). *Metab., Clin. Exp.* **9**, 905.

Ben-Ishay, D., Viskoper, R. J., and Menczel, J. (1972). *Isr. J. Med. Sci.* **8**, 495.

Benoit, F. L., Theil, G. B., and Watten, R. H. (1963). *Metab., Clin. Exp.* **12**, 1072.

Bernstein, D. S., Wachman, A., and Hattner, R. S. (1970). *In* "Osteoporosis" (U. S. Barzel, ed.), p. 207. Grune & Stratton, New York.

Bernstein, M., Yamahiro, H. S., and Reynolds, T. B. (1965). *J. Clin. Endocrinol.* **25**, 895.
Berthaux, P., Paupe, J., and Nguyen-the-Minh (1960). *C. R. Seances Soc. Biol. Ses. Fil.* **154**, 1759.
Bijvoet, O. L. M. (1969). *Clin. Sci.* **37**, 23.
Bijvoet, O. L. M. (1972). *Folia Med. Neerl.* **15**, 84.
Bijvoet, O. L. M. (1973). *Hard Tissue Growth, Repair Remineralization, Ciba Found. Symp., 1972*, p. 432.
Bijvoet, O. L. M., and De Vries, H. R. (1974). *Lancet* **1**, 1283.
Bijvoet, O. L. M., and Froeling, P. G. A. M. (1973a). *Proc. Int. Congr. Endocrinol., 4th, 1972* Excerpta Med. Found. Int. Congr. Ser. No. 273, p. 474.
Bijvoet, O. L. M., and Froeling, P. G. A. M. (1973b). *In* "Clinical Aspects of Metabolic Bone Disease" (B. Frame, A. M. Parfitt, and H. Duncan, eds.), Int. Congr. Ser. No. 270, p. 184. Excerpta Med. Found., Amsterdam.
Bijvoet, O. L. M., and Majoor, C. L. H. (1965). *Clin. Chim. Acta* **11**, 181.
Bijvoet, O. L. M., and Morgan, D. B. (1971). *In* "Phosphate et métabolisme phosphocalcique" (D. J. Hioco, ed.), p. 153. L'Espansion Scientifique Française, Paris.
Bijvoet, O. L. M., and Van der Sluys Veer, J. (1968). *Folia Med. Neerl.* **11**, 161.
Bijvoet, O. L. M., and Van der Sluys Veer, J. (1972). *Clin. Endocrinol. Metab.* **1**, 217.
Bijvoet, O. L. M., Jansen, A. P., Prenen, H., and Majoor, C. L. H. (1964). *In* "Water and Electrolyte Metabolism" (J. de Graeff and B. Leynse, eds.), Vol. 2, p. 151. Elsevier, Amsterdam.
Bijvoet, O. L. M., Van der Sluys Veer, J., and Jansen, A. P. (1968). *Lancet* **1**, 876.
Bijvoet, O. L. M., Morgan, D. B., and Fourman, P. (1969). *Clin. Chim. Acta* **26**, 15.
Bijvoet, O. L. M., Van der Sluys Veer, J., Wildiers, J., and Smeenk, D. (1970). *Calcitonin, Proc. Int. Symp., 2nd, 1969* p. 531.
Bijvoet, O. L. M., Van der Sluys Veer, J., de Vries, H. R., and Van Koppen, A. I. J. (1971). *N. Engl. J. Med.* **284**, 681.
Bijvoet, O. L. M., Van der Sluys Veer, J., Greven, H. M., and Schellekens, A. P. M. (1972). *In* "Calcium, Parathyroid Hormone and the Calcitonins" (R. V. Talmage and P. L. Munson, eds.), Int. Congr. Ser. No. 243, p. 284. Excerpta Med. Found., Amsterdam.
Bijvoet, O. L. M., Nollen, A. J. G., Slooff, T. J. J. H., and Feith, R. (1974). *Acta Orthop. Scand.* **45**, 926.
Birke, T. J., Robinson, R. R., and Clapp, J. R. (1972). *Kidney* **1**, 16.
Birkenhager, W. H., Hellendoorn, H. B. A., and Gerbrandy, J. (1957). *Ned. Tijdschr. Geneesk.* **101**, 1294.
Birkenhager, W. H., Hellendoorn, H. B. A., and Gerbrandy, J. (1959). *Clin. Sci.* **18**, 45.
Blythe, W. B., Gittelman, H. J., and Welt, L. G. (1968). *Am. J. Physiol.* **214**, 52.
Bones, G., Newton, M., and Rieselbach, R. E. (1973). *Kidney Int.* **3**, 24.
Boudry, J. F., Trockler, U., Bonjour, J. P., and Fleisch, H. (1973). *34th Abstr., 7th Meet. Eur. Soc. Clin. Invest.* p. 47.
Brain, R. T., Kay, H. D., and Marshall, P. G. (1928). *Biochem. J.* **22**, 628.
Bricker, N. S. (1969). *Arch. Intern. Med.* **124**, 292.
Bricker, N. S., Khahr, S., Parkerson, M., and Schultze, G. (1965). *Medicine (Baltimore)* **44**, 263.
Brickman, A. S., Massry, S. G., and Coburn, J. W. (1972). *J. Clin. Invest.* **51**, 945.
Briscoe, A. M., and Ragan, C. (1966). *Metab., Clin. Exp.* **15**, 1002.
Brodehl, J., and Gellissen, K. (1966). *Klin. Wochenschr.* **44**, 171.
Brodehl, J., Kaas, W. P., and Weber, H. P. (1971). *Pediatr. Res.* **5**, 591.
Bronner, F., and Thompson, D. D. (1961). *J. Physiol. (London)* **157**, 232.
Brunette, M. G., Taleb, L., and Carriere, S. (1973). *Am. J. Physiol.* **225**, 1076.

Buchanan, G. D. (1961). *In* "The Parathyroids" (R. O. Greep and R. V. Talmage, eds.), p. 334. Thomas, Springfield, Illinois.

Buckle, R. M. (1969). *Br. Med. J.* **2**, 789.

Butler, A. M., Wilson, J. L., and Farler, S. (1936). *J. Pediatr.* **8**, 489.

Campbell, J. A., and Webster, T. A. (1921). *Biochem. J.* **15**, 660.

Canary, J. J., and Kyle, J. H. (1959). *J. Clin. Invest.* **38**, 994.

Canary, J. J., Mintz, D., Prezio, J., and Meloni, C. (1964). *Clin. Res.* **12**, 263.

Cattaneo, C., Martini, F., and Modico, A. (1964). *Acta Endocrinol. (Copenhagen)* **45**, 203.

Chalmers, T. M., Adams, P., Adams, J. E., Hill, L. F., Truscott, B., and Smellie, W. A. B. (1972). *In* "Rein et calcium" (D. J. Hioco, ed.), p. 295. Sandoz Editions, Paris.

Chambers, E. L., Gordan, G. S., Goldman, L., and Reifenstein, E. C. (1956). *J. Clin. Endocrinol. Metab.* **16**, 1507.

Charbon, G. A., and Hoekstra, M. H. (1963). *Arch. Int. Pharmacodyn. Ther.* **141**, 1.

Charbon, G. A., Hoekstra, M. H., and Kool, D. S. (1963). *Acta Physiol. Pharmacol. Neerl.* **12**, 48.

Chase, L. R., and Aurbach, G. D. (1967). *Proc. Natl. Acad. Sci. U.S.A.* **58**, 518.

Chen, P. S., and Neuman, W. F. (1955). *Am. J. Physiol.* **180**, 623.

Chu, H. I., Liu, S. H., Yu, T. F., Hsu, H. C., Cheng, T. Y., and Chao, H. C. (1940). *J. Clin. Invest.* **19**, 349.

Clapp, J. R., Nottebohm, G. A., and Robinson, R. R. (1971). *Am. J. Physiol.* **220**, 1355.

Cochran, M., and Nordin, B. E. C. (1971). *Clin. Sci.* **40**, 305.

Coe, F. L., Canterbury, J., and Reiss, E. (1971). *Trans. Assoc. Am. Physicians* **84**, 152.

Cohen, J. J., Berglund, F., and Lotspeich, W. D. (1956). *Am. J. Physiol.* **184**, 91.

Collip, J. B. (1925). *J. Biol. Chem.* **63**, 395.

Cooke, R. E., and Kleeman, C. R. (1950). *Yale J. Biol. Med.* **23**, 199.

Copp, D. H. (1960). *Metab., Clin. Exp.* **9**, 680.

Copp, D. H., Cameron, E. C., Cheney, B. A., Davidson, A. G. F., and Henze, K. G. (1962). *Endocrinology* **70**, 638.

Cortelyou, J. R., Hibner-Qwerko, A., and Mulroy, J. (1960). *Endocrinology* **66**, 441.

Corvilain, J. (1972). *J. Clin. Endocrinol. Metab.* **34**, 452.

Corvilain, J., and Abramov, M. (1962). *J. Clin. Invest.* **41**, 1230.

Crawford, J. D., Osborne, M. M., Talbot, N. B., Terry, M. L., and Morrill, M. F. (1950). *J. Clin. Invest.* **29**, 1448.

Cushing, A. R. (1917). "The Secretion of Urine." Longmans and Green, London.

Cuthbertson, D. P. (1929). *Biochem. J.* **23**, 1328.

Darmady, E. M., and Stranack, F. (1957). *Br. Med. Bull.* **13**, 21.

Daves, B. B., Kedes, L. H., and Field, J. B. (1966). *Metab., Clin. Exp.* **15**, 482.

Daves, D. R., Dent, C. E., and Wilcox, A. (1956), *Br. Med. J.* **2**, 1133.

Davis, R. H., Morgan, D. B., and Rivlin, R. S. (1970). *Clin. Sci.* **39**, 1.

Dean, R. F. A., and McCance, R. A. (1948). *J. Physiol. (London)* **107**, 182.

Deitrick, J. E., Whedon, G. D., and Shorr, E. (1948). *Am. J. Med.* **4**, 3.

Delling, G., and Donath, K. (1973). *Virchows Arch. A* **358**, 321.

Demartini, F. E., Briscoe, A. M., and Ragan, C. (1967). *Proc. Soc. Exp. Biol. Med.* **124**, 320.

Dent, C. E. (1969). *Proc. R. Soc. Med.* **63**, 401.

Dent, C. E., and Stamp. T. C. B. (1971). *Q. J. Med.* **40**, 303.

DeRouffignac, C., Morel, F., Moss, N., and Roinel, M. (1973). *Pfluegers Arch.* **344**, 309.

Dewonck, G., Back, Z. M., and Barac, G. (1963). *C. R. Seances Soc. Biol. Ses Fil.* **157**, 897.

Dirks, J. M., Cirksena, W. J., and Berliner, R. W. (1965). *J. Clin. Invest.* **44**, 1160.

Dirks, J. M., Cirksena, W. J., and Berliner, R. W. (1966). *J. Clin. Invest.* **45**, 1875.

Dohan, P. H., Yamashita, K., Larsen, R., Davis, B., Deftos, L., and Field, J. B. (1971). *Clin. Res.* **19**, 474.

Donaldson, I. A., and Nassim, J. R. (1954). *Br. Med. J.* **1**, 1228.

Dossetor, J. B., Gorman, H. M., and Beck, J. C. (1963). *Metab., Clin. Exp.* **12**, 1083.

Drake, T. G., Albright, F., and Castleman, B. (1937). *J. Clin. Invest.* **16**, 203.

Drammond, K. N., and Michael, A. F. (1964). *Nature (London)* **201**, 1333.

Drezner, M., Neelon, F. A., and Lebovitz, H. E. (1973). *N. Engl. J. Med.* **289**, 1056.

Duarte, C. G., and Watson, J. F. (1967). *Am. J. Physiol.* **212**, 1355.

Dunning, M. F., and Plum, F. (1957). *Arch. Intern. Med.* **99**, 716.

Edwards, B. R., Baer, R. G., Sutton, R. A. L., and Dirks, J. H. (1973). *J. Clin. Invest.* **52**, 2418.

Edwards, N. A., and Hodgkinson, A. (1965). *Clin. Sci.* **29**, 143.

Ehrig, U., Harrison, J. E., and Wilson, D. R. (1974). *Metab., Clin. Exp.* **23**, 139.

Eisenberg, E. (1965). *J. Clin. Invest.* **44**, 942.

Eisenberg, E. (1968a). *J. Clin. Endocrinol. Metab.* **28**, 651.

Eisenberg, E. (1968b). *In* "Parathyroid Hormone and Thyrocalcitonin (Calcitonin)" (R. V. Talmage and L. F. Bélanger, eds.), Int. Congr. Ser. No. 159, p. 465. Excerpta Med. Found., Amsterdam.

Eisinger, A. J., Jones, M. F., Barraclough, M. A., and McSwiney, R. R. (1970). *Clin. Sci.* **39**, 687.

Eknoyan, G., Suki, W. N., and Martinex-Maldonado, M. (1970). *J. Lab. Clin. Med.* **76**, 257.

Ellsworth, R. (1932). *J. Clin. Invest.* **11**, 1011.

Ellsworth, R., and Howard, J. E. (1934). *Bull. Johns Hopkins Hosp.* **55**, 296.

Ellsworth, R., and Nicholson, W. M. (1935). *J. Clin. Invest.* **14**, 823.

Engfeldt, B., Hjerdquist, S. O., and Strandh, J. R. E. (1954). *Acta Endocrinol. (Copenhagen)* **15**, 119.

Epstein, F. H. (1968). *Am. J. Med.* **45**, 700.

Erdheim, J. (1907). *Sitzungsber. Akad. Wiss. Wien., Math.-Naturwiss. Kl., Abt.* **116**, 311.

Farlop, M., and Brazeau, P. (1967). *J. Clin. Invest.* **47**, 983.

Farquharson, R. F., Salter, W. T., Tibetts, D. M., and Aub, J. C. (1931). *J. Clin. Invest.* **10**, 221.

Fauley, G. B., Freeman, S., Ivy, S. C., Atkinson, A. J., and Wigodsky, H. S. (1941). *Arch. Intern. Med.* **67**, 563.

Fernandez, P. C., and Puschett, J. B. (1973). *Am. J. Physiol.* **225**, 954.

Finn, W. F., Cerilli, G. J., and Ferris, T. F. (1970). *N. Engl. J. Med.* **283**, 1450.

Flocks, R. H. (1939). *J. Am. Med. Assoc.* **114**, 1466.

Foulks, J. G. (1955). *Can. J. Biochem. Physiol.* **33**, 638.

Frick, A. (1969). *Pfluegers Arch.* **313**, 106.

Frick, A. (1971). *Pfluegers Arch.* **325**, 1.

Frick, A., Rumrich, G., Ullrich, K. J., and Lassiter, W. E. (1965). *Pfluegers Arch.* **286**, 109.

Friis, T., Hahnemann, S., and Weeke, E. (1968). *Acta Med. Scand.* **183**, 497.

Froeling, P. G. A. M., and Bijvoet, O. L. M. (1974). *Neth. J. Med.* **17**, 174.

Fülgraff, G., and Heidenreich, O. (1973). *Naunyn-Schmiedebergs Arch. Pharmacol.* **276**, 243.

Gaillard, P. J. (1961). *In* "The Parathyroids" (R. O. Greep and R. V. Talmage, eds.), p. 20. Thomas, Springfield, Illinois.

Gallagher, J. C., and Nordin, B. E. C. (1973). *In* "Ageing and Estrogens. Frontiers of Hormone Research" (P. A. van Keep and C. Lauritzen, eds.), p. 98. Karger, Basel.

Gantt, C. L., and Carter, W. J. (1964). *Can. Med. Assoc. J.* **90**, 287.

Garcia, D. A., and Yendt, E. R. (1970). *Can. Med. Assoc. J.* **103**, 473.

Gekle, D. (1971). *Pfluegers Arch, ***323**, 96.

Gekle, D., Stroder, J., and Rostock, D. (1971). *Pediatr. Res.* **5**, 40.

Gill, J. R., Jr., Bell, N. H., and Bartter, F. C. (1967). *J. Appl. Physiol.* **22**, 136.

Glorieux, F., and Scriver, C. R. (1972). *Science* **175**, 997.

Glorieux, F. H., Scriver, C. R., Holick, M. F., and DeLuca, H. F. (1973). *Lancet* **2**, 287.

Gold, L. W., Massry, S. G., Arieff, A. J., and Coburn, J. W. (1970). *J. Clin. Invest.* **49**, 1073.

Gold, L. W., Massry, S. G., Arieff, A. I., and Coburn, J. W. (1973). *J. Clin. Invest.* **52**, 2556.

Goldberg, M., McCurdy, D. K., Folz, E. L., and Bluemle, L. W. (1964). *J. Clin. Invest.* **43**, 201.

Goldman, R., and Bassett, S. M. (1958). *J. Clin. Endocrinol. Metab.* **18**, 981.

Goldman, R., Bassett, S., and Duncan, G. B. (1954). *J. Clin. Invest.* **33**, 1623.

Goldsmith, R. S., Jr., Siemsen, A. W., Mason, A. D., Jr., and Forland, M. (1965). *J. Clin. Endocrinol.* **25**, 1649.

Gordan, G. S., Loken, H. F., Blum, A., and Teal, J. S. (1962). *Metab., Clin. Exp.* **11**, 94.

Gough, J., Duguid, J. B., and Davies, D. R. (1933). *Br. J. Exp. Pathol.* **14**, 137.

Gran, F. C. (1960). *Acta Physiol. Scand.* **50**, 132.

Gray, S. P., Morris, J. E. W., and Brooks, C. J. (1973). *Clin. Sci. Mol. Med.* **45**, 751.

Greenwald, I. (1911). *Am. J. Physiol.* **28**, 103. .

Greenwald, I., and Gross, J. (1925). *J. Biol. Chem.* **66**, 217.

Grollman, A. P., Walker, W., Harrison, H. C., and Harrison, H. E. (1963). *Am. J. Physiol.* **205**, 697.

Haas, H. G., Dambacher, N. A., Guncaga, J., and Lauffenburger, T. (1971). *J. Clin. Invest.* **50**, 2689.

Halver, B. (1967). *Acta Med. Scand.* **182**, 737.

Halver, B. (1968). *Acta Med. Scand.* **184**, 311.

Halver, B. K., Wolthers, K., and Svane, H. (1968). *Acta Med. Scand.* **184**, 307.

Hanna, S., Harrison, M. T., MacIntyre, I., and Fraser, R. (1961). *Br. Med. J.* **2**, 12.

Hanna, S., Alcock, N., Lazarus, B., and Mullan, B. (1963). *J. Lab. Clin. Med.* **61**, 220.

Harrison, A. R. (1959). *Br. J. Urol.* **31**, 298.

Harrison, A. R., and Rose, G. A. (1968). *Clin. Sci.* **34**, 343.

Harrison, H. E., and Harrison, H. C. (1941). *J. Clin. Invest.* **20**, 47.

Heaton, F. W. (1965). *Clin. Sci.* **28**, 543.

Heaton, F. W., and Hodgkinson, A. (1963). *Clin. Chim. Acta* **8**, 246.

Hebert, C. S., Rouge, D., Eknoyan, G., Martinez-Maldonado, M., and Suki, W. N. (1972). *Kidney Int.* **2**, 247.

Heersche, N. M., Marcus, R., and Aurbach, G. D. (1974). *Endocrinology* **94**, 241.

Heggeness, F. W. (1959). *J. Nutr.* **69**, 142.

Heidland, A., Hennemann, H., Hensler, R., Heidbreder, E., and Gekle, K. (1971). *Klin. Wochenscher.* **41**, 1121.

Hellman, D. E., Baird, H. R., and Bartter, F. C. (1964). *Am. J. Physiol.* **207**, 89.

Hellman, D. E., Au, W. Y. W., and Bartter, F. C. (1965). *Am. J. Physiol.* **209**, 643.

Henneman, P. H., Carrol, E. L., and Dempsey, E. F. (1954). *J. Clin. Invest.* **33**, 941.

Henneman, P. H., Dempsey, E. F., Carroll, E. L., and Albright, F. (1956). *J. Clin. Invest.* **35**, 1229.

Henneman, P. H., Benedict, P. H., Forbes, A. P., and Dudley, H. R. (1958). *N. Engl. J. Med.* **259**, 802.

Hernandez, T., and Coulson, R. A. (1956). *Fed. Proc., Fed. Am. Soc. Exp. Biol.* **15**, 91.

Heynen, G., and Franchimont, P. (1974). *Eur. J. Clin. Invest.* **4**, 213.

Higgins, B. A., Nassim, J. R., Collins, J., and Hilb, A. (1964). *Clin. Sci.* **27**, 457.

Hodgkinson, A., and Pyrah, L. N. (1958). *Br. J. Surg.* **46**, 10.

Hodgkinson, A., and Heaton, F. W. (1965). *Clin. Chim. Acta* **11**, 354.

Hornum, I., and Transbøl, I. (1973). *Acta Med. Scand.* **193**, 325.

Howard, P. J., Wilde, W. S., and Malvin, R. L. (1959). *Am. J. Physiol.* **197**, 337.

Huth, E. J., Webster, G. D., Jr., and Elkinton, J. R. (1960). *Am. J. Med.* **29**, 1960.

Hyde, R. D., Vaughan Jones, R., McSwiney, R. R., and Prunty, F. T. G. (1960). *Lancet* **1**, 250.

Ingbar, S. H., Kass, E. G., Burnett, C. H., Relmann, A. S., Burrows, B. A., and Sissons, J. H. (1951), *J. Lab. Clin. Med.* **38**, 533.

Issekutz, B., Jr., Blizzard, J. J., Birkhead, N. C., and Rodahl, L. (1966). *J. Appl. Physiol.* **21**, 1013.

Jackson, W. P. U., Hoffenberg, R., Linder, G. C., and Irwin, L. (1956). *J. Clin. Endocrinol. Metab.* **16**, 1043.

Jones, J. H., Peters, K. D., Morgan, D. B., Coles, G. A., and Mallick, N. P. (1967). *Q. J. Med.* **36**, 301.

Jørgensen, F. S., and Nielsen, S. P. (1972). *Acta Pharmacol. Toxicol.* **31**, 521.

Jørgensen, F. S., and Transbøl, I. (1974). *Acta Med. Scand.* **195**, 33.

Jowsey, J. (1968). *In* "Parathyroid Hormone and Thyrocalcitonin (Calcitonin)," (R. V. Talmage and L. F. Bélanger, eds.), Int. Congr. Ser. No. 159, p. 137. Excerpta Med. Found., Amsterdam.

Jowsey, J., and Balambranamiam, P. (1972). *Clin. Sci.* **42**, 289.

Jowsey, J., and Riggs, B. L. (1970). *Acta Endocrinol. (Copenhagen)* **63**, 21.

Jowsey, J., and Simons, G. W. (1968). *Nature (London)* **217**, 1277.

Jubiz, W., Canterbury, J. M., Reiss, E., and Tyler, F. H. (1972). *J. Clin. Invest.* **51**, 2040.

Kaminski, N. I., Broadus, A. E., Hardman, J. G., Jones, D. J., Jr., Ball, J. H., Sutherland, E. W., and Liddle, G. W. (1970). *J. Clin. Invest.* **49**, 2387.

Kaplan, E. L., Hill, B. J., Locke, S., Toth, D. N., and Peskin, G. W. (1971). *J. Lab. Clin. Med.* **78**, 814.

Kaplan, E. L., Peskin, G. W., and Jaffee, B. M. (1972). *Surgery* **72**, 53.

Kaye, M. (1974). *J. Clin. Invest.* **53**, 256.

Kildeberg, P., Engel, K., and Winters, R. W. (1969). *Acta Paediatr. Scand.* **58**, 321.

Kleeman, C. R., and Cooke, R. E. (1951). *J. Lab. Clin. Med.* **38**, 112.

Kleeman, C. R., Bernstein, D., Dowling, T. T., and Maxwell, M. H. (1960). *Acta Endocrinol. (Copenhagen)*, Suppl. **51** 493.

Kleeman, C. R., Bernstein, D., Rockney, R., Dowling, J. T., and Maxwell, M. H. (1961). *Yale J. Biol. Med.* **34**, 1.

Kleeman, C. R., Bohannan, J., Bernstein, D., Ling, S., and Maxwell, M. H. (1964). *Proc. Soc. Exp. Biol. Med.* **115**, 29.

Kleeman, C. R., Massry, S. G., Coburn, J. W., and Popovtzer, M. M. (1970). *Clin. Orthop. Relat. Res.* **68**, 210.

Kleeman, C. R., Massry, S. G., and Coburn, J. W. (1971). *Calif. Med.* **114**, 16.

Klotz, H. P., and Kanovitz, D. (1966). *Sem. Hop.* **42**, 3095.

Knox, F. G., Wright, F. S., Howards, S. S., and Berliner, R. W. (1969). *Am. J. Physiol.* **217**, 192.

Knox, F. G., Schneider, E. G., Willis, L. R., Strandhoy, J. W., Ott, E., Cuche, J. L., Goldsmith, R. S., and Arnaud, C. D. (1974). *J. Clin. Invest.* **53**, 501.

Kyle, L. H., Schaaf, M., and Canary, J. J. (1958). *Am. J. Med.* **24**, 240.

Kyle, L. H., Canary, J. J., Mintz, D. H., and De Leon, A. (1962). *J. Clin. Endocrinol. Metab.* **22**, 52.

Laake, H. (1960). *Acta Endocrinol. (Copenhagen)* **34**, 60.

Lafferty, F. W., and Pearson, O. H. (1963). *J. Clin. Endocrinol. Metab.* **23**, 891.

Lamberg, B. A., and Kuhlback, B. (1959). *Scand. J. Clin. Lab. Invest.* **11**, 351.

Lambert, P. P., and Corvilain, J. (1964). *In* "Hormones and the Kidney" (P. C. Williams, ed.), p. 139. Academic Press, New York.

Lassiter, W. E., Gottschalk, C. W., and Mylle, M. (1963). *Am. J. Physiol.* **204**, 771.

Lavender, A. R., and Pullman, T. N. (1963). *Am. J. Physiol.* **205**, 1025.

LeGrimellec, C., Roinel, N., and Morel, F. (1974). *Pfluegers Arch.* **346**, 171 and 189.

Lemann, J., Jr., and Lennon, E. J. (1972). *Kidney Int.* **1**, 275.

Lemann, J., Jr., Litzow, J. R., and Lennon, E. J. (1966). *J. Clin. Invest.* **45**, 1608.

Lemann, J., Jr., Litzow, J. R., and Lennon, E. J. (1967). *J. Clin. Invest.* **46**, 1318.

Lemann, J., Jr., Litzow, J. R., and Lennon, E. J. (1969). *N. Engl. J. Med.* **280**, 232.

Lemann, J., Jr., Piering, W. F., and Lennon, E. J. (1970). *Nephron* **7**, 117.

Levinsky, N. G., and Davidson, D. D. (1957). *Am. J. Physiol.* **191**, 530.

Liberman, U. A., Sperling, O., Astmon, A., Frank, M., Modan, M., and de Vries, A. (1968). *J. Clin. Invest.* **47**, 2580.

Lichtwitz, A., DeSeze, S., Hioco, D. J., Miravet, L., Lanham, O., and Parlier, R. (1963). *Presse Med.* **71**, 107.

Lightwood, R. (1935). *Arch. Dis. Child.* **10**, 205.

Lightwood, R., Payne, W. W., and Black, J. A. (1953). *Pediatrics* **12**, 628.

Lindeman, R. D., Adler, S., Yiengst, M. J., and Beard, E. S. (1967). *J. Lab. Clin. Med.* **70**, 236.

Lotz, M., Zisman, E., and Bartter, F. C. (1968). *N. Engl. J. Med.* **278**, 409.

Lowe, C. E., Bird, E. D., and Thomas, W. C. (1962). *J. Clin. Endocrinol. Metab.* **22**, 261.

Ludwig, C. (1844). *In* "Handwörterbuch der Physiologie mit Rucksicht auf physiologische Pathologie" (R. Wagner, ed.), Vol. 2, p. 629. Biegweg, Braunschweig.

Lutwak, L., Whedon, G. D., Lachance, P. A., Reid, J. M., and Lipscomb, H. S. (1969). *J. Clin. Endocrinol. Metab.* **29**, 1140.

MacIntyre, I. (1963). *Sci. Basis Med.* p. 216.

MacIntyre, I.; Boss, S., and Troughton, V. A. (1963). *Nature (London)* **198**, 1058.

McCance, R. A., and Widdowson, M. E. (1942). *J. Physiol. (London)* **101**, 350.

McCann, W. S. (1928). *J. Am. Med. Assoc.* **90**, 249.

McCrory, W. W., Forman, C. W., McNamara, H., and Barnett, H. L. (1950). *Am. J. Dis. Child.* **80**, 512.

McGeown, M. G. (1961). *Proc. R. Soc. Med.* **54**, 642.

McGeown, M. G. (1964). *In* "Hormones and the Kidney" (P. C. Williams, ed.), p. 146. Academic Press, New York.

McLean, F. C., and Hinricks, M. A. (1938). *Am. J. Physiol.* **21**, 580.

McSherry, E., Sebastian, A., and Morris, R. C. (1972). *J. Clin. Invest.* **51**, 499.

Makler, R. F., and Stanbury, S. W. (1956). *Q. J. Med.* **25**, 21.

Malm, O. J. (1953). *Scand. J. Clin. Lab. Invest.* **5**, 75.

Malvin, R. L., and Lotspeich, W. D. (1956). *Am. J. Physiol.* **187**, 51.

Malvin, R. L., Wilde, W. S., and Sullivan, L. P. (1958a). *Am. J. Physiol.* **187**, 51.

Malvin, R. L., Wilde, W. S., and Sullivan, L. P. (1958b). *Am. J. Physiol.* **194**, 135.

Mankin, H. J. (1974). *J. Bone Joint Surg., Am. Vol.* **56**, 352.

Marshall, E. K., Jr., and Grafflin, A. L. (1933). *Proc. Soc. Exp. Biol. Med.* **31**, 44.

Massry, S. G., and Kleeman, C. R. (1972). *J. Lab. Clin. Med.* **80**, 654.

Massry, S. G., Coburn, J. W., Chapman, L. W., and Kleeman, C. R. (1967). *Am. J. Physiol.* **213**, 1218.

Massry, S. G., Coburn, J. W., Chapman, L. W., and Kleeman, C. R. (1965a). *Am. J. Physiol.* **214**, 1403.

Massry, S. G., Coburn, J. W., Chapman, L. W., and Kleeman, C. R. (1968b). *J. Lab. Clin. Med.* **71**, 212.

Massry, S. G., Coburn, J. W., and Kleeman, C. R. (1969). *J. Clin. Invest.* **48**, 1237.

Massry, S. G., Coburn, J. W., and Kleeman, C. R. (1970). *J. Clin. Invest.* **49**, 1619.

Massry, S. G., Friedler, R. M., and Coburn, J. W. (1973). *Arch. Intern. Med.* **131**, 828.

Melson, G. L., Chase, L. R., and Aurbach, G. D. (1970). *Endocrinology* **86**, 511.

Michael, A. F., and Drammond, K. N. (1967). *Can. J. Physiol. Pharmacol.* **45**, 103.

Milne, M. D. (1951). *Clin. Sci.* **10**, 471.

Milne, M. D., Stanbury, S. W., and Thomson, A. E. (1952). *Q. J. Med.* **21**, 61.

Minkin, C., and Jennings, C. M. (1972). *Science* **176**, 1031.

Mioni, G., d'Angelo, A., Ossi, E., Bertaglia, E., Marconi, G., and Maschio, G. (1971). *Rev. Eur. Etud. Clin. Biol.* **16**, 881.

Molinatti, G. M., Camanni, F., and Olivetti, M. (1960). *Acta Endocrinol. (Copenhagen)* **34**, 323.

Morey, E. R., and Kenney, A. D. (1964). *Endocrinology* **75**, 78.

Morgan, D. B. (1973). "Osteomalacia, Renal Osteodystrophy and Osteoporosis." Thomas, Springfield, Illinois.

Morgan, D. B., Rivlin, R. S., and Davis, R. H. (1972). *Am. J. Clin. Nutr.* **25**, 652.

Morris, R. C., Jr. (1969). *N. Engl. J. Med.* **281**, 1405.

Morrissey, J. F., Ochoa, M., Jr., Lotspech, W. D., and Waterhouse, C. (1963). *Ann. Intern. Med.* **58**, 159.

Mostellar, M. E., and Tuttle, E. P., Jr. (1964). *J. Clin. Invest.* **43**, 138.

Muldowney, F. P., Freaney, R., and McGeeny, D. (1968). *Q. J. Med.* **37**, 517.

Muldowney, F. P., Carrol, D. V., Donohoe, J. F., and Freaney, R. (1971). *Q. J. Med.* **160**, 487.

Muldowney, F. P., Donohoe, J. F., Carroll, D. V., Powell, D., and Freaney, R. (1972). *Q. J. Med.* **163**, 321.

Muller, H. (1969). *Lancet* **1**, 449.

Murad, F., and Pak, C. Y. C. (1972). *N. Engl. J. Med.* **286**, 1382.

Murad, F., Brewer, H. B., Jr., and Vaughan, M. (1970). *Proc. Natl. Acad. Sci. U.S.A.* **65**, 446.

Murdaugh, H. V., Jr., and Robinson, R. R. (1960). *Am. J. Physiol.* **189**, 571.

Myers, W. P. L., Rothschild, E. O., and Lawrence, W., Jr. (1964). *In* "Bone and Tooth" (H. J. J. Blackwood, ed.), p. 193. Pergamon, Oxford.

Nash, M. A., Torrado, A. D., Greifer, I., Spitzer, A., and Edelmann, C. M. (1972). *J. Pediatr.* **80**, 738.

Nassim, J. R., and Higgins, B. A. (1965). *Br. Med. J.* **1**, 675.

Nassim, J. R., Saville, P. D., and Mulligan, L. (1956). *Clin. Sci.* **15**, 367.

Neuman, W. F., and Neuman, M. W. (1957). *Am. J. Med.* **22**, 123.

Neuman, W. F., and Ramp, W. K. (1971). *In* "Cellular Mechanisms for Calcium Transfer and Homeostasis" (G. Nichols, Jr. and R. H. Wasserman, eds.), p. 197. Academic Press, New York.

Ney, R. L., Kelly, G., and Bartter, F. C. (1968). *Endocrinology* **82**, 760.

Nicholson, T. F., and Shepherd, G. W. (1959). *Can. J. Biochem. Physiol.* **37**, 103.

Nordin, B. E. C. (1960). *Clin. Sci.* **19**, 311.

Nordin, B. E. C., and Bulusu, L. (1968). *Postgrad. Med. J.* **44**, 93.

Nordin, B. E. C., and Fraser, R. (1960). *Lancet* **1**, 947.

Nordin, B. E. C., and Peacock, M. (1969). *Lancet* **2**, 1280.

Nordin, B. E. C., and Smith, D. A. (1965). "Diagnostic Procedures in Disorders of Calcium Metabolism." Churchill, London.

Nordin, B. E. C., Young, M. M., Bulusu, L., and Horshman, A. (1970). *In* "Osteoporosis (U. S. Barzel ed.), p. 47. Grune & Stratton, New York.

Nordin, B. E. C., Peacock, M., and Wilkinson, R. (1972a). *Clin. Endocrinol. Metab.* **1,** 169.

Nordin, B. E. C., Peacock, M., and Wilkinson, R. (1972b). *In* "Calcium, Parathyroid Hormone and the Calcitonins" (R. V. Talmage and P. L. Munson, eds.), Int. Congr. Ser. No. 243. p. 263, Excerpta Med. Found., Amsterdam.

Nunziata, V., Reiner, M., Nadarajah, A., Woodhouse, N. J. Y., Fisher, M., and Joplin, G. F. (1971). *Isr. J. Sci.* **7,** 388.

Ollayos, R. W., and Winkler, A. W. (1943). *J. Clin. Invest.* **22,** 147.

Omdahl, J. L., and DeLuca, H. F. (1973). *Physiol. Rev.* **53,** 327.

Paillard, F., Ardaillou, F., Malendin, H., Fillastre, J. P., and Prior, S. (1972). *J. Lab. Clin. Med.* **80,** 200.

Pak, C. Y. C., East, D., Sanzenbacher, L., Ruskin, B., and Cox, J. (1972a). *Arch. Intern. Med.* **129,** 48.

Pak, C. Y. C., East, D. A., Sanzenbacher, L. J., Delea, C. S., and Bartter, F. C. (1972b). *J. Clin. Endocrinol. Metab.* **35,** 261.

Palmer, F. J., Nelson, J. C., and Bacchers, H. (1974). *Ann. Intern. Med.* **80,** 200.

Pang, P. K. T. (1971). *J. Exp. Zool.* **178,** 89.

Pang, P. K. T. (1973). *Am. Zool.* **13,** 775.

Parfitt, A. M. (1969). *Clin. Sci.* **36,** 267.

Parfitt, A. M. (1972). *J. Clin. Invest.* **51,** 1879.

Parsons, V., and Anderson, J. (1964). *Clin. Sci.* **27,** 313.

Pascale, L. R., Dubin, A., and Hoffman, W. S. (1954). *Metab., Clin. Exp.* **3,** 462.

Patrick, G., and Stirling, C. (1973). *Arch. Int. Physiol. Biochim.* **81,** 453.

Paunier, L., Rey, J. P., and Wyss, M. (1969–1970). *Helv. Med. Acta* **35,** 504.

Peacock, M., and Nordin, B. E. C. (1968a). *J. Clin. Pathol.* **21,** 353.

Peacock, M., and Nordin, B. E. C. (1968b). *In* "Renal Stone Research Symposium" (A. Hodgkinson and B. E. C. Nordin, eds.), p. 253. Churchill, London.

Peacock, M., and Nordin, B. E. C. (1973). *Hard Tissue Growth, Repair Remineralization, Ciba Found. Symp., 1972* p. 409.

Peacock, M., Robertson, W. G., and Nordin, B. E. C. (1969). *Lancet* **1,** 384.

Pechet, M. M. (1966). *Proc. Pan-Am. Congr. Endocrinol., 6th, 1965* Excerpta Med. Found. Int. Congr. Ser. No. 112, p. 179.

Pechet, M. M., Bowers, B., and Bartter, F. C. (1959). *J. Clin. Invest.* **38,** 691.

Phang, J. M., Berman, M., Finerman, G. A., Neer, R. M., and Rosenberg, L. E. (1969). *J. Clin. Invest.* **48,** 67.

Pickleman, J. R., Straus, F. H., Forland, M., and Paloyan, E. (1969). *Metab., Clin. Exp.* **18,** 867.

Pitts, R. F., and Alexander, R. S. (1944). *Am. J. Physiol.* **142,** 648.

Popovtzer, M. M., Massry, S. G., Coburn, J. W., and Kleeman, C. R. (1969). *J. Lab. Clin. Med.* **73,** 763.

Popovtzer, M. M., Schainuck, L. I., Massry, S. G., and Kleeman, C. R. (1970). *Clin. Sci.* **38,** 297.

Popovtzer, M. M., Pinggera, W. F., Hutt, M. P., Robinette, J., Halgrimson, C. G., and Starzl, T. E. (1972). *J. Clin. Endocrinol. Metab.* **35,** 213.

Popovtzer, M. M., Robinette, J. B., DeLuca, H. F., and Holick, M. F. (1974). *J. Clin. Invest.* **53,** 913.

Poulos, P. P. (1957). *J. Lab. Clin. Med.* **49,** 253.

Prader, A., Illig, R., and Uehlinger, E. (1959). *Helv. Paediatr. Acta* **14,** 554.

Pronove, P., and Bartter, F. C. (1961). *Metab., Clin. Exp.* **10,** 349.

Pronovo, P., Bell, N. H., and Bartter, F. C. (1961). *Metab., Clin. Exp.* **10,** 364.

Pullman, T. N., Lavender, A. R., Aho, I., and Rasmussen, H. (1960). *Endocrinology* **67,** 570.

Pullman, T. N., Lavender, A. R., and Aho, I. (1967). *Metab., Clin. Exp.* **16,** 358.

Puschett, J. B., and Goldberg, M. (1969). *J. Lab. Clin. Med.* **73,** 956.

Puschett, J. B., Moranz, J., and Kurnick, W. S. (1972a). *J. Clin. Invest.* **51,** 373.

Puschett, J. B., Fernandez, P. C., Boyle, I. T., Gray, R. W., Omdahl, J. L., and DeLuca, H. F. (1972b). *Proc. Soc. Exp. Biol. Med.* **141,** 379.

Puschett, J. B., Beck, W. S., Jr., Jelonek, A., and Fernandez, P. C. (1974). *J. Clin. Invest.* **53,** 756.

Raisz, L. G. (1965). *J. Clin. Invest.* **44,** 103.

Raisz, L. G. (1972). *In* "Clinical Disorders of Fluid and Electrolyte Metabolism" (M. H. Maxwell and C. R. Kleeman, eds.), p. 375. McGraw-Hill, New York.

Raisz, L. G., Trummel, C. L., and Simmons, H. (1972). *Endocrinology* **90,** 744.

Rasmussen, H. (1972). *Clin. Endocrinol. Metab.* **1,** 3.

Rasmussen, H., Arnaud, C., and Hawker, C. (1964). *Science* **144,** 1019.

Rastegas, A., Agus, Z., Connor, T. B., and Goldberg, M. (1972). *Kidney Int.* **2,** 279.

Recker, R. R., Hassing, G. S., Lan, J. R., and Saville, P. D. (1973). *J. Lab. Clin. Invest.* **81,** 258.

Reifenstein, E. C., and Albright, F. (1947). *J. Clin. Invest.* **26,** 24.

Reiss, E., and Canterbury, J. M. (1971). *Am. J. Med.* **50,** 679.

Reiss, E., Canterbury, J. M., and Kanter, A. (1969). *Arch. Intern. Med.* **124,** 417.

Reiss, E., Canterbury, J. M., Bercovitz, M. A., and Kaplan, E. L. (1970). *J. Clin. Invest.* **49,** 2146.

Reynolds, T. B., Lanman, H., and Tupikova, N. (1960). *Arch. Intern. Med.* **106,** 48.

Robbins, C. L. (1937). *J. Clin. Invest.* **16,** 682.

Roberts, K. E., and Pitts, R. F. (1953). *Endocrinology* **52,** 318.

Robertson, D. R. (1972). *In* "Calcium, Parathyroid Hormone and the Calcitonins" (R. V. Talmage and P. L. Munson, eds.), Int. Congr. Ser. No. 243, p. 21. Excerpta Med. Found., Amsterdam.

Robertson, J. D. (1942). *Lancet* **1,** 672.

Robertson, W. G., and Morgan, D. B. (1972). *Clin. Chim. Acta* **37,** 503.

Robinson, B. H. B., Marsh, E. B., Jr., Duckett, J. W., Jr., and Walser, M. (1962). *J. Clin. Invest.* **41,** 1394.

Robinson, C. J., Martin, T. J., and MacIntyre, I. (1966). *Lancet* **2,** 83.

Rodahl, K., Birkhead, N. C., Blizzard, J. J., Issekutz, B., Jr., and Pruett, E. D. R. (1966). *Nord. Med.* **75,** 182.

Rodriguez, H. J., Walls, J., Yates, J., and Klahr, S. (1974). *J. Clin. Invest.* **53,** 122.

Rodriguez-Soriano, J., and Edelman, C. M., Jr. (1969). *Annu. Rev. Med.* **20,** 363.

Roelfsema, F., Van der Sluys Veer, J., and Smeenk, D. (1970). *J. Endocrinol.* **48,** IX.

Sakai, D., and Enomoto, Y. (1964). *Arch. Int. Pharmacodyn. Ther.* **151,** 358.

Salassa, R. M., Joney, J., and Arnaud, C. D. (1970). *N. Engl. J. Med.* **283,** 65.

Schaaf, M., and Kyle, L. H. (1954). *Am. J. Med. Sci.* **228,** 262.

Schmid, E., von Bubnoff, M., and Taugner, R. (1956). *Naunyn-Schmiedebergs Arch. Exp. Pathol. Pharmakol.* **228,** 207.

Schneider, E. G., Strandhoy, J. W., Willis, L. R., and Knox, F. G. (1973). *Kidney Int.* **4,** 369.

Schneider, R. W., and Corcoran, A. (1950). *J. Lab. Clin. Med.* **36,** 985.

Schwarz, G. (1964). "Pseudohypoparathyreoidismus und Pseudo-pseudohypoparathyreoidismus." Springer-Verlag, Berlin and New York.

Seldin, D. W., Eknoyan, G., Suki, W. N., and Rector, F. C., Jr. (1966). *Ann. N.Y. Acad. Sci.* **139,** 328.

Seldin, D. W., Carter, N. W., and Rector, F. C. (1971). *In* "Diseases of the Kidneys" (M. Strauss and L. G. Welt, eds.), p. 211. Little, Brown, Boston, Massachusetts.

Shannon, J. A., and Fisher, S. (1938). *Am. J. Physiol.* **122**, 765.

Shelling, D. H. (1935). "The Parathyroids in Health and Disease." Mosby, St. Louis, Missouri.

Shorr, E. (1945). *J. Urol.* **53**, 507.

Short, E. M., Binder, H. J., and Rosenberg, L. E. (1973). *Science* **179**, 700.

Silva, O. L., Snider, R. H., and Becker, K. L. (1974). *Clin. Chem.* **20**, 337.

Singer, F. R., Woodhouse, N. J. Y., Parkinson, D. K., and Joplin, G. F. (1969). *Clin. Sci.* **37**, 181.

Sjöberg, M. E. (1969). *Horm. Metab. Res.* **1**, 136.

Slatopolsky, E., and Bricker, N. S. (1973). *Kidney Int.* **4**, 141.

Slatopolsky, E., Robson, A. M., Elkan, I., and Bricker, N. S. (1968). *J. Clin. Invest.* **47**, 1865.

Slatopolsky, E., Caglar, S., Pennel, J. P., Taggart, D. D., Canterbury, J. M., and Bricker, N. S. (1971). *J. Clin. Invest.* **50**, 492.

Slatopolsky, E., Caglar, S., Gradowska, L., Canterbury, J., Reiss, E., and Bricker, N. S. (1972). *Kidney Int.* **2**, 147.

Smith, D. A., Fraser, S. A., and Wilson, G. M. (1973). *Clin. Endocrinol. Metab.* **2**, 333.

Smith, H. W. (1956). "Principles of Renal Physiology." Oxford Univ. Press, London and New York.

Smith, H. W., Goldring, W., Chasis, H., Ranges, H. A., and Bradley, S. E. (1943). *J. Mt. Sinai Hosp.* **10**, 59.

Sotornik, I., Adamicka, V., Kocvara, S., and Schuck, O. (1972). *Nephron* **9**, 318.

Spornitz, U. M., and Frick, A. (1973). *Pfluegers Arch.* **340**, 161.

Stalder, G., Schmidt, R., and Gerstner, I. (1957). *Ann. Paediatr.* **189**, 293.

Stamp, T. C., and Stacey, T. E. (1970). *Clin. Sci.* **39**, 506.

Stanbury, S. W. (1972a). *Clin. Endocrinol. Metab.* **1**, 239.

Stanbury, S. W. (1972b). *Clin. Endocrinol. Metab.* **1**, 267.

Stanbury, S. W., Lumb, G. A., and Nicholson, W. F. (1960). *Lancet* **1**, 793.

Steele, T. H. (1970). *Metab., Clin. Exp.* **19**, 129.

Stote, R. M., Smith, L. H., Wilson, D., Dube, W. J., Goldsmit, R. S., and Arnaud, C. (1972). *Ann. Intern. Med.* **77**, 587.

Strickler, J. C., Thompson, D. D., Klose, R. M., and Giebisch, G. (1964). *J. Clin. Invest.* **43**, 1596.

Suki, W. N., Rector, F. C., Jr., and Seldin, D. W. (1965). *J. Clin. Invest.* **44**, 1458.

Suki, W. N., Hull, A. R., Rector, F. C., and Seldin, D. W. (1967). *Clin. Res.* **15**, 78.

Suki, W. N., Yium, J. J., Minden, M. V., Saller-Hebert, C., Eknoyan, G., and Martinez-Maldonado, M. (1970). *N. Engl. J. Med.* **283**, 236.

Talmage, R. V. (1956–1957). *Ann. N.Y. Acad. Sci.* **64**, 326.

Talmage, R. V., and Kraintz, F. W. (1954). *Proc. Soc. Exp. Biol. Med.* **87**, 263.

Talmage, R. V., Kraintz, F. W., Frost, R. C., and Kraintz, L. (1953). *Endocrinology* **52**, 318.

Talmage, R. V., Kraintz, F. W., and Buchanan, G. D. (1955). *Proc. Soc. Exp. Biol. Med.* **88**, 600.

Talso, P. J., and Carballo, A. J. (1960). *Ann. N.Y. Acad. Sci.* **88**, 822.

Tambyah, J. A., and Lim, M. K. L. (1969). *Br. Med. J.* **1**, 751.

Tashian, A. H., Jr., and Melvin, K. E. W. (1968). *N. Engl. J. Med.* **279**, 279.

Taugner, R., Bubnoff, M. V., and Braun, W. (1953). *Pfluegers Arch. Gesamte Physiol. Menschen Tiere* **258**, 133.

Taugner, R., van Egidy, H., Iravany, J., and Taugner, G. (1960). *Naunyn-Schmiedebergs Arch. Exp. Pathol. Pharmakol.* **238**, 419.

Thalassinos, N. C., Lesse, B., Latham, S. C., and Joplin, G. F. (1970). *Arch. Dis. Child.* **45**, 269.

Thompson, D. D., and Hiatt, H. H. (1957). *J. Clin. Invest.* **36**, 566.

Thwaites, M. Z., and Trounce, J. R. (1972). *Int. J. Clin. Pharmacol., Ther. Toxicol.* **6**, 48.

Vainsel, M. (1973). *Biomedicine* **18**, 112.

Van der Sluys Veer, J., Birkenhager, J. C., and Smeenk, D. (1966). *Calcif. Tissues 1966, Proc. Eur. Symp., 4th, 1966* p. 96.

Van der Sluys Veer, J., Birkenhager, J. C., and Smeenk, D. (1967). *Calcif. Tissues 1967 Proc. Eur. Symp., 5th, 1967* p. 201.

Verbanck, M., and Toppet, N. (1961). *Rev. Fr. Etud. Clin. Biol.* **6**, 239.

Verfecke, A. (1898). *Arch. Int. Pharmacodyn.* **4**, 81.

Walker, B. R., Hoppe, R. C., and Alexander, F. (1972). *Clin. Pharmacol. Ther.* **13**, 245.

Walser, M. (1961a). *J. Clin. Invest.* **40**, 723.

Walser, M. (1961b). *Am. J. Physiol.* **200**, 1099.

Walser, M. (1969). *Miner. Metab.* **3**, 235.

Walser, M., and Trounce, J. R. (1961). *Biochem. Pharmacol.* **8**, 157.

Walton, R. J., and Bijvoet, O. L. M. (1975). *Lancet* **2**, 309.

Warte, L. C. (1972). *Endocrinology* **91**, 1160.

Wesson, L. G., Jr. (1962). *J. Lab. Clin. Med.* **59**, 630.

Wesson, L. G., Jr. (1964). *Medicine (Baltimore)* **43**, 547.

Wesson, L. G., Jr. (1973). *Kidney Int.* **4**, 236.

Wesson, L. G., Jr., and Lauler, P. D. (1959). *Proc. Soc. Exp. Biol. Med.* **101**, 235.

West, C. D., and Rapaport, S. (1949). *Proc. Soc. Exp. Biol. Med.* **71**, 322.

Whedon, G. D., and Shorr, E. (1957). *J. Clin. Invest.* **36**, 966.

Whittembury, G., and Proverbio, F. (1969). *Pfluegers Arch.* **316**, 1.

Widrow, S. H., and Levinsky. N. G. (1962). *J. Clin. Invest.* **41**, 2151.

Wilbur, K. M. (1973). *Hard Tissue Growth, Repair Remineralization, Ciba Found. Symp., 1972* p. 7.

Wilder, R. M., Higgins, G. M., and Sheard, C. (1934). *Ann. Int. Med.* **7**, 1059.

Wills, M. R. (1970a). *Lancet* **2**, 802.

Wills, M. R. (1970b). *Ann. Clin. Biochem.* **7**, 136.

Wills, M. R. (1971). *J. Clin. Pathol.* **24**, 219.

Wills, M. R., and McGowan, G. K. (1963). *J. Bone Joint. Surg.* **45B**, 799.

Wills, M. R., Gill, J. R., and Bartter, F. C. (1969). *Clin. Sci.* **37**, 621.

Woodhouse, N. J. Y. (1972). *Clin. Endocrinol. Metb.* **1**, 125.

Wrong, O., and Davies, H. E. F. (1959). *Quart. J. Med.* **28**, 259.

Yamahiro, H. S., and Reynolds, T. B. (1962). *Metabolism* **11**, 213.

Yendt, E. R., Gagne, R. J. A., and Cohanim, M. (1966). *Am. J. Med. Sci.* **231**, 449.

3

Alkaline Phosphatase and Metabolic Bone Disorders

SOLOMON POSEN, CORALIE CORNISH, AND
MICHAEL KLEEREKOPER

I. HISTORICAL

The presence of alkaline phosphatase in mammalian skeletal tissue and the high alkaline phosphatase activity in the plasma of patients with skeletal disorders were described in the 1920's (Robison, 1923; Kay, 1929). Despite innumerable publications since that time (Fishman and Ghosh, 1967; Posen, 1967; Kaplan, 1972), our basic understanding of skeletal alkaline phosphatase has not progressed appreciably. Admittedly, our methods of assay have become somewhat more sophisticated owing to the introduction of substrates (Bessey *et al.*, 1946; Cornish *et al.*, 1970) and buffers (Wilson *et al.*, 1964) that were not available to the early investigators. Moreover, we have become aware of several disorders that were not recognized or, like dialysis bone disease, did not exist in 1929. However, as Table I shows, the "advances" in our knowledge of skeletal alkaline phosphatase since the days of Robison and Kay are small in number and insignificant in their implications. We still do not know

TABLE I

Chronological Order of Some of the Advances in Our Knowledge of Skeletal Alkaline Phosphatase (AP) since 1923[a]

Reference	Findings
Robison (1923)	Presence of phosphatase in bone
Robison and Soames (1924)	Optimum pH on alkaline side of neutral
Kay (1929)	Enhanced AP activity in plasma of patients with skeletal disorders
Gomori (1943)	Histochemical demonstration of AP in bone
Rathbun (1948)	Hypophosphatasia
Bakwin and Eiger (1956)	Familial hyperphosphatasia
Schlamowitz (1958)	Antiskeletal AP antibody
Hodson *et al.* (1962)	Starch gel electrophoresis of skeletal AP
Posen *et al.* (1965b)	Use of denaturation procedures to characterize circulating skeletal AP
Eaton and Moss (1968)	Purification of skeletal AP
Gothlin and Ericsson (1971)	Localization of skeletal AP on cell walls

[a] Advances involving alkaline phosphatase in general are not listed here.

whether alkaline phosphatase is released into the circulation from living or disintegrating cells (Hekkelman, 1970; Hill *et al.*, 1972), and we still do not understand the function of this enzyme. The dialyzable factor that stimulates alkaline phosphatase in bone culture (Martin and DeLuca, 1969) has not yet been identified. This relative lack of progress may be contrasted with the considerable advances in our knowledge of alkaline phosphatases from *E. coli* (Torriani, 1960; Simpson and Vallee, 1968; Schlesinger *et al.*, 1969; Reid and Wilson, 1971; Lazdunski *et al.*, 1971; Taylor and Coleman, 1972; Kelly *et al.*, 1973) and from nonskeletal mammalian tissues (Wachsmuth and Hiwada, 1974; Cathala *et al.*, 1975).

II. ALKALINE PHOSPHATASE AND CALCIFICATION

The hypothesis concerning a cause and effect relationship between alkaline phosphatase and tissue calcification was first put forward by Robison and Soames in 1924. Essentially, this hypothesis stated that phosphatase in osteoblasts and cartilage cells hydrolyzes circulating phosphate esters with a resulting increase in inorganic phosphate ions in the vicinity of the phosphatase-producing cells. This in turn was said to cause the solubility product of various calcium phosphate compounds to be exceeded, with a resulting deposition of hydroxyapatite and similar compounds. Histochemical studies subsequently introduced by Gomori (1943) showed a close relationship between phosphatase-positive cartilage and calcification. This finding was later confirmed by electron microscopy (Matsuzawa and Anderson, 1971). The transformation of fibroblasts into osteogenic tissue was found to be accompanied by a local rise in alkaline phosphatase (Reddi and Huggins, 1972).

Numerous objections were raised against Robison's theory almost as soon as it was published (Shipley *et al.*, 1926). Phosphatase is present in noncalcifying tissues, including the cartilaginous skeleton of elasmobranchs (Bodansky *et al.*, 1931). The pH optimum is "unphysiological." The concentration of naturally occurring substrates is totally inadequate to account for the rise in inorganic phosphate at calcification sites (Posner, 1969). High phosphatase activities do not appear to lead to high concentrations of inorganic phosphate (Siffert, 1951). Calcification fails to occur in ricketic bone and in bone implants of diphosphonate-treated animals (Strates *et al.*, 1971) even though phosphatase is abundant. Kay who was skeptical of Robinson's calcification theory suggested as early as 1926 that "phosphatase activity may be merely the fortuitous result of a particular type of molecular configuration of frequent occurrence in the cell" (Kay, 1926).

TABLE II

The p-Nitrophenylphosphatase and Inorganic Pyrophosphatase Activities of an
Extract Prepared from Fetal Bones during Various States of Purification[a,b]

Stage of purification	Total p-nitrophenyl-phosphatase activity	Total inorganic pyrophosphatase activity
Crude homogenate (fetal bones)	275	48
Butanol extract (aqueous layer)	604	14
Ethanol precipitate (66%)	816	90
Ethanol supernatant (66%)	40	4
Dialyzed material (after ethanol precipitation)	772	109
Fraction 39 (DEAE cellulose)	48	4

[a] From Cornish (1973).

[b] While the p-nitrophenylphosphatase : inorganic pyrophosphatase ratios are not identical at all stages, there is nevertheless a reasonable correlation between the two activities. Activities for each substrate are expressed in μmoles of substrate hydrolyzed per minute at 37°C.

The theory concerning the calcifying role of alkaline phosphatase acquired a new lease on life when it was suggested (Fleisch and Neuman, 1961) that the function of skeletal alkaline phosphatase consisted of "the destruction of an inhibitor" to the mineralization process. It was subsequently established* that pyrophosphate could serve as a substrate to mammalian alkaline phosphatases (Cox and Griffin, 1965; Fernley and Walker, 1967; Eaton and Moss, 1967) including skeletal alkaline phosphatase† (Table II). It was also shown that inorganic pyrophosphate, which was present in bone (Perkins and Walker, 1958), converted hydroxyapatite crystals into "inert" material (Fleisch et al., 1966), preventing both mineral deposition and mineral resorption. Protagonists of the calcification function of alkaline phosphatase now argued that this enzyme diminished the concentration of inorganic pyrophosphate or other calcification inhibitors, allowing the deposition of calcium phosphate salts. In support of this hypothesis was the observation that patients with

* Kay (1928), whose writing were in many ways far ahead of his time, stated that inorganic pyrophosphate was hydrolyzed by mammalian alkaline phosphatases. This was subsequently denied (Morton, 1955; Kuhlman, 1965). Fernley and Walker (1967) showed that the reported discrepancies were largely due to differences in assay methods.

† The identity between alkaline phosphatase and inorganic pyrophosphatase is not universally accepted (Alcock and Shils, 1969). The reported discrepancies in the pH optima of pyrophosphatases remain unexplained (Alcock and Shils, 1969).

hypophosphatasia excreted abnormally large amounts of pyrophosphate in their urine (Russell, 1965), allegedly because of their inability to hydrolyze this material enzymically. In spite of many objections, and in spite of the presence of alkaline phosphatase and pyrophosphatase in noncalcifying tissues, the role of this enzyme in calcification continues to exercise the imagination of a large number of workers (Solomon *et al.*, 1966; Jibril, 1967; Johnson and Alkek, 1970; Granda and Posner, 1971; Streifler *et al.*, 1972; Kuftinec and Miller, 1972).

III. LOCALIZATION AND PURIFICATION OF SKELETAL ALKALINE PHOSPHATASE

The localization of skeletal alkaline phosphatase in various parts of bone, its association with different cells, and its intracellular distribution have been studied by a variety of methods. Infants' ribs separated into periosteum "bone," "marrow," and cartilage showed most of the alkaline phosphatase activity to be derived from bone (Cornish, 1973). Serial sections through calcifying epiphyses of a number of species showed a progressive increase in alkaline phosphatase activity from unorganized cartilage through proliferating and hypertrophic cartilage to primitive spongiosa (Kuhlman, 1965; Granda and Posner, 1971).

Osteoblasts and osteocytes are rich in alkaline phosphatase but contain little acid phosphatase. The reverse is true of osteoclasts (Burstone, 1960; Jeffree, 1970). The intracellular distribution of skeletal alkaline phosphatase has been studied by means of differential ultracentrifugation (Vaes and Jacques, 1965b). Unlike acid phosphatase, which is associated with the light mitochondrial fraction, alkaline phosphatase if found in the "microsomal" and supernatant fractions. There is some evidence that, like other alkaline phosphatases, skeletal alkaline phosphatase is associated with cell membranes (Gothlin and Ericsson, 1971).

Alkaline phosphatases from various mammalian sources have been purified to high degrees of specific activity (Morton, 1954; Trubowitz *et al.*, 1961; J. K. Smith *et al.*, 1968; Wachsmuth and Hiwada, 1974; Cathala *et al.*, 1975), and some have actually been prepared in crystalline form (Harkness, 1968). Investigations into skeletal alkaline phosphatase have been hindered by its apparent instability and by the relatively low specific activity of bone extracts. Moreover, it is difficult to obtain skeletal tissue uncontaminated by marrow (Wergedal, 1969).

Grossberg *et al.* (1961) and Eaton and Moss (1968) who purified skeletal alkaline phosphatase by means of DEAE-cellulose column chromatography, found that most of the enzymatic material was eluted in a single peak. Makinen and Knuuttila (1972) who also used DEAE-cellulose column chromatography found that skeletal alkaline phosphatase was not homogenous in their system. Cornish (1973) showed that major differences in elution patterns from DEAE-cellulose columns could be produced by relatively slight variations in technique (Fig. 1–3).

Bone alkaline phosphatase tends to "smear" during electrophoretic procedures (Boyer, 1963, Walker and Pollard, 1971) suggesting molecular heterogeneity. This may result from differences between the amino acid sequences of enzymes produced by different individuals or at different sites by the same individual. It may result from secondary modification (*in vivo*) of enzyme structure after synthesis (Natori and Garen, 1970) or from *in vitro* changes induced by purification procedures (Chang and Moog, 1972a,b). Genetic heterogeneity, such as Boyer (1961) and Robson and Harris (1965, 1967) found for human placental alkaline phosphatase, has not been demonstrated in relation to human skeletal alkaline phosphatase.

In the absence of pure preparations (let alone an amino acid sequence),

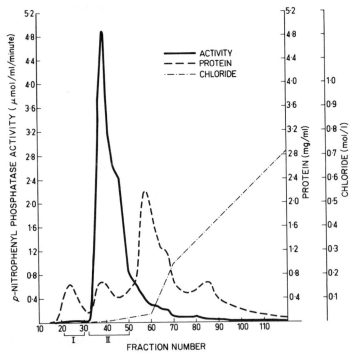

Fig. 1. DEAE-cellulose chromatography of human skeletal alkaline phosphatse treated by butanol extraction and ethanol precipitation. Column dimensions, 100×2.64 cm; sample volume, 80 ml; fraction sizes, 4 ml; linear NaCl gradient, $0–1\ M$ in $0.01\ M$ Tris HCl, pH 7.5. The enzyme appears relatively homogeneous with 56% of the activity of the starting material eluting in fractions 32–48. (From Cornish, 1973.)

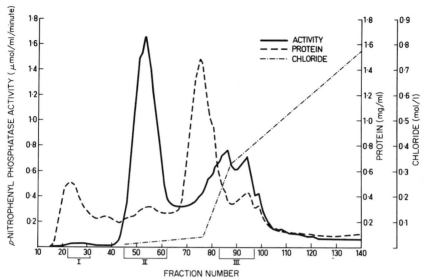

Fig. 2. Same procedure as in Fig. 1 except that the ethanol precipitate had been kept at 4°C for 8 weeks before being dissolved in the starting buffer. (From Cornish, 1973.)

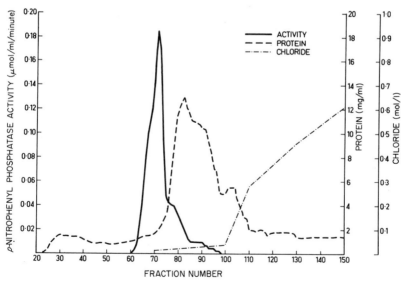

Fig. 3. Same column and same procedure as in Figs. 1 and 2. The starting material was serum from a patient with Paget's disease (total activity 275 KA units/100 ml) freshly precipitated with 66% ethanol and redissolved in starting buffer. As in Fig. 1, most of the enzymatic activity appeared in a single, early, peak. (From Cornish, 1973.)

skeletal alkaline phosphatase has to be distinguished from other alkaline phosphatases by various nonspecific features. These include its propensity to denaturation by physical and chemical agents (Posen *et al.*, 1965b; Birkett *et al.*, 1967; Horne *et al.*, 1968; Small, 1969; Ratliff *et al.*, 1972); its migration on starch gel (Boyer, 1963), cellulose acetate (Rhone and Mizuno, 1972) and polyacrylamide (I. Smith *et al.*, 1968; Kaplan and Rogers, 1969); its response to inhibitors (Fishman and Ghosh, 1967) and activators (Posen *et al.*, 1969); and its precipitation by antibodies.

Most of the above features of skeletal alkaline phosphatase are not truly "characteristic." As Fig. 4 shows, electrophoretic patterns change during storage. Heat stability is affected by dilution (Cornish *et al.*, 1970), by pH changes (Moss *et al.*, 1972), and by purification procedures. Thus in some experiments the material eluted from DEAE-cellulose in the first main peak (designated peak II in Fig. 2) was relatively heat resistant, while the second main peak (designated peak III in Fig. 2), particularly in its descending limb, showed the "characteristic" heat lability of the starting material (C. Cornish and S. Posen, unpublished). Antibodies prepared against various human skeletal alkaline phosphatase preparations cross-react with material obtained from human hepatic tissue (Table III).

Attempts have been made to characterize the kinetic properties, particularly the Michaelis constant, of skeletal alkaline phosphatase (Moss *et al.*, 1961; Landau and Schlamowitz, 1961; Moss and King, 1962; Makinen and Paunio, 1970), but as long as only semipurified skeletal phosphatase is available, the results of kinetic studies are likely to vary from one prepara-

TABLE III

Differences between "Hepatic" Alkaline Phosphatase[a] and "Biliary" Alkaline Phosphatase[b]

Properties	Hepatic	Biliary
Mean percentage activity remaining after 15 minutes at 56°C	15	70
Mean percentage activity precipitated after 4 days incubation with antihuman bone alkaline phosphatase antiserum	91	19
Migration on polyacrylamide (I. Smith *et al.*, 1968; Johnson *et al.*, 1972) starch gel (Price *et al.*, 1972) or cellulose acetate (S. Posen, unpublished)	Most anodal of all alkaline phosphatases	More cathodal than intestinal AP
Elution from G200 Sephadex column (Estborn, 1964)	With 7 S proteins	With 19 S proteins

[a] "Hepatic" material was extracted from human livers.

[b] "Biliary" material was obtained from contents of gallbladders or from T tubes draining the common bile duct.

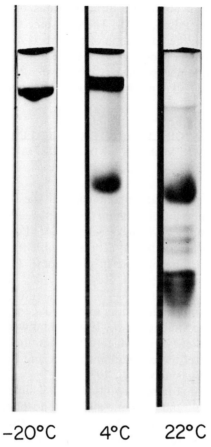

Fig. 4. Polyacrylamide electrophoresis of alkaline phosphate extracted from infants' ribs in Tris HCl, 0.01 M, PH 7.5 and kept for 38 days at various temperatures. Electrophoresis was performed according to the method of I. Smith, *et al.* (1968) while enzyme activity was demonstrated according to the method of Epstein *et al.* (1967).

tion to the next. At any rate, one wonders about the meaning of experiments involving Michaelis constants when one is dealing with a group of enzymes with pH optima that vary with substrate concentration (Morton, 1957). It has been claimed (Makinen and Paunio, 1970) that adenosine phosphates and glyceryl phosphates constitute "poorer" substrates for human skeletal phosphates than the aryl phosphates.

The techniques of gel filtration (Dunne *et al.*, 1967; Fennelly *et al.*, 1969) and isoelectric focusing (Latner *et al.*, 1971), while useful in purification procedures, do not isolate skeletal alkaline phosphatase from other alkaline phosphatases.

Very little is known about the turnover rates of circulating skeletal alkaline phosphatase (Posen, 1970). There is some evidence that this enzyme disappears from the circulation of patients (Franseen and McLean, 1935) or infused subjects (Posen et al., 1965a) at a somewhat faster rate than placental alkaline phosphatase (Clubb et al., 1965) and more slowly than infused intestinal alkaline phosphatase (Saini and Posen, 1969).

IV. TISSUE SOURCES OF CIRCULATING ALKALINE PHOSPHATASES IN NORMAL AND ABNORMAL SUBJECTS

Several alkaline phosphatase-containing tissues are known to deliver their enzymes into the circulation (Posen et al., 1973). The placenta is largely (McMaster et al., 1964; Birkett et al., 1966; Posen et al., 1969) if not entirely (Biswas and Hindocha, 1972) responsible for the increase in maternal serum alkaline phosphatase in pregnancy. The small intestine is largely (Kleerekoper et al., 1970; Reynoso et al., 1971), if not entirely (Walker et al., 1971) responsible for the rise in serum alkaline phosphatase after fat ingestion. Malignant tumors may produce alkaline phosphatases (Fishman et al., 1968; Stolbach et al., 1969), and it would appear that such ectopically produced enzymes, which vary from tumor to tumor (Warnes et al., 1972), may enter the circulation (Jacoby and Bagshawe, 1971; Jennings et al., 1972; Higashino et al., 1972).

There is evidence that in man two types of alkaline phosphatase ("bile alkaline phosphatase" and "hepatic alkaline phosphatase") are found in the hepatobiliary system and that the two differ from one another in a variety of parameters (Table III). The material circulating in patients with hepatobiliary disease is probably of biliary rather than hepatic origin (Posen et al., 1965b; Small, 1969), though there is some evidence to the contrary (Pope and Cooperband, 1966). Variant alkaline phosphatase produced by primary hepatomas (Warnock and Reisman, 1969; Higashino et al., 1972) has been described in the circulation of patients with this disorder (Higashino et al., 1972).

Other human tissues that contain alkaline phosphatase include the kidney (Boyer, 1963) and leukocytes (Trubowitz et al., 1961; Bottomley et al., 1969), but there is no convincing evidence that either contributes to serum alkaline phosphatase to any extent.

The evidence that alkaline phosphatase in the circulation of subjects with increased osteoblastic activity is of skeletal origin is reasonably conclusive (Posen, 1967). Serum alkaline phosphatase in patients with skeletal disorders correlates to some extent with bone turnover as measured by other parameters (Klein *et al.*, 1964, Cerda *et al.*, 1970), though such a correlation cannot be demonstrated in individual patients (Shifrin, 1970). The circulating alkaline phosphatase in patients with bone disorders resembles bone alkaline phosphatase in its sensitivity to heat (Posen *et al.*, 1965b; Fitzgerald *et al.*, 1969), to EDTA (Conyers *et al.*, 1967), and to urea (Horne *et al.*, 1968). While it has been claimed on immunological grounds (Sussman, 1970) that the circulating alkaline phosphatase in Paget's disease is of hepatic origin, this is not the general consensus of workers in the field (Kaplan, 1972).

The tissue source of circulating alkaline phosphatase in normal subjects has not been established with certainty. Heat denaturation (Posen *et al.*, 1965b; Fitzgerald *et al.*, 1969; Ohlen *et al.*, 1971) and urea denaturation (Horne *et al.*, 1968) suggest that serum alkaline phosphatase in normal adults consists of a mixture of skeletal and nonskeletal materials. Immunological studies (Schlamowitz, 1958; Schlamowitz and Bodansky, 1959) (Table IV) confirm this view and suggest that in some normal subjects up to 20% of circulating alkaline phosphatase is of intestinal origin (Posen *et al.*, 1967; Kleerekoper *et al.*, 1970). Electrophoretic migration patterns have been variously interpreted. They suggested a hepatic origin to some workers (Hodson *et al.*, 1962; Haije and De Jong, 1963; I. Smith *et al.*, 1968), while the evidence was regarded as equivocal by others (Fritsche and Adams-Park, 1972). Green *et al.* (1972), who used both polyacrylamide and starch gel, concluded that normal sera contained skeletal as well as hepatobiliary material.

Serum alkaline phosphatase from normal children resembles serum al-

TABLE IV

Precipitation of Alkaline Phosphatase (AP) from Sera of Various Patients by Antiskeletal Alkaline Phosphatase Antiserum[a]

Type of patient	Number of patients	Mean total serum AP (KA units/100 ml)	Mean percent precipitated by anti-skeletal phosphatase antibody
Normal adults	10	9.0	58.9
Normal children	10	28.1	66.2[b]
Hepatobiliary diseases	10	175.7	53.7[b]
Skeletal diseases	10	149.0	81.4[c]

[a] Antiserum precipitated 85.6% of its antigen under identical conditions.
[b] Not significantly different from normal adults or from each other.
[c] Significantly greater ($p < 0.01$) than precipitation in 3 other groups of sera.

kaline phosphatase from adults with skeletal disorders in relation to heat and urea denaturation (Horne *et al.*, 1968; Cornish *et al.*, 1970). Patients with mongolism (trisomy 21) whose leukocyte alkaline phosphatase is elevated (Alter *et al.*, 1963) have normal plasma alkaline phosphatase activities (Schuppisser *et al.*, 1967) and quantitatively normal alkaline phosphatase in their platelets (Tangheroni *et al.*, 1971) and fibroblasts (Cox, 1965).

The various methods for the inhibition or denaturation of circulating alkaline phosphatase may be performed on a routine basis. Indeed, automated methods are described for heat inactivation (Small, 1969; Jennings *et al.*, 1972) and urea inactivation (Horne *et al.*, 1968) as well as for phenylalanine and homoarginine inhibition (Fishman and Green, 1967; Anstiss *et al.*, 1971).

It is possible, on the basis of differential inhibition or inactivation, or on the basis of electrophoretic studies, to state that in a given serum, the alkaline phosphatase is predominantly of skeletal origin. However, when total serum alkaline phosphatase activities are normal or near normal such maneuvers are unlikely to be helpful (Winkelman *et al.*, 1972), even though it is theoretically possible for a normal total activity to hide a high intestinal, placental, or skeletal component. Current methods are not sufficiently precise (Moss *et al.*, 1972), and normal values not sufficiently well worked out for a laboratory to come out with statements such as "This patient's serum alkaline phosphatase is abnormally elevated. It contains 95 I.U. of alkaline phosphatase per liter, 68 of these units are of skeletal origin." Even in the presence of proven skeletal disorders (Garrick *et al.*, 1971; Pratley *et al.*, 1973), we have found isoenzymic studies disappointing in the presence of normal total serum alkaline phosphatase activities.

Information concerning the tissue sources of circulating alkaline phosphatase may be clinically useful in patients with double pathology (for example, in patients with Paget's disease as well as jaundice) and in patients with serum alkaline phosphatase elevation, in the absence of demonstrable pathology (Posen *et al.*, 1965b).

V. METHODS OF ASSAY: NORMAL VALUES

Enzymes are proteins whose presence is detected by their ability to catalyze certain reactions *in vitro*. They are, therefore, not quantitated in absolute units (such as weight per volume) but in units of activity—so many micromoles of reaction product released per unit of time. The enzymatic reaction obviously depends on conditions of assay, such as pH, substrate concentration, type and concentration of buffer, presence of inhibitors and activators, and temperature of incubation. Various assay methods gave rise to various "units" (Table V), such as those described by Bodansky (1933), King and Armstrong (1934), Shinowara *et al.* (1942), and Bessey *et al.* (1946). It is, in general, possible to "translate" one type of unit into another (Schwartz *et al.*, 1960; Deren *et al.*, 1964; Cornish *et al.*, 1970), and many laboratories report their results in one type of unit while actually using a procedure involving different units (see Table V). An international committee is currently attempting to standardize procedures and to provide reference material for quality control.

The most widely employed method of assay at this point in time appears to be that of Bessey *et al.* (1946) with transphosphorylating buffer (Wilson *et al.*, 1964) as automated by Morgenstern *et al.* (1965). The methods of King and Armstrong (1934), as modified by Kind and King (1954), and the method of Bodansky (1933) have also been automated (Marsh *et al.*, 1959; Tietz and Green, 1964). Some authors (Newfield, 1968; Cornish, 1973) obtained higher results with automated than with manual methods, even

TABLE V

Some of the More Commonly Employed "Units" in the Measurement of
Alkaline Phosphatase

Unit	Reference	Substrate	Reputed "normal range" (adults)	Approximate multiplication factor to convert to Bodansky units[a]
Bodansky	Bodansky (1933)	β-Glycero-phosphate	1.5–4.0	1
King–Armstrong	King and Armstrong (1934)	Phenyl phosphate	4–20[b]	0.34
Bessey–Lowry	Bessey *et al.* (1946)	*p*-Nitrophenyl phosphate	0.8–2.3	1.8
International	Bowers and McComb (1966)	*p*-Nitrophenyl phosphate	6–110[c]	0.04

[a] For a discussion concerning the difficulties of converting from one unit to another see Deren *et al.* (1964), Kaplan (1972), and McComb *et al.* (1977).

[b] See Table VI.

[c] Observed range in 248 apparently normal blood donors. Bowers and McComb (1966) use a buffer which enhances the reaction and hence they observe higher activities than those reported by workers not employing such buffers.

when all other variables had apparently been eliminated. Morgenstern *et al.* (1965) did not note such a discrepancy.

Continuous spectrophotometric methods (Bowers and McComb, 1966; Massod *et al.*, 1970) are not as yet widely employed. However, such methods will probably come into increasing use, particularly since their methodology and precision have been worked out in greater detail than those of other methods (McComb and Bowers, 1972). New instruments are now becoming available, specifically designed for continuous assays.

Alkaline phosphatase activities in serum samples submitted to a laboratory are liable to increase with dilution (Schwartz *et al.*, 1960; Gelb *et al.*, 1962) and with storage at room or refrigerator temperature (Bodansky, 1932, 1933; Kaplan and Narahara, 1953). Activity in serum samples and in commercial reference material is also liable to increase after reconstitution of lyophilized material (Brojer and Moss, 1971; Massion and Frankenfeld, 1972). It is therefore recommended that when serial estimations of serum alkaline phosphatase activities are to be made on a patient, all sera be kept deep frozen until the last specimen has been collected. The assays are then carried out together on the same day. No significant differences are discernible between the activities of serum and plasma (Bodansky, 1933; Breuer and Stucky, 1975), so that both are acceptable for alkaline phosphatase estimation. Blood should not be collected in tubes containing EDTA, which inactivates skeletal alkaline phosphatase irreversibly (Conyers *et al.*, 1967).

Patients are not required to fast for alkaline phosphatase determinations. Admittedly, large quantities of fat taken by mouth cause increases in serum alkaline phosphatase activity (Kleerekoper *et al.*, 1970). However, such increases are relatively slight, while the fat loads required to produce them are quite "unphysiological." Hemolysis has no effect on serum alkaline phosphatase activities (Brydon and Roberts, 1972).

Since the introduction of multiphasic screening tests, it has been realized that normal adults have a wider range of serum alkaline phosphatase activities than was formerly recognized (Reed *et al.*, 1972). Ranges of 2.0–3.5 Bodansky units (Jaffe and Bodansky, 1943) or 3–13 King–Armstrong units (Dent and Harper, 1962) are unrealistic, as there are many otherwise normal individuals whose serum alkaline phosphatase activities exceed the upper limits of these ranges (Flood *et al.*, 1937; Morgan *et al.*, 1965; Green *et al.*, 1972). There is some evidence that, as in the case of other enzymes (Thomson, 1968), serum alkaline phosphatase activities are not normally distributed about a mean but are skewed to the right (Wootton *et al.*, 1951; Morgan *et al.*, 1965; Roberts, 1967; Keating *et al.*, 1969; Posen, 1970; Hosenfeld and Drossler, 1970). Qualitatively, the circulating material among such "high normals" is similar to that found in patients with serum alkaline phosphatase activities in the "normal" range.

Large numbers of serum alkaline phosphatase ranges have been published for normal subjects by different workers using a variety of methods (Keating *et al.,* 1969; Sereny and McLaughlin, 1970; Reed *et al.,* 1972; Green *et al.,* 1972). Many investigators publish only 95% confidence limits (Roberts, 1967; Ohlen, 1971). It should be emphasized that most laboratories introduce subtle changes into published methods so that it is very difficult to make any meaningful comparisons between papers published by different groups.

It is generally agreed that men have higher serum alkaline phosphatase activities than women (see Table VI) (Clark and Beck, 1950; Dent and Harper, 1962; Tietz *et al.,* 1972; Reed *et al.,* 1972) and that apparently normal individuals over the age of 50 have higher mean serum alkaline phosphatases than young adults (Keating *et al.,* 1969; Ambler *et al.,* 1970; Reed *et al.,* 1972). The reason for this age-related change has not been satisfactorily investigated. It is feasible that the mean values among the older age groups are influenced by patients with symptomless osteomalacia or symptomless Paget's disease.

Normal children and adolescents have higher serum alkaline phosphatase activities than normal adults (Bodansky and Jaffe, 1934a, b; Clark and Beck, 1950; Cornish *et al.,* 1970; Sereny and McLaughlin, 1970; Belfield and Goldberg, 1971). Similar age-related changes are seen in other

TABLE VI

Serum Alkaline Phosphatase Activity in 179 Clinically Normal
Subjects of Various Ages[a]

Age group	No. in group	Mean serum alkaline phosphatase	Range
Neonates	28	17.52	7–28
0–2	11	34.04	15–60
3–10	28	27.74	14–39
12–13	17	32.20	15–58
20–50 (Male)	51	9.95	5–20
20–50 (Female)	44	7.59	4–12

[a] The results are expressed in King–Armstrong units per 100 ml even when the estimations were performed by a different method (Cornish *et al.,* 1970). As noted by other workers (Clark and Beck, 1950; Belfield and Goldberg, 1971) the "pubertal rise" is unimpressive when mean values are considered.

species (Wolff *et al.*, 1970). The abrupt rises in serum alkaline phosphatase in neonates of various species (Bodansky, 1934; Healy, 1971; Tumbleson and Kalish, 1972) do not appear to be related to any skeletal changes. These rises are discussed in detail elsewhere (McComb *et al.*, 1977).

Table VI shows the serum alkaline phosphatase activities in normal individuals of different age groups as measured in our laboratory. Cord blood has a mean alkaline phosphatase activity 1.7 times that of normal adult males (Kitchener *et al.*, 1965). There is relatively little change in mean values throughout childhood (Cornish *et al.*, 1970), and the pubertal or prepubertal spurt which is marked in some children is unimpressive when mean values are considered. These findings are in general agreement with the classic studies of Bondansky and Jaffe (1934a) and those of Clark and Beck (1950).

VI. THE DIAGNOSTIC VALUE OF SERUM ALKALINE PHOSPHATASE DETERMINATIONS IN SKELETAL DISORDERS

Many skeletal disorders are associated with elevations of serum alkaline phosphatase activity. They all share one feature—the presence of increased osteoblastic activity with or without associated bone destruction. Purely destructive processes* presumably do not cause an increase in the production of alkaline phosphatase at the site of the lesions, and they do not give rise to an increase in circulating alkaline phosphatase (Bodansky and Jaffe, 1934a). Qualitative differences between alkaline phosphatases circulating in various skeletal disorders have not been reported.

A. Hyperparathyroidism

Hyperparathyroidism was one of the earliest skeletal disorders described as a cause of serum alkaline phosphatase elevation (Kay, 1929, 1930, 1932). A positive correlation exists between the degree of skeletal involvement, and serum alkaline phosphatase acitivity (Pyrah *et al.*, 1966; Lloyd, 1968; Purnell *et al.*, 1971; Kleerekoper *et al.*, 1974). Unlike the close correlation seen in calcium-depleted hens between parathyroid gland weights and serum alkaline phosphatase activities (Hurwitz and

---

* Multiple myeloma does not cause an increase in serum alkaline phosphatase, even in those rare instances where the bone lesions are sclerotic (Case Records of the Massachusetts General Hospital, 1972), presumably because osteoblastic activity in these instances is low. The Hand–Schüller–Christian disease may be associated with elevated serum alkaline phosphatase activities especially during times of skeletal reossification (Avioli *et al.*, 1963).

Griminger, 1961), the correlation between these two parameters is a very loose one in human primary hyperparathyroidism (Lloyd, 1968; Purnell *et al.*, 1971; Kleerekoper *et al.*, 1974).

Most patients with this disorder have normal serum alkaline phosphatase activities (Dent, 1962b) even when skeletal histology (Fig. 5) is abnormal (Pratley *et al.*, 1973). On the other hand, (as noted in Chapter 1, Volume II), if serum alkaline phosphatase activity is elevated, there is likely to be radiological as well as histological evidence of parathyroid osteopathy (Gordan *et al.*, 1962; Dent, 1962b; Pratley *et al.*, 1973). After successful removal of a parathyroid adenoma, serum alkaline phosphatase may rise in the postoperative period (Albright and Reifenstein, 1948), presumably because of an increase in osteoblastic activity associated with the repair of macroscopic or microscopic cystic lesions.

B. Paget's Disease

The elevation of serum alkaline phosphatase in this disorder was described many years ago (Kay, 1929). Since then there have been relatively few advances in the diagnostic uses of serum alkaline phosphatase estimation in Paget's disease (Nagant de Deuxchaines and Krane, 1964), except (as noted on Volume II, Chapter 5) for the assessment of progress during various therapeutic regimens (Ryan *et al.*, 1969; Haddad *et al.*, 1970). A sudden increase in serum alkaline phosphatase activity in this disorder has been described in association with the development of osteogenic sarcoma (Woodard, 1959), though neither event is necessarily accompanied by the other (Porretta *et al.*, 1957; Woodard, 1959). No qualitative differences have been described between alkaline phosphatase circulating in patients with Paget's disease and alkaline phosphatase circulating in patients with other bone disorders.

Patients with Paget's disease have some of the highest serum alkaline phosphatase activities on record (Fig. 6). High levels of circulating skeletal alkaline phosphatase in patients with Paget's disease do not influence the disappearance rate of infused placental alkaline phosphatase (Posen, 1966).

C. Osteomalacia and Rickets*

The histological changes of rickets and osteomalacia have been described in association with a variety of disorders (Arnstein *et al.*, 1967; Dent *et al.*, 1970; Garrick *et al.*, 1971; Salassa *et al.*, 1970; Parfitt, 1972a). For reasons detailed in Chapters 4 and 5, patients with such changes

---

* The terms osteomalacia and rickets are not synonymous. Rickets is a disorder of ossifying cartilage; osteomalacia refers to a lack of mineralization in bone (Parfitt, 1972a).

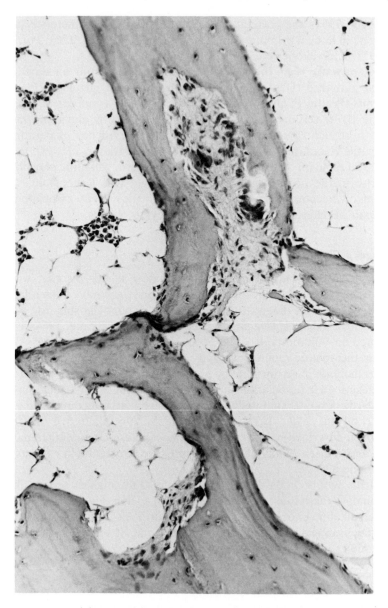

Fig. 5. Iliac crest biopsy from a 56-year-old housewife with primary hyperplasia of all four parathyroid glands. Her serum calcium was constantly around 13.5 mg per 100 ml, the immunoassayable PTH was 1.5 ng/ml (Kleerekoper *et al.*, 1974), while the BUN and serum creatinine were normal. The skeletal X rays were normal as was the serum alkaline phosphatase (before and after parathyroidectomy). Iliac crest biopsy showed numerous areas of parathyroid osteopathy. One such area is shown in this micrograph. Hematoxylin and eosin. ×128.

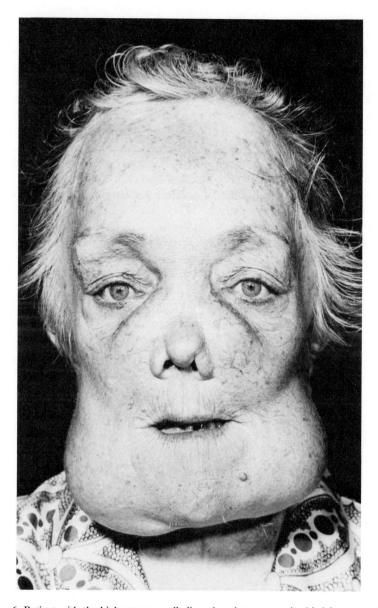

Fig. 6. Patient with the highest serum alkaline phosphatase seen in this laboratory, 1330 KA units per 100 ml as measured by the automated phenyl phosphate method of Marsh *et al.* (1959) modified by Kitchener *et al.* (1965). There was extensive involvement of most of the skeleton by Paget's disease. The grotesque appearance is due predominantly to enlargement, of the calvarium, mandible, and parts of the maxilla. This patient's formalin-stable serum acid phosphatase was repeatedly elevated to 8 KA units per 100 ml (approximately four times the upper limit of normal).

develop increased osteoblastic activity so that increased quantities of alkaline phosphatase are delivered into the circulation (Bodansky and Jaffe, 1934b). Treatment of osteomalacia with vitamin D (Barnes and Carpenter, 1937; Chalmers *et al.*, 1967), with phosphate (Nagant de Deuxchaisnes and Krane, 1967), and possibly by means of phytate withdrawal (Wills *et al.*, 1972) may temporarily enhance osteoblastic activity with increases in serum alkaline phosphatase activities (Fig. 7). Such increases usually disappear within a few months of the initiation of adequate therapy (Swan and Cooke, 1971).

Histological osteomalacia (Fig. 8), radiological osteomalacia and even symptomatic osteomalacia (Nagant de Deuxchaisnes and Krane, 1967) may be present in the absence of serum alkaline phosphatase elevation (Harris *et al.*, 1969; Garrick *et al.*, 1971).

Since the association between antiepileptic medication and osteomalacia was first reported (Kruse, 1968), there have been several pa-

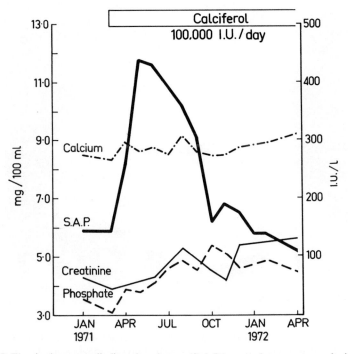

Fig. 7. The rise in serum alkaline phosphatase (S.A.P.) seen when an osteomalacic patient is treated with ergocalciferol. These data were obtained in a 64-year-old woman with relatively mild, stable renal failure (Ingham *et al.*, 1974) and an osteoid index (Garrick *et al.*, 1971) of 6.8%. After 18 months of ergocalciferol treatment, the osteoid index was 1.4%.

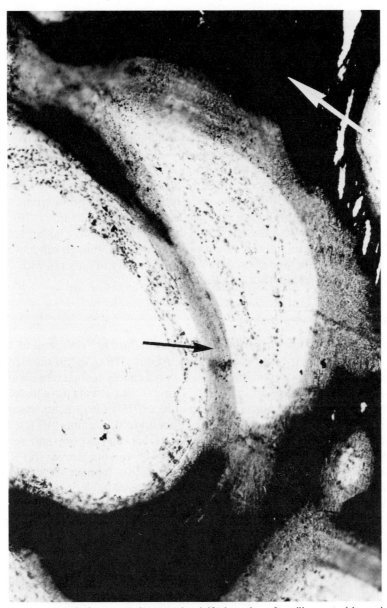

Fig. 8. Osteomalacia as seen in an undecalcified section of an iliac crest biopsy in the absence of serum alkaline phosphatase elevation. The patient was a 60-year-old woman with gluten-induced enteropathy. The osteoid index (Garrick *et al.*, 1971) was approximately 25%, while the serum alkaline phosphatase was 11 KA units/100 ml. The black arrow points to an area of uncalcified osteoid, the white arrow to calcified bone. Von Kossa's stain and toluidine blue, ×43.

pers supporting this observation (Dent *et al.*, 1970; Genuth *et al.*, 1972; Tolman *et al.*, 1975; Crosley *et al.*, 1975). The prevalence of drug-induced osteomalacia is at present unknown. There are patients taking long-term anticonvulsants whose iliac crest biopsies show no evidence of osteomalacia (S. Posen and J. P. Ingham, unpublished).

Serum alkaline phosphatase elevation has been reported in patients receiving anticonvulsants, and, in at least two patients (Genuth *et al.*, 1972; Taitz, 1973), heat inactivation suggested a skeletal source for the circulating enzyme. Hahn *et al.* (1972) claimed, on the basis of electrophoretic studies, that anticonvulsant medication caused an elevation of both the hepatic and the skeletal isoenzymes in the circulation and that the rise in the circulating hepatic isoenzyme occurred before any rise in circulating skeletal alkaline phosphatase was detectable. Kazamatsuri (1970) reported that, as a group, epileptics on hydantoin therapy have higher serum alkaline phosphatase activities than normal controls, though other workers found serum alkaline phosphatase elevation only in patients with concomitant hypocalcemia (Sotaniemi *et al.*, 1972).

D. Azotemic Osteodystrophy

The skeletal changes associated with renal failure are reviewed in Volume II, Chapter 2 in considerable detail. About 10% (4/46) of unselected patients with end stage renal failure have abnormally high serum alkaline phosphatase activities (Katz *et al.*, 1969), and these patients have histological evidence of osteomalacia (Ingham *et al.*, 1973). There is an apparent lack of correlation between circulating parathyroid hormone (PTH), histological and radiological evidence of hyperparathyroidism, and serum alkaline phosphatase in patients with azotemic osteodystrophy (O'Riordan *et al.*, 1970; M. Kleerekoper, unpublished). Ingham *et al.* (1974) studied a group of patients with relatively mild renal failure but disproportionately severe skeletal symptoms. These patients all showed histological osteomalacia and 12/14 had elevated serum alkaline phosphatase activities.

Prolonged hemodialysis is not generally associated with serum alkaline phosphatase elevation except in the presence of severe osteomalacia and/or osteitis fibrosa (Mahony *et al.*, 1976). A rising serum alkaline phosphatase in a normocalcemic patient receiving chronic dialysis is, therefore, regarded as one of the indications for withdrawal of aluminum hydroxide, for vitamin D therapy, or for parathyroidectomy provided the alkaline phosphatase is of skeletal origin (see Volume II, Chapter 2). Hyperparathyroidism may persist after a successful renal transplantation

(Parfitt, 1972b), but serum alkaline phosphatase elevation is uncommon and, when present, is usually due to nonskeletal material (Kleerekoper *et al.*, 1975).

E. Skeletal Metastases: Hypercalcemia of Malignancy

The determination of serum alkaline phosphatase activity is unsatisfactory for the detection of skeletal metastases (Galasko, 1972). It has recently been claimed (Galasko, 1972) that a transient rise in serum alkaline phosphatase following the initiation of therapy may indicate regression of skeletal metastases but, as a rise in serum alkaline phosphatase may also be associated with the relentless progression of metastatic disease, this test is obviously of limited predictive value.

A reciprocal relationship between the degree of hypercalcemia and serum alkaline phosphatase activity was reported in one study of hypercalcemia associated with carcinoma of the breast (Griboff *et al.*, 1954). We have observed one patient with a bronchial carcinoma, a serum calcium of 17.0 mg per 100 ml and a serum alkaline phosphatase of 19 KA units per 100 ml. Seven days after the commencement of phosphate therapy the serum alkaline phosphatase (which had not changed during the first few days of treatment) has risen to 39 KA units per 100 ml. In the presence of hepatic as well as skeletal metastases and in view of the possible ectopic production of alkaline phosphatase in this clinical situation (Fishman *et al.*, 1968), careful documentation of the source of circulating alkaline phosphatase is required before any conclusions can be drawn concerning a relationship between hypercalcemia of malignancy and osteoblastic activity.

F. Fibrous Dysplasia

Polyostotic fibrous dysplasia (Fig. 9) whether accompanied by endocrine abnormalities (Albright *et al.*, 1937; Benedict, 1962; Ehrig and Wilson, 1972) or not, is associated with elevated serum alkaline phosphatase activities in many cases (Firat and Stutzman, 1968). As in other diffuse abnormalities involving the skeleton, there is a poor correlation between the degree of involvement as shown by skeletal X rays and the serum alkaline phosphatase activity (McIntosh *et al.*, 1962). A recent review of 12 cases of sarcomatous change in fibrous dysplasia (Huvos *et al.*, 1972) makes no mention of changes in serum alkaline phosphatase in these patients. Osteomalacia has been described in association with this condition (Dent and Gertner, 1976).

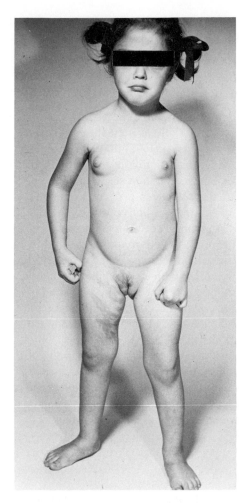

Fig. 9. This 3-year-old girl with characteristic "Coast of Maine" pigmentation on the right thigh, precocious puberty, and radiological lesions consistent with polyostotic fibrous dysplasia had a serum alkaline phosphatase of 121 KA units per 100 ml on the day this photograph was taken. The circulating material behaved like skeletal alkaline phosphatase on heat denaturation.

G. Familial Hyperphosphatasemia

In recent years, several patients have been reported (particularly among families of Puerto Rican origin) suffering from grotesque skeletal deformities, histological evidence of poor cortical bone formation, and high serum alkaline phosphatase activities (Bakwin *et al.,* 1964; Stemmerman,

1966; Jett and Frost, 1968; Eyring and Eisenberg, 1968; Thompson *et al.*, 1969; Mitsudo, 1971). The bones in these patients show much cellular and enzymatic activity, and abnormal amino acids are excreted in the urine. The disease appears to be inherited as an autosomal recessive. Its relationship with "juvenile Paget's disease" (Woodhouse *et al.*, 1972) is uncertain. Specimens of serum alkaline phosphatase from the two children described by Eyring and Eisenberg (1968) behaved like serum alkaline phosphatase from other patients with skeletal disorders in their electrophoretic migration and in their susceptibility to denaturation by heat and urea (S. Posen, unpublished). Another syndrome of familial hyperphosphatasemia (Mabry *et al.*, 1970) appears unrelated to skeletal disorders, and the circulating enzyme behaves like biliary material on heat denaturation.

H. Thyrotoxicosis

Minor serum alkaline phosphatase elevations occur in patients with thyrotoxicosis (Kay, 1930; Bodansky and Jaffe, 1934a; Cassar and Joseph, 1969), and further rises may occur when this condition is treated (Cook *et al.*, 1959). Heat denaturation suggests a predominantly skeletal origin for the circulating enzyme (Richter and Ohlen, 1971), and this is in keeping with the finding (Fleisher *et al.*, 1965) that enzymes of hepatic origin are generally not elevated in hyperthyroidism (see Volume II, Chapter 4 for details). Spectacular rises in serum alkaline phosphatase activity have not been reported in thyrotoxic patients even in the presence of hypercalcemia (Parfitt and Dent, 1970).

I. Hypophosphatasia

This condition is characterized by radiological and histological features resembling rickets (Fraser, 1957; Currarino *et al.*, 1957), but differs from vitamin D deficiency and familial hypophosphatemia (Parfitt, 1972a) by the presence of craniostenosis, dental abnormalities (Pimstone *et al.*, 1966), and excretion in the urine of abnormal quantities of phosphoethanolamine (Rasmussen, 1968) and inorganic pyrophosphate (Russell, 1965). Alkaline phosphatase activities in sera of affected individuals and their heterzygous relatives are usually low. Alkaline phosphatase is present in nonskeletal tissues in normal amounts (Danovitch *et al.*, 1968; Heizer and Laster, 1969), and intestinal alkaline phosphatase may be shown to enter the circulation in response to appropriate stimuli (Rasmussen, 1968; Warshaw *et al.*, 1971).

None of the above features are diagnostic. Craniostenosis has been reported in other forms of rickets (Reilly *et al.*, 1964), while some patients with hypophosphatasia excrete normal amounts of pyrophosphate (Russell, 1965). However, taken together, the various features form a distinct syndrome, which probably represents at least one nosological entity (Rasmussen, 1968). Qualitative studies concerning alkaline phosphatase obtained from skeletal tissue of patients with hypophosphatasia have not been reported.

It has been claimed (Rathbun et al., 1961) that the full-blown syndrome of hypophosphatasia is inherited as an autosomal recessive, but that heterozygotes have low serum alkaline phosphatase activities as well as elevated urinary ethanolamine excretion. An inspection of published genetic data shows that a number of so called carriers as well as a few affected individuals had serum alkaline phosphatase activities within normal limits (Rathbun et al., 1961; Pimstone et al., 1966).

"Pseudohypophosphatasia" (Scriver and Cameron, 1969), which consists of the clinical features of hypophosphatasia in patients with normal serum alkaline phosphatase activities, may or may not represent a distinct entity.

J. Extraskeletal Calcification and Ossification

Several conditions, unrelated to demonstrable abnormalities of calcium metabolism, are associated with extraskeletal calcification. These include scleroderma, myositis ossificans, calcinosis universalis, and local tissue damage such as papillary necrosis of the kidney. These heterogenous disorders are not associated with known abnormalities of serum alkaline phosphatase (Bodansky and Jaffe, 1934a; Lutwak, 1964).

Furman et al. (1970) recently reported elevated serum alkaline phosphatase activities in paraplegic patients with extensive para-articular ossification. Some positive correlation was believed to exist between the activity of serum alkaline phosphatase and the progression of the disease.

K. Skeletal Disorders with Normal Serum Alkaline
Phosphatase Activities

The various skeletal dysplasias have recently been classified in a rational manner (McKusick and Scott, 1971). Most of these such as achondroplasia (Fig. 10), hypochondroplasia (Beals, 1969), the various spondyloepiphyseal dysplasias, osteopetrosis (Johnston et al., 1968), hyperostosis corticalis (Van Buchem et al., 1962), pycnodystostosis (Giedion and Zachmann, 1968; Elmore, 1967), and osteogenesis imperfecta (Bodansky and Jaffe, 1934a; Cattell and Clayton, 1968) are not associated with major elevations of serum alkaline phosphatase activity. Burgert et al. (1965) in a rather incomplete report, claimed that a patient with carti-

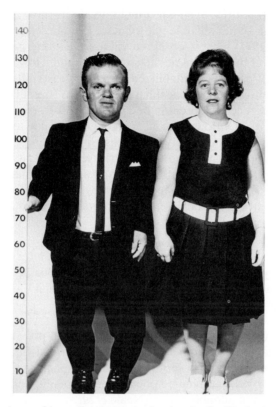

Fig. 10. Two types of bone disorders in husband and wife. The husband (aged 27) has achondroplasia, the wife (aged 31) has familial hypophosphatemic vitamin D resistant rickets. Serum alkaline phosphatase was normal in both patients on the day this photograph was taken in spite of the fact that the ricketic patient had Looser zones and an osteoid index (Garrick *et al.*, 1971) of approximately 10%.

lage hair hypoplasia had spectular elevations of serum alkaline phosphatase. The majority of patients with this disorder have normal serum alkaline phosphatase activities (McKusick *et al.*, 1965). Osteoporosis does not lead to serum alkaline phosphatase elevation (Bodansky and Jaffe, 1934a; Cooke, 1955), and the administration of therapeutic doses of fluoride appears to be without effect (Rich *et al.*, 1964).

The alkaline phosphatase activity of fracture callus is usually greater than that of normal bone (Gudmundson and Semb, 1971). The claim has been made (Semb *et al.*, 1971) that experimental fractures in the rat result in a rise in serum alkaline phosphatase within 24 hours. As a large proportion of circulating alkaline phosphatase in this species is of intestinal origin (Saini and Posen, 1969), results obtained in the rat are not usually applicable to other species.

In humans, fractures, even when multiple, do not give rise to spectacular elevations in serum alkaline phosphatase (Bodansky and Jaffe, 1934a). Hodkinson's (1971) highest observed value in geriatric patients suffering from fractures of the femoral neck was 30 KA units. Howard *et al.* (1945), who studied 17 patients immobilized in plaster casts after various fractures, found serum alkaline phosphatase activities "remarkably unaltered during convalescence," except in one patient whose serum alkaline phosphatase rose from 4.4 Bodansky units on the second day to 36.5 Bodansky units on the twenty-fourth day. The extensive literature concerning the effect of immobilization on the skeleton (Rose, 1966; Lutwak *et al.*, 1969) is largely devoid of any studies relating to alkaline phosphatase. Lawrence and Loeffler (1973) reported a single patient with immobilization hypercalcemia in whom a reciprocal relationship was observed between serum calcium and serum alkaline phosphatase.

L. Temporary Skeletal Alkaline Phosphatase Elevation in the Serum of Subjects without Evidence of Skeletal Pathology

We recently evaluated an 18-month-old girl who presented because of "irritable behavior." A number of tests were performed, but all of them gave normal results except for a serum alkaline phosphatase of 2900 I.U./liter (540 KA units by the automated phenyl phosphate method). There was no history of albumin administration (Neale *et al.*, 1963; Mackie *et al.*, 1971) and no clinical or biochemical evidence of hepatic dysfunction (Gutman, 1959; Kaplan, 1972). The serum was subjected to heat denaturation and electrophoresis, and the alkaline phosphatase was found to behave like the enzyme in the circulation of patients with skeletal disorders. Roentgenographic examination failed to reveal any skeletal abnormality. The alkaline phosphatase elevation and the skeletal origin of the enzyme were confirmed on a second occasion (10 days after the first). Six weeks after the second test the serum alkaline phosphatase was checked for a third time and, on this occasion, it was normal. The child has been clinically and biochemically well since then. No explanation is currently available for this state of affairs, which is not unique (Posen *et al.*, 1977).

Stephen and Stephenson (1971) reported several apparently healthy children with transient serum alkaline phosphatase elevations to "more than 100" KA units, while Asanti *et al.* (1966) reported similarly elevated levels in apparently healthy Finnish infants. One may speculate about a sudden stimulus to osteoblastic activity or a sudden interference with whatever mechanism normally controls the removal of alkaline phosphatase from the circulation. It is even possible that we were dealing with an as yet unrecognized viral disease similar to that causing serum lactate dehydrogenase elevation* in the mouse (Mahy, 1964; Mahy and Rowson, 1965).

M. Long-Term Skeletal Alkaline Phosphatase Elevation in the Serum of Subjects without Skeletal Pathology

A considerable increase in serum alkaline phosphatase occurs in some individuals around the time of the pubertal growth spurt. (Bodansky and Jaffe, 1934a; Sereny and McLaughlin, 1970). Longitudinal studies are not available on large populations so that "upper limits of normal" at this age have not been delineated with certainty (see Table VI). One of the authors (S. P.) has seen one boy aged 14 years with a serum alkaline phosphatase of 58 KA units per 100 ml. The enzyme behaved like skeletal material on heat denaturation; there was no clinical or radiological evidence of skeletal pathology; and 6 months later the activity had fallen to 36 KA units per 100 ml. Bauer and De Vino (1970) report a normal 12-year-old boy with a serum alkaline phosphatase of 300 IU/liter, while Werner et al. (1970) found an alkaline phosphatase activity of 348 IU/liter in a 12-year-old male visitor to the San Francisco Health Fair. Because of the lack of data on normal subjects, it is difficult to evaluate reports purporting to show an association between serum alkaline phosphatase "elevation" and this or that syndrome (Kaplan et al., 1968).

More problematical (and more common) is the following type of patient: A 50-year-old symptomless university professor had 12 serum parameters estimated during a demonstration of multichannel biochemical equipment. All tests were normal except for a serum alkaline phosphatase of 45 KA units per 100 ml. Heat inactivation (Posen et al., 1965b) and polyacrylamide electrophoresis (I. Smith et al., 1968) suggested a mixture of skeletal and nonskeletal material. This man has remained well for 4 years since the tests were performed, but his serum alkaline phosphatase remains elevated.

The inspection of "normal values" found by other workers suggests that such cases are not rare, though there appears to be some reluctance to publish observed ranges (Budinger and Weller, 1970; Craig and Bartholomew, 1970).

---

* The Riley virus elevates serum lactate dehydrogenase (LDH) in the mouse by two mechanisms: (1) an increase in the delivery rate of slow moving LDH, and (2) a diminution in the clearance rate of this isoenzyme (Notkins and Scheele, 1964). Serum alkaline phosphatase elevations due to diminished clearance rates have not been described in humans.

VII. ALKALINE PHOSPHATASE ELEVATIONS IN EXTRASKELETAL DISORDERS

A number of clinical conditions are associated with serum alkaline phosphatase elevations in the absence of pregnancy and in the absence of demonstrable hepatobiliary disease. None of these is associated with demonstrable skeletal disease, and the tissue sources of the circulating enzyme(s) are currently unknown. Only a few selected disorders are mentioned here. A systematic classification is presented elsewhere (McComb *et al.,* 1977).

A. Hypernephroma

There are several cases on record (Durocher, 1969) of patients with hypernephromas whose elevated serum alkaline phosphatase activities returned to normal after removal of the tumor. Suspected tissue sources of the circulating enzyme include the tumor and the liver, but no conclusive studies are available.

B. Pulmonary Embolus

There are several studies claiming that patients with recent episodes of pulmonary infarction have elevated serum alkaline phosphatase activities (Dijkman and Kloppenborg, 1966; Lum and Gambino, 1972). Such elevations, which are rarely spectacular, disappear within a few weeks of the pulmonary episode. Studies concerning the tissue source of circulating alkaline phosphatase(s) in this condition have not been conclusive. There have been no studies to determine whether serum alkaline phosphatase elevations in patients with pulmonary embolis are associated with any alterations in alkaline phosphatase turnover (Posen, 1970).

C. Myocardial Infarction

Statements have appeared suggesting that some patients with myocardial infarction have elevated alkaline phosphatase activities in serum (Ewen and Griffiths, 1971) and urine (Dietz *et al.,* 1967). The prevalence of these biochemical abnormalities and their relation to "sick livers" and "sick kidneys" in such patients have not been adequately documented.

D. Pernicious Anemia

A rise in serum alkaline phosphatase was reported in patients with pernicious anemia after the initiation of treatment with vitamin B_{12} (Van

Dommelen and Klaassen, 1964). This finding (which does not appear to have been confirmed) remains unexplained.

E. Milk-Alkali Syndrome

Wenger *et al.* (1957) reported an increase in serum alkaline phosphatase in this syndrome, particularly during the recovery phase. They speculated that "elevated alkaline phosphatase apparently is related to the readjustment of calcium and phosphorus stores in bone." No studies appear to have been performed to investigate the tissue of origin of serum alkaline phosphatase in the milk-alkali syndrome.

VIII. "STOP-GO" DECISIONS BASED ON SERUM ALKALINE PHOSPHATASE

The determination of serum alkaline phosphatase has a well-defined place in the investigation of hepatobiliary disorders. When the serum alkaline phosphatase exceeds a certain arbitrary activity (e.g. 30 KA units per 100 ml) and it is established that the phosphatase is of biliary origin, a clinician has to think carefully about ways and means of visualizing the biliary tract. There may be some controversy concerning the advantages of 5-nucleotidase over alkaline phosphatase isoenzyme determination in suspected biliary obstruction (Hill and Sammons, 1967; Connell and Dinwoodie, 1970; Belfield and Goldberg, 1971), but there can be no doubt concerning the important and possibly sinister implications of total serum alkaline phosphatase elevation in this situation.

By the time circulating skeletal alkaline phosphatase activity is significantly elevated, bone disease is usually diagnosable by other means (particularly by X rays or scintiscans). Nevertheless, the estimation of this enzyme is useful in a number of clinical situations: (1) As noted in Chapter 6, patients with suspected osteoporosis with elevated circulating skeletal alkaline phosphatase activity should be subjected to bone biopsy for the exclusion of osteomalacia. (2) In patients with Paget's disease who are being treated with cytotoxic agents or calcitonin, circulating skeletal alkaline phosphatase is one of the few parameters available for the objective evaluation of therapy. Similarly, serial alkaline phosphatase determinations are useful in the assessment of therapy in osteomalacia (Harris *et al.*, 1969) and hyperparathyroidism (Dent, 1962a). (3) In children with suspected rickets, a low or normal serum alkaline phosphatase raises the question of hypophosphatasia or metaphysial dysplasia (Stickler *et al.*, 1972). (4) In patients receiving chronic hemodialysis, a rising serum alkaline phosphatase of skeletal origin is usually associated with progressive skeletal disease (see Volume II, Chapter 2).

IX. ACID PHOSPHATASE

Acid phosphatase has been measured quantitatively in bone tissue (Vaes and Jacques, 1965a), and its intracellular distribution has been described (Vaes and Jacques, 1965b). Although acid and alkaline phosphatases catalyze the hydrolysis of many common substrates, there is little evidence that these enzymes share any other properties. Localization studies in skeletal and nonskeletal tissues have tended to confirm the view that cells or subcellular structures endowed with intense alkaline phosphatase activity may be devoid of acid phosphatase activity.

The dissociation between sites of acid and alkaline phosphatase activities has been demonstrated in fracture callus (Takada, 1966) and in the tibial diaphysis of the rat (Wergedal and Baylink, 1969). Most histochemical studies of bone tissue report a positive reaction for acid phosphatase in osteoclasts with little or no reaction for alkaline phosphatase in these cells (Burstone, 1960; Fullmer, 1966). Studies at the ultrastructural level have revealed acid phosphatase activity in the pericanalicular dense bodies of the lysosomes (Goldfischer et al., 1964) and alkaline phosphatase activity on the plasma membrane of osteoblasts (Gothlin and Ericsson, 1971).

Skeletal acid phosphatase activity increases at times of parathyroid-induced bone resorption both in the intact rat and in tissue culture (Mills et al., 1966; Vaes, 1968). It increases during ossification (Jibril, 1967) and during calcification of bone implants (Buring and Semb, 1970). Kuftinec and Miller (1972) showed three periods of maximum acid phosphatase activity during a longitudinal study of bone growth. These peaks of activity occurred concurrently with changes in protein synthesis and were unrelated to the peaks of alkaline phosphatase activity. There is thus considerable evidence (1) that acid phosphatase is present in bone and (2) that it is different in almost every respect from alkaline phosphatase.

Skeletal acid phosphatase may enter the circulation together with other nonprostatic acid phosphatases (Dow and Whitaker, 1970). Osteopetrosis (Johnston et al., 1968), familial hyperphosphatasia (Thompson et al., 1969), Paget's disease (Fig. 6), and hyperparathyroidism (Fig. 11) may all be associated with an elevation of serum acid phosphatase presumably of skeletal origin. No specific tests are currently available to distinguish skeletal acid phosphatase from other acid phosphatases. Indeed, even tests allegedly specific for the detection of prostatic acid phosphatase (Dow and Whitaker, 1970) occasionally reveal the "prostatic" isoenzyme

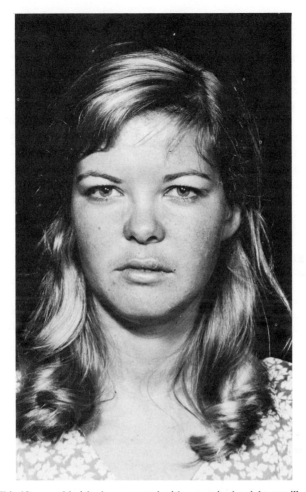

Fig. 11. This 19-year-old girl who presented with a cyst in the right maxilla was found to suffer from primary hyperparathyroidism (Pratley *et al.*, 1973). Her preoperative serum alkaline phosphatase was approximately 1/20 that of the patient shown in Fig. 6. The formalin-stable acid phosphatase was higher than that of the patient in Fig. 6 (12 KA units per 100 ml, approximately six times the upper limits of normal).

in females (Fig. 11) or in males who have undergone a total prostatectomy (Dow and Whitaker, 1970). The estimation of serum acid phosphatase is, therefore, not very helpful in the diagnosis of skeletal disorders other than those associated with extensive prostatic metastases. No correlation has been demonstrated between circulating alkaline phosphatase and circulating acid phosphatase (Grundig *et al.*, 1970) (Figs. 6 and 11).

X. CONCLUSIONS

Over a period of more than four decades the estimation of serum phosphatase, especially alkaline phosphatase, has become one of the most frequently performed tests in clinical biochemistry. Alkaline phosphatases derive from a number of tissue sources (Posen *et al.*, 1973), so that the activity in a given specimen of serum at a given point in time reflects several production rates as well as several biological decay rates (Posen, 1970). Skeletal alkaline phosphatase activity in the circulation rises only when there is a considerable increase in osteoblastic activity, and sometimes not even then. So long as these facts are kept in mind, alkaline phosphatase estimations will continue to have a place in the diagnosis of metabolic bone disorders.

ACKNOWLEDGMENTS

This work was supported by the National Health and Medical Research Council of Australia, the Australian Kidney Foundation, and the New South Wales State Cancer Council. Gai Hume, Sandra Smith, Maureen Murphy, and Deborah Reynolds gave valuable secretarial assistance. Dr. Robert McComb read the manuscript and made many helpful suggestions.

REFERENCES

Albright, F., and Reifenstein, E. C. (1948). "The Parathyroid Glands and Metabolic Bone Disease," p. 108. Williams & Wilkins, Baltimore, Maryland.
Albright, F., Butler, A. M., Hampton, A. D., and Smith, P. (1937). *N. Engl. J. Med.* **216,** 727.
Alcock, N. W., and Shils, M. E. (1969). *Biochem. J.* **112,** 505.
Alter, A. A., Lee, S. L., Pourfar, M., and Dobkin, G. (1963). *Blood* **22,** 165.
Ambler, J., Green, A. G., and Pulvertaft, C. N. (1970). *Gut* **11,** 255.
Anstiss, C. L., Green, S., and Fishman, W. H. (1971). *Clin. Chim. Acta* **33,** 279.
Arnstein, A. R., Frame, B., and Frost, H. M. (1967). *Ann. Intern. Med.* **67,** 1296.
Asanti, R., Hultin, H., and Visakorpi, J. K. (1966). *Ann. Paediatr. Fenn.* **212,** 139.
Avioli, L. V., Lasersohn, J. T., and Lopresti, J. M. (1963). *Medicine (Baltimore)* **42,** 119.
Bakwin, H., and Eiger, M. S. (1956). *J. Pediatr.* **40,** 558.
Bakwin, H., Golden, A., and Fox, S. (1964). *Am. J. Roentgenol., Radium Ther. Nucl. Med.* [N.S.] **91,** 609.
Barnes, D. J., and Carpenter, M. D. (1937). *J. Pediatr.* **10,** 596.
Bauer, S., and De Vino, T. (1970). *Adv. Autom. Anal., Technicon Int. Congr., 1969* Vol. 3, pp. 31–42.
Beals, R. K. (1969). *J. Bone Joint Surg. Am.* Vol. **51,** 728.
Belfield, A., and Goldberg, D. M. (1971). *Arch. Dis. Child.* **46,** 842.
Benedict, P. H. (1962). *Metab., Clin. Exp.* **11,** 30.
Bessey, C. A., Lowry, O. H., and Brock, M. J. (1946). *J. Biol. Chem.* **164,** 321.
Birkett, D. J., Done, J., Neale, F. C., and Posen, S. (1966). *Br. Med. J.* **1,** 1210.

Birkett, D. J., Conyers, R. A. J., Neale, F. C., Posen, S., and Brudenell-Woods, J. (1967). *Arch. Biochem.* **121,** 470.

Biswas, S., and Hindocha, P. (1972). *Clin. Chim. Acta* **38,** 455.

Bodansky, A. (1932). *Proc. Soc. Exp. Biol. Med.* **29,** 1292.

Bodansky, A. (1933). *J. Biol. Chem.* **101,** 93.

Bodansky, A. (1934). *J. Biol. Chem.* **104,** 717.

Bodansky, A., and Jaffe, H. L. (1934a). *Arch. Intern. Med.* **54,** 88.

Bodansky, A., and Jaffe, H. L. (1934b). *Am. J. Dis. Child.* **48,** 1268.

Bodansky, O., Bakwin, R. N., and Bakwin, H. (1931). *J. Biol. Chem.* **94,** 551.

Bottomley, R. H., Lovig, C. A., Holt, R., and Griffin, M. J. (1969). *Cancer Res.* **29,** 1866.

Bowers, G. N., and McComb, R. B. (1966). *Clin. Chem.* **12,** 70.

Boyer, S. H. (1961). *Science* **134,** 1002.

Boyer, S. H. (1963). *Ann. N.Y. Acad. Sci.* **103,** 938.

Breuer, J., and Stucky, W. (1975). *Z. Klin. Chem. Klin. Biochem.* **13,** 355.

Brojer, B., and Moss, D. W. (1971). *Clin. Chim. Acta* **35,** 511.

Brydon, W. G., and Roberts, L. B. (1972). *Clin. Chim. Acta* **41,** 435.

Budinger, J. M., and Weller, C. (1970). *Adv. Autom. Anal., Technicon Int. Congr., 1969* Vol. 3, pp. 23–24.

Burgert, E. O., Dower, J. C., and Tauxe, W. N. (1965). *J. Pediatr.* **67,** 711.

Buring, K., and Semb, H. (1970). *Calcif. Tissue Res.* **4,** Suppl., 102.

Burstone, M. S. (1960). *Ann. N.Y. Acad. Sci.* **85,** 431.

Case Records of the Massachusetts General Hospital (1972). *N. Engl. J. Med.* **287,** 138.

Cassar, J., and Joseph, S. (1969). *Clin. Chim. Acta* **23,** 33.

Cathala, G., Brunel, C., Chappelet-Tordo, D., and Lazdunski, M. (1975). *J. Biol. Chem.* **250,** 6046.

Cattell, H. S., and Clayton, B. (1968). *J. Bone Joint Surg., Amer. Vol.* **50,** 123.

Cerda, J. J., Toskes, P. P., Shopa, N. A., and Wilkinson, J. H. (1970). *Clin. Chim. Acta.* **27,** 437.

Chalmers, J., Conacher, W. D. H., Gardner, D. L., and Scott, P. J. (1967). *J. Bone Joint Surg., Br. Vol.* **49,** 403.

Chang, C. H., and Moog, F. (1972a). *Biochim. Biophys. Acta* **258,** 154.

Chang, C. H., and Moog, F. (1972b). *Biochim. Biophys. Acta* **258,** 166.

Clark, L. C., and Beck, E. (1950). *J. Pediatr.* **36,** 335.

Clubb, J. S., Neale, F. C., and Posen, S. (1965). *J. Lab. Clin. Med.* **66,** 493.

Connell, M. D., and Dinwoodie, A. J. (1970). *Clin. Chim. Acta* **30,** 235.

Conyers, R. A. J., Birkett, D. J., Neale, F. C., Posen, S., and Brudenell-Woods, J. (1967). *Biochim. Biophys. Acta* **139,** 636.

Cook, P. B., Nassim, J. R., and Collins, J. (1959). *Quart. J. Med.* **28,** 505.

Cooke, A. M. (1959). *Lancet* **1,** 929.

Cornish, C. J. (1973). M. Sc. Thesis, University of Sydney, Sydney Australia.

Cornish, C. J., Neale, F. C., and Posen, S. (1970). *Am. J. Clin. Pathol.* **53,** 68.

Cox, R. P. (1965). *Exp. Cell. Res.* **37,** 690.

Cox, R. P., and Griffin, M. J. (1965). *Lancet* **2,** 1018.

Craig, J. L., and Bartholomew, M. D. (1970). *Adv. Auto. Ana. Technicon Int. Congr., 1969* Vol. 3, pp. 105–109.

Crosley, C. J., Chee, C., and Berman, P. N. (1975). *Pediatrics* **56,** 52.

Currarino, G., Neuhauser, E. B. D., Reyerbach, G. C., and Sobel, E. H. (1957). *Am. J. Roentgenol., Radium Ther. Nucl. Med.* [N.S.] **78,** 392.

Danovitch, S. H., Baer, P. N., and Laster, L. (1968). *N. Engl. J. Med.* **278,** 1253.

Dent, C. E. (1962a). *Br. Med. J.* **2,** 1419.

Dent, C. E. (1962b). *Br. Med. J.* **2,** 1495.

Dent, C. E., and Gertner, J. M. (1976). *Quart. J. Med.* **45,** 411.

Dent, C. E., and Harper, C. M. (1962). *Lancet* **1,** 559.

Dent, C. E., Richens, A., Rowe, D. J. F., and Stamp, T. C. B. (1970). *Br. Med. J.* **4,** 69.

Deren, J. J., Williams, L. A., Muench, H., Chalmers, T., and Zamchek, N. (1964). *N. Engl. J. Med.* **270,** 1277.

Dietz, A. A., Hodges, L. K., and Foxworthy, D. T. (1967). *Clin. Chem.* **13,** 359.

Dijkman, J. H., and Kloppenborg, P. W. C. (1966). *Acta Med. Scand.* **180,** 273.

Dow, D., and Whitaker, R. H. (1970). *Br. Med. J.* **4,** 470.

Dunne, J., Fennelly, J. J., and McGreeney, K. (1967). *Cancer* **20,** 71.

Durocher, J. R. (1969). *N. Engl. J. Med.* **281,** 1369.

Eaton, R. H., and Moss, D. W. (1967). *Enzymologia* **35,** 168.

Eaton, R. H., and Moss, D. W. (1968). *Enzymologia* **35,** 31.

Ehrig, V., and Wilson, D. R. (1972). *Ann. Intern. Med* **77,** 234.

Elmore, S. M. (1967). *J. Bone Joint Surg., Vol.* **49,** 153.

Epstein, E., Wolf, P. I., Horwitz, J. P., and Zak, B. (1967). *Am. J. Clin. Nutr.* **48,** 530.

Estborn, B. (1964). *Z. Klin. Chem.* **2,** 53.

Ewen, L. M., and Griffiths, J. (1971). *Am. J. Clin. Pathol.* **56,** 614.

Eyring, E. J., and Eisenberg, E. (1968). *J. Bone Joint Surg., Am. Vol.* **50,** 1099.

Fennelly, J. J., Fitzgerald, M. X., and McGeeney, K. (1969). *Gut* **10,** 45.

Fernley, H. M., and Walker, P. G. (1967). *Biochem. J.* **104,** 1011.

Firat, D., and Stutzman, L. (1968). *Am. J. Med.* **44,** 421.

Fishman, W. H., and Ghosh, N. K. (1967). *Adv. Clin. Chem.* **10,** 255.

Fishman, W. H., and Green, S. (1967). *Enzymologia* **33,** 89.

Fishman, W. H., Inglis, N. I., Stolbach, L. L., and Krant, M. J. (1968). *Cancer Res.* **28,** 150.

Fitzgerald, M. X. M., Fennelly, J. J., and McGeeney, K. (1969). *Am. J. Clin. Pathol.* **51,** 194.

Fleisch, H., and Neuman, W. F. (1961). *Am. J. Physiol.* **200,** 1296.

Fleisch, H., Russell, R. G. G., and Straumann, F. (1966). *Nature (London)* **212,** 901.

Fleisher, G. A., McConahey, W. M., and Pankow, M. (1965). *Mayo Clin. Proc.* **40,** 300.

Flood, C. A., Gutman, E. B., and Gutman, A. B. (1937). *Arch. Intern. Med.* **59,** 981.

Franseen, C. C., and McLean, R. (1935). *Am. J. Cancer* **24,** 299.

Fraser, D. (1957). *Am. J. Med.* **22,** 730.

Fritsche, H. A., and Adams-Park, H. R. (1972). *Clin. Chem.* **18,** 417.

Fullmer, H. M. (1966). *Clin. Orthop.* **48,** 285.

Furman, R., Nicholas, J. J., and Jivoff, L. (1970). *J. Bone Joint Surg., Am. Vol.* **52,** 1131.

Galasko, C. S. (1972). *Ann. R. Coll. Surg. Engl.* **50,** 3.

Garrick, R., Ireland, A. W., and Posen, S. (1971). *Ann. Intern. Med.* **75,** 221.

Gelb, D., West, M., and Zimmerman, H. J. (1962). *Am. J. Clin. Pathol.* **38,** 198.

Genuth, S. M., Klein, L., Rabinovich, S., and King, K. C. (1972). *J. Clin. Endocrinol. Metab.* **35,** 378.

Giedion, A., and Zachmann, M. (1966). *Helv. Paediat. Acta* **21,** 612.

Goldfischer, S., Essner, E., and Novikoff, A. B. (1964). *J. Histochem. Cytochem.* **12,** 72.

Gomori, G. (1943). *Am. J. Pathol.* **19,** 197.

Gordan, G. S., Eisenberg, E., Loken, H. F., Gardner, B., and Hayashida, T. (1962). *Recent Prog. Horm. Res.* **18,** 297.

Gothlin, G., and Ericsson, J. L. E. (1971). *Isr. J. Med. Sci.* **7,** 488.

Granda, J. L., and Posner, A. S. (1971). *Clin. Orthop.* **74,** 269.

Green, S., Cantor, F., Inglis, N. R., and Fishman, W. H. (1972). *Am. J. Clin. Pathol.* **57,** 52.

Griboff, S. I., Herrmann, J. B., Smelin, A., and Moss, J. (1954). *J. Clin. Endocrinol. Metab.* **14,** 378.

Grossberg, A. L., Harris, E. G., and Schlamowitz, M. (1961). *Arch. Biochem. Biophys.* **93,** 267.

Grundig, E., Czitober, H., and Maruna, R. F. L. (1970). *Clin. Chim. Acta* **30**, 331.
Gudmundson, C., and Semb, H. (1971). *Acta Orthop. Scand.* **42**, 18.
Gutman, A. B. (1959). *Am. J. Med.* **27**, 875.
Haddad, J. G., Birge, S. J., and Avioli, L. V. (1970). *N. Engl. J. Med.* **283**, 549.
Hahn, T. J., Hendin, B. A., Scharp, C. R., and Haddad, J. G. (1972). *N. Engl. J. Med.* **287**, 900.
Haije, W. G., and De Jong, M. (1963). *Clin. Chim. Acta* **8**, 620.
Harkness, D. R. (1968). *Arch. Biochem. Biophys.* **126**, 503.
Harris, O. D., Warner, M., and Cooke, W. T. (1969). *Gut* **10**, 655.
Healy, P. J. (1971). *Clin. Chim. Acta* **33**, 437.
Heizer, W. D., and Laster, L. (1969). *J. Clin. Invest.* **48**, 210.
Hekkelman, J. W. (1970). *Calcif. Tissue Res.* **4**, Suppl., 73.
Higashino, K., Hashinotsume, M., Kang, K. Y., Takahashi, Y., and Yamamura, Y. (1972). *Clin. Chim. Acta* **40**, 67.
Hill, J. L., Delgado, F., Norton, L. W., and Eiseman, B. (1972). *J. Bone Joint Surg., Am. Vol.* **54**, 109.
Hill, P. G., and Sammons, H. G. (1967). *Q. J. Med.* **36**, 457.
Hodkinson, H. M. (1971). *Gerontol. Clin.* **13**, 153.
Hodson, A. W., Latner, A. L., and Raine, L. (1962). *Clin. Chim. Acta* **7**, 255.
Horne, M., Cornish, C. J., and Posen, S. (1968). *J. Lab. Clin. Med.* **72**, 905.
Hosenfeld, D. and Drossler, E. (1970). *Acta Genet. Med. Gemellol.* **19**, 122.
Howard, J. E., Parson, W., and Bigham, R. S. (1945). *Bull. Johns Hopkins Hosp.* **77**, 291.
Hurwitz, S., and Griminger, P. (1961). *J. Nutr.* **73**, 177.
Huvos, A. G., Higinbotham, N. L., and Miller, T. R. (1972). *J. Bone Joint Surg., Am. Vol.* **54**, 1047.
Ingham, J. P., Stewart, J. H., and Posen, S. (1973). *Br. Med. J.* **2**, 745.
Ingham, J. P., Kleerekoper, M. Stewart, J. H., and Posen, S. (1974). *Med. J. Aust.* **1**, 873.
Jacoby, B., and Bagshawe, K. D. (1971). *Clin. Chim. Acta* **35**, 473.
Jaffe, H. L., and Bodansky, A. (1943). *Bull. N. Y. Acad. Med.* [2] **19**, 831.
Jeffree, G. M. (1970). *Histochem. J.* **2**, 231.
Jennings, R. C., Brocklehurst, D., and Hirst, M. (1972). *J. Clin. Pathol.* **25**, 349.
Jett, S., and Frost, H. M. (1968). *Henry Ford Hosp. Med. J.* **6**, 325.
Jibril, A. O. (1967). *Biochim. Biophys. Acta* **141**, 605.
Johnson, R. B., Ellingboe, K., and Gibbs, P. (1972). *Clin. Chem.* **18**, 110.
Johnson, W. C., and Alkek, D. S. (1970). *Clin. Orthop. Relat. Res.* **69**, 75.
Johnston, C. C., Lavy, N., Lord, T., Velios, F., Merritt, A. D., and Deiss, W. P. (1968). *Medicine (Baltimore)* **47**, 148.
Kaplan, A., and Narahara, A. (1953). *J. Lab. Clin. Med.* **41**, 819.
Kaplan, M. M. (1972). *Gastroenterology* **62**, 452.
Kaplan, M. M., and Rogers, L. (1969). *Lancet* **2**, 1029.
Kaplan, M. S., Opitz, J. M., and Gossett, F. R. (1968). *Am. J. Dis. Child.* **116**, 359.
Katz, A. I., Hampers, C. L., and Merrill, J. B. (1969). *Medicine (Baltimore)* **48**, 333.
Kay, H. D. (1926). *Biochem. J.* **20**, 791.
Kay, H. D. (1928). *Biochem. J.* **22**, 1446.
Kay, H. D. (1929). *Br. J. Exp. Pathol.* **10**, 253.
Kay, H. D. (1930). *J. Biol. Chem.* **89**, 249.
Kay, H. D. (1932). *Physiol. Rev.* **12**, 384.
Kazamatsuri, H. (1970). *N. Engl. J. Med.* **283**, 1411.
Keating, F. R., Jones, J. D., Elveback, L. R., and Randall, R. V. (1969). *J. Lab. Clin. Med.* **73**, 825.
Kelley, P. M. Neumann, P. A. Shriefer, K., Cancedda, F., Schlesinger, M. J., and Bradshaw, R. A. (1973). *Biochemistry* **12**, 3499.

Kind, P. R. N., and King, E. J. (1954). *J. Clin. Pathol.* **7,** 322.

King, E. J., and Armstrong, A. R. (1934). *Can. Med. Assoc. J.* **31,** 376.

Kitchener, P. N., Neale, F. C., Posen, S., and Brudenell-Woods, J. B. (1965). *Am. J. Clin. Pathol.* **44,** 654.

Kleerekoper, M., Horne, M., Cornish, C. J., and Posen, S. (1970). *Clin. Sci.* **38,** 339.

Kleerekoper, M., Ingham, J. P., McCarthy, S. W., and Posen, S. (1974). *Clin. Chem.* **20,** 369.

Kleerekoper, M., Ibels, L. S., Ingham, J. P., McCarthy, S. W., Mahony, J. F., Stewart, J. H., and Posen, S. (1975). *Brit. Med. J.* **3,** 680.

Klein, B., Read, P. A., and Babson, A. L. (1960). *Clin. Chem.* **6,** 269.

Klein, L., Lafferty, F. W., Pearson, O. H., and Curtiss, P. H. (1964). *Metab., Clin. Exp.* **13,** 272.

Kruse, R. (1968). *Monatsschr. Kinderheilkd.* **116,** 378.

Kuftinec, M. M., and Miller, S. A. (1972). *Calcif. Tissue Res.* **9,** 173.

Kuhlman, R. E. (1965). *J. Bone Joint Surg., Am. Vol.* **47,** 545.

Landau, W., and Schlamowitz, M. (1961). *Arch. Biochem. Biophys.* **95,** 474.

Latner, A. L., Parsons, M., and Skillen, A. W. (1971). *Enzymologia* **40,** 1.

Lawrence, G. O., and Loeffler, R. G. (1973). *J. Bone Joint Surg., Am. Vol.* **55,** 87.

Lazdunski, M., Petitclerc, C., Chappelet, D., and Lazdunski, C. (1971). *Eur. J. Biochem.* **20,** 124.

Lloyd, H. M. (1968). *Medicine (Baltimore)* **47,** 53.

Lum, G., and Gambino, S. R. (1972). *N. Engl. J. Med.* **287,** 361.

Lutwak, L. (1964). *Am. J. Med.* **37,** 269.

Lutwak, L., Whedon, G. D., Lachance, P. A., Reid, J. M., and Lipscomb, H. S. (1969). *J. Clin. Endocrinol. Metab.* **29,** 1140.

Mabry, C. C., Bautista, A., Kirk, R. F. H., Dubilier, L. D., Braunstein, H., and Koepke, J. A. (1970). *J. Pediatr.* **77,** 74.

McComb, R. B., and Bowers, G. N. (1972). *Clin. Chem.* **18,** 97.

McComb, R. B., Bowers, G. N., and Posen, S. (1977). "Alkaline Phosphatase." CRC Publishers. Cleveland, Ohio (in press).

McIntosh, H. D., Miller, D. E., Gleason, W. L., and Goldner, J. L. (1962). *Am. J. Med.* **32,** 393.

Mackie, J. A., Arvan, D. A., Mullen, J. L., and Rawnsley, H. M. (1971). *Am. J. Surg.* **121,** 57.

McKusick, V. A., and Scott, C. I. (1971). *J. Bone Joint Surg., Am. Vol.* **53,** 978.

McKusick, V. A., Eldridge, R., Hostetler, J. A., Ruangwit, U., and Egeland, J. A. (1965). *Bull. Johns Hopkins Hosp.* **116,** 285.

McMaster, Y., Tennant, R., Clubb, J. S., Neale, F. C., and Posen, S. (1964). *J. Obstet. Gynaecol. Br. Commonw.* **71,** 735.

Mahony, J. F., Hayes, J. M., Ingham, J. P., and Posen, S. (1976). *Brit. Med. J.* **3,** 142.

Mahy, B. W. J. (1964). *Virology* **24,** 481.

Mahy, B. W. J., and Rowson, K. E. K. (1965). *Science* **149,** 756.

Makinen, K. K., and Knuuttila, M. L. (1972). *Calcif. Tissue Res.* **9,** 28.

Makinen, K. K., and Paunio, I. K. (1970). *Acta Chem. Scand.* **24,** 3770.

Marsh, W. H., Fingerhut, B., and Kirsch, E. (1959). *Clin. Chem.* **5,** 119.

Martin, S. B., and DeLuca, H. F. (1969). *Arch. Biochem. Biophys.* **129,** 202.

Massion, C. G., and Frankenfeld, J. K. (1972). *Clin. Chem.* **18,** 366.

Massod, M. F., Werner, K. R., and McGuire, S. L. (1970). *Am. J. Clin. Pathol.* **54,** 110.

Matsuzawa, T., and Anderson, H. C. (1971). *J. Histochem. Cytochem.* **12,** 801.

Mills, B. G., Mallett, M., and Bavetta, L. A. (1966). *Proc. Soc. Exp. Biol. Med.* **121,** 1052.

Mitsudo, S. M. (1971). *J. Bone Joint Surg., Am. Vol.* **53,** 303.

Morgan, D. B., Paterson, O. R., Woods, C. G., Pulvertaft, C. N., and Fourman, P. (1965). *Lancet* **2**, 1085.

Morgenstern, S., Kessler, G., Auerbach, J., Flor, R. V., and Klein, B. (1965). *Clin. Chem.* **11**, 876.

Morton, R. K. (1954). *Biochem. J.* **57**, 595.

Morton, R. K. (1955). *Biochem. J.* **61**, 232.

Morton, R. K. (1957). *Biochem. J.* **65**, 674.

Moss, D. W., and King, E. J. (1962). *Biochem. J.* **84**, 192.

Moss, D. W., Campbell, D. M., Anagnostou-Kakaras, E., and King, E. J. (1961). *Biochem. J.* **81**, 441

Moss, D. W., Shakespeare, M. J., and Thomas, D. M. (1972). *Clin. Chim. Acta* **40**, 35.

Nagant de Deuxchaisnes, C., and Krane, S. M. (1964). *Medicine (Baltimore)* **43**, 233.

Nagant de Deuxchaisnes, C., and Krane, S. M. (1967). *Am. J. Med.* **43**, 508.

Natori, S., and Garen, A. (1970). *J. Mol. Biol.* **49**, 577.

Neale, F. C., Clubb, J. S., and Posen, S. (1963). *Med. J. Aust.* **2**, 684.

Newfield, O. E. (1968). *Med. J. Aust.* **1**, 545.

Notkins, A. L., and Scheele, C. (1964). *J. Natl. Cancer Inst.* **33**, 741.

Ohlen, J., Pause, H., and Richter, J. (1971). *Eur. J. Clin. Invest.* **1**, 445.

O'Riordan, J. L. H., Page, J., Kerr, D. N. S., Walls, J., Moorhead, J., Crockett, R. E., Franz, H., and Ritz, E. (1970). *Q. J. Med.* **39**, 359.

Parfitt, A. M. (1972a). *Orthop. Clin. N. Am.* **3**, 653.

Parfitt, A. M. (1972b). *Orthop. Clin. N. Am.* **3**, 681.

Parfitt, A. M., and Dent, C. E. (1970). *Q. J. Med.* **39**, 171.

Perkins, H. R., Walker, P. G. (1958). *J. Bone Joint Surg., Br. Vol.* **40**, 333.

Pimstone, B., Eisenberg, E., and Silverman, S. (1966). *Ann. Intern. Med.* **65**, 722.

Pope, C. E., and Cooperband, S. R. (1966). *Gastroenterology* **50**, 631.

Porretta, C. A., Dahlin, D. C., and Janes, J. M. (1957) *J. Bone Joint Surg., Am. Vol.* **39**, 1314.

Posen, S. (1966). M. D. Thesis, University of Adelaide, Australia.

Posen, S. (1967). *Ann. Intern. Med.* **67**, 183.

Posen, S. (1970). *Clin. Chem.* **16**, 71.

Posen, S., Clubb, J. S., Neale, F. C., and Hotchkis, D. (1965a). *J. Lab. Clin. Med.* **65**, 530.

Posen, S., Neale, F. C., and Clubb, J. S. (1965b). *Ann. Intern. Med.* **62**, 1234.

Posen, S., Neale, F. C., Birkett, D. J., and Brudenell-Woods, J. (1967). *Am. J. Clin. Pathol.* **48**, 81.

Posen, S., Cornish, C. J., Horne, M., and Saini, P. K. (1969). *Ann. N.Y. Acad. Sci.* **166**, 733.

Posen, S., Kleerekoper, M., and Cornish, C. (1973). *In* "Clinical Aspects of Metabolic Bone Disease" (B. Frame, A. M. Parfitt, and H. Duncan, eds.), Int. Congr. Ser. No. 270, p. 74.

Posen, S., Lee, C., Vines, R., Kilham, H., Latham, S., and Keefe, J. F. (1977). *Clin. Chem.* (in press).

Posner, A. S. (1969). *Physiol. Rev.* **49**, 760.

Pratley, S. K., Posen, S., and Reeve, T. S. (1973). *Med. J. Aust.* **1**, 421.

Price, C. P., Hill, P. G., and Sammons, H. G. (1972). *J. Clin. Pathol.* **25**, 149.

Purnell, D. C., Smith, L. H., Scholz, D. A., Elveback, L. R., and Arnaud, C. D. (1971). *Am. J. Med.* **50**, 670.

Pyrah, L. N., Hodgkinson, A., and Anderson, C. K. (1966). *Br. J. Surg.* **53**, 245.

Rasmussen, K. (1968). M. D. Thesis, University of Aarhus, Denmark.

Rathbun, J. C. (1948). *J. Dis. Child.* **75**, 822.

Rathbun, J. C., MacDonald, J. W., Robinson, H. M. C., and Wanklin, J. M. (1961). *Arch. Dis. Child.* **36**, 540.

Ratliff, C. R., Hall, F. F., Culp, T. W., Gevedon, R. E., and Westfall, C. L. (1972). *Am. J. Gastroenterol.* **38,** 22.

Reddi, A. H., and Huggins, C. B. (1972). *Proc. Soc. Exp. Biol. Med.* **140,** 807.

Reed, A. H., Cannon, D. C., Winkelman, J. W., Bhasin, Y. P., Henry, R. J., and Pileggi, V. J. (1972). *Clin. Chem.* **18,** 57.

Reid, T. W., and Wilson, I. B. (1971). *Biochemistry* **10,** 380.

Reilly, B. J., Leeming, J. M., and Fraser, D. (1964). *J. Pediatr.* **64,** 396.

Reynoso, G., Elias, E. G., and Mittelman, A. (1971). *Am. J. Clin. Pathol.* **56,** 707.

Rhone, D. P., and Mizuno, F. M. (1972). *Clin. Chem.* **18,** 662.

Rich, C., Ensinck, J., and Ivanovich, P. (1964). *J. Clin. Invest.* **43,** 545.

Richter, J., and Ohlen, J. (1971). *Dtsch. Med. Wochenschr.* **96,** 196.

Roberts, L. B. (1967). *Clin. Chim. Acta* **16,** 69.

Robison, R. (1923). *Biochem. J.* **17,** 286.

Robison, R., and Soames, K. M. (1924). *Biochem. J.* **18,** 740.

Robson, E. B., and Harris, H. (1965). *Nature (London)* **207,** 1257.

Robson, E. B., and Harris, H. (1967). *Ann. Hum. Genet.* **30,** 219.

Rose, G. A. (1966). *Br. J. Surg.* **53,** 769.

Russell, R. G. G. (1965). *Lancet* **2,** 461.

Ryan, W. G., Schwartz, T. B., and Perlia, C. P. (1969). *Ann. Intern. Med.* **70,** 549.

Saini, P. K., and Posen, S. (1969). *Biochim. Biophys. Acta* **177,** 50.

Salassa, R. M., Jowsey, J., and Arnaud, C. D. (1970). *N. Engl. J. Med.* **283,** 65.

Schlamowitz, M. (1958). *Ann. N. Y. Acad. Sci.* **75,** 373.

Schlamowitz, M., and Bodansky, O. (1959). *J. Biol. Chem.* **234,** 1433.

Schlesinger, M. J., Reynolds, J. A., and Schlesinger, S. (1969). *Ann. N. Y. Acad. Sci.* **166,** 368.

Schuppisser, R., Joss, E., and Richterich, R. (1967). *Schweiz. Med. Wochenschr.* **97,** 1540.

Schwartz, M. K., Kressler, G., and Bodansky, O. (1960). *Am. J. Clin. Pathol.* **33,** 275.

Scriver, C. R., and Cameron, D. (1969). *N. Engl. J. Med.* **281,** 604.

Semb, T. H., Gudmundson, C. R., Westlin, N. E., and Hallander, L. B. (1971). *Clin. Chim. Acta* **31,** 375.

Sereny, G., and McLaughlin, L. (1970). *Can. Med. Assoc. J.* **102,** 1400.

Shifrin, L. Z. (1970). *Clin. Orthop. Relat. Res.* **70,** 212.

Shinowara, G. Y., Jones, L. M., and Reinhart, H. L. (1942). *J. Biol. Chem.* **142,** 921.

Shipley, P. G., Kramer, B., and Howland, J. (1920). *Biochem. J.* **20,** 379.

Siffert, R. S. (1951). *J. Exp. Med.* **93,** 415.

Simpson, R. T., and Vallee, B. L. (1968). *Biochemistry* **7,** 4343.

Small, C. W. (1969). *Clin. Chim. Acta* **23,** 347.

Smith, I., Lightstone, P. J., and Perry, J. D. (1968). *Clin. Chim. Acta* **19,** 499.

Smith, J. K., Eaton, R. H., Whitby, L. G., and Moss, D. W. (1968). *Anal. Biochem.* **23,** 84.

Solomon, R. D., Nadkarni, B. B., and Richardson, L. (1966). *Arch. Pathol.* **82,** 60.

Sotaniemi, E. A., Hakkarainen, H. K., Puranen, J. A., and Lahti, R. O. (1972). *Ann. Intern. Med.* **77,** 389.

Stemmerman, G. N. (1966). *Am. J. Pathol.* **48,** 641.

Stephen, J. M. L., and Stephenson, P. (1971). *Arch. Dis. Child.* **46,** 185.

Stickler, G. B., Maher, F. T., Hunt, J. C., Burke, E. C., and Rosevear, J. W. (1962). *Pediatrics* **29,** 996.

Stolbach, L. L., Krant, M. J., and Fishman, W. H. (1969). *N. Engl. J. Med.* **281,** 757.

Strates, B., Firschein, H. E., and Urist, M. R. (1971). *Biochim. Biophys. Acta* **244,** 121.

Streifler, C., Orenstein, A., and Harell, A. (1972). *Acta Endocrinol. (Copenhagen)* **70,** 676.

Sussman, H. H. (1970). *Clin. Chim. Acta* **27,** 121.

Swan, C. H. J., and Cooke, W. T. (1971). *Lancet* **2**, 456.

Taitz, L. S. (1973). *Proc. R. Soc. Med.* **66**, 220.

Takada, K. (1966). *Acta Histochem.* **23**, 53.

Tangheroni, W., Cao, A., Lungarotti, S., Coppa, G., De Virgiliis, S., and Furbetta, M. (1971). *Clin. Chim. Acta* **35**, 165

Taylor, J. S., and Coleman, J. E. (1972). *Proc. Natl. Acad. Sci. U.S.A.* **69**, 859.

Thompson, R. C., Gaull, G. E., Horwitz, S. J., and Schenk, R. K. (1969). *Am. J. Med.* **47**, 209.

Thomson, W. H. S. (1968). *Clin. Chim. Acta* **21**, 469.

Tietz, N. W., and Green, A. (1964). *Clin. Chim. Acta* **9**, 392.

Tietz, N. W., Weinstock, A., and Wills, D. (1972). *Proc. Int. Sem. Workshop. Enzymol., Chicago 1972*.

Tolman, K. G. Jubiz, W., Sannella, J. J., Madsen, J. A., Belsey, R. E. Goldsmith, R. S., and Freston, J. W. (1975). *Pediatrics* **56**, 45.

Torriani, A. (1960). *Biochim. Biophys. Acta* **38**, 460.

Trubowitz, S., Feldman, D., Morgenstern, S. W., and Hunt, V. M. (1961). *Biochem. J.* **80**, 369.

Tumbleson, M., and Kalish, P. R. (1972). *Can. J. Comp. Med.* **36**, 202.

Vaes, G. (1968). *J. Cell Biol.* **39**, 676.

Vaes, G., and Jacques, P. (1965a). *Biochem. J.* **97**, 380.

Vaes, G., and Jacques, P. (1965b). *Biochem. J.* **97**, 389.

Van Buchem, F. S. P., Hadders, H. W., Hansen, J. F., and Worldring, M. G. (1962). *Am. J. Med.* **33**, 387.

Van Dommelen, C. K. V., and Klaassen, C. H. L. (1964). *N. Engl. J. Med.* **271**, 541.

Wachsmuth, E. D., and Hiwada, K. (1974). *Biochem. J.* **141**, 273.

Walker, A. W., and Pollard, A. C. (1971). *Clin. Chim. Acta* **34**, 19.

Walker, B. A., Eze, L. C., Tweedie, M. C. K., and Price Evans, D. A. (1971). *Clin. Chim. Acta* **35**, 433.

Warnes, T. W., Timperley, W. R., Hine, P., and Kay, G. (1972). *Gut* **13**, 513.

Warnock, M. L., and Reisman, R. (1969). *Clin. Chim. Acta* **24**, 5.

Warshaw, J. B., Littlefield, J. W., Fishman, W. H., Inglis, N. R., and Stolbach, L. L. (1971). *J. Clin. Invest.* **50**, 2137.

Wenger, J., Kirsner, J. B., and Palmer, W. L. (1957). *Gastroenterology* **33**, 745.

Wergedal, J. E. (1969). *Calcif. Tissue Res.* **3**, 55.

Wergedal, J. F., and Baylink, D. J. (1969). *J. Histochem. Cytochem.* **17**, 799.

Werner, M., Tolls, R. E., Hultin, J. V., and Mellecker, J. (1970). *Z. Klin. Chem. Klin. Biochem.* **8**, 105.

Wills, M. R., Day, R. C., Phillips, J. B., and Bateman, E. C. (1970). *Lancet* **1**, 771.

Wilson, I. B., Dayan, J., and Cyr, K. (1964). *J. Biol. Chem.* **239**, 4182.

Winkelman, J., Nadler, S., Demetriou, J., and Pileggi, V. J. (1972). *Am. J. Clin. Pathol.* **57**, 625.

Wolff, W. A., Tumbleson, M. E., and Littleton, C. A. (1970). *Adv. Autom. Anal. Technicon Int. Congr. 1969* Vol. 3, pp. 179–185.

Woodard, H. Q. (1959). *Cancer* **12**, 1226.

Woodhouse, N. J. Y., Fisher, M. T., Sigurdsson, G., Joplin, G. F., and MacIntyre, I. (1972). *Br. Med. J.* **4**, 267.

Wootton, I. D. P., King, E. J., and Smith, J. M. (1951). *Br. Med. Bull.* **7**, 307.

4

The Diagnostic Value of Bone Biopsies

PAUL D. BYERS

I. INTRODUCTION

The architecture and structure of bone are established by growth, ossification, and remodeling. After growth ceases, the cellular activities of remodeling continue, now more as a turnover function, although the former is still possible locally on demand. Disturbance of growth, ossification, remodeling, and turnover form the pathogenesis of metabolic bone disease. All but endochondral growth are cellular activities on surfaces either of the cartilage lattice of the growth plate or of bone (osteonal, trabecular, periosteal, endosteal). Aspects of these activities can be identified in a biopsy and interpreted in physiological terms, which is the value of the biopsy. Some can be measured, and the values used to define boundaries between health and disease and between diseases. Quantitation helps in making value judgements, that is a diagnosis, and indicates the probabilities that the properties of an individual case lie within one or another of those boundaries. It is the variability within and between individuals which may limit the value of a bone biopsy.

II. GROWTH

Growth and ossification can be segregated for descriptive purposes. Nevertheless, they form an integrated cycle of events to which the remodeling activity is related. Interference with any part will disturb the whole. Tissue formation during growth is mainly through the agency of cartilage, which forms the anlage of most bones. Here growth is interstitial, meaning that the daughters of a cell's division secrete new matrix around themselves thereby expanding the tissue. However, some bones are formed in mesenchymal tissue (mainly flat bones, such as the skull, and hence membranous bone formation), in which cells differentiate into osteoblasts. They secrete osteoid onto surfaces. This constitutes growth by apposition (the first surface is the initial osteoid secreted into the mesenchymal interstitium); this is the second method by which bones grow.

The term "center of ossification" describes each site in the cartilage model at which ossification starts; most bones have several sites, appearing at different intervals of time. They are usually referred to as "primary," "secondary," or even "tertiary" centers of ossification. In long bones, the primary center is in the shaft, and the secondary, in the epiphyses. The primary center of ossification is initiated by vascular penetration in the midregion of the model after a periosteal collar of bone has developed around the site by membrane bone formation. The latter both strengthens the site and provides for circumferential expansion by appositional growth. The marrow cavity created in the ossification center by remodeling expands laterally by resorption of the inner surface of the cortex, and expands longitudinally by a rate of ossification that is greater than the rate of longitudinal growth. When the ossifying face has reached a critical point, rates of ossification and growth become equal. In the case of tubular bones, this is well demonstrated at the metaphyseal–epiphyseal junction. The epiphyses of the tubular bones become (secondary) ossification centers, and there the ossification front advances in all directions. When only a cartilage plate separates the two opposing fronts at the metaphyseal–epiphyseal junction, the epiphyseal side ceases to function. By that time, the remaining epiphyseal cartilage has become a hemisphere with an inner face for growth and an outer one for articulation. Thus, one can picture two cartilage plates increasing in diameter and growing away from each other at either end of an expanding bony tube, carrying with them on their flat inactive outer faces, expanding spheres of ossifying cartilage. The bony product of the growing ossifying cartilage is undergoing constant remodeling to achieve and maintain the appropriate architecture; for some periods of time at some sites, periosteal tissue can be wholly devoted to bone resorption; this is seen most obviously at the metaphyseal cone. The cessation of growth is marked by the conversion into bone of all epiphyseal plate cartilage, which precludes any further growth here, and by the formation of a subchondral plate beneath the articular cartilage. The latter retains some growth potential, manifested by osteophyte formation, on the one hand, and by growth of limb length in patients with acromegaly, on the other. The periosteum, of course, always retains its bone-forming (and resorbing) potential.

III. OSSIFICATION

Ossifying cartilage is oriented from the zones of cell proliferation and of matrix formation. The increase in matrix advances the proliferative zone, leaving the new formed tissue to undergo progressive developments preparatory for the vascular penetration that inseminates the surfaces with osteoblasts and osteoclasts. The developments are cell migration to form columns oriented in the axis of growth, enlargement and death of the columnar cells, coincidental mineralization of the intercolumnar matrix, and thinning of the matrix membranes between lacunae of each column. The membranes are disrupted by the growing vessels creating a complex of tubes, the "cartilage lattice," that provides the surfaces needed for osteoblastic and osteoclastic activity. The rate of upward growth of the capillaries equals the senescence of the cells just beyond, which is equal in turn to the hypertrophy of cells in the zone above, to the columnation of cells above that, and to the proliferation and matrix production of the cells above that. Penetrating vessels are followed successively by osteoblasts laying down osteoid, by osteoid mineralization, and by remodeling of the whole tissue (calcified cartilage core and overlying bone) through osteoclastic resorption and osteoblastic reformation. These activities take place at coordinated rates. Growth and ossification can be conceived of as centrifugal horizontal bands of activity, each using the resultant of the previous band for its own function in preparing for the one that follows. The process starts with proliferating cells and ends with bone that is remodeled during growth and turned over during adult life. Even though the rates are related, the dimensions are variable, although relatively constant. As will be noted later, rates can, under appropriate circumstances, be determined for some bone activities, but there is at present no convenient or useful way to do so for diagnostic purposes in growth plates. The dimensions and cell numbers are more accessible, but there are no generally available standards for use in diagnostic work. As is the case in much histological diagnosis, observations are assessed against accumulated personal knowledge, illustrations in textbooks, and the control histological sections of the laboratory.

Much is unknown about the growth plate. Electron microscopy has added to detailed knowledge of the cells (Robinson and Cameron, 1956; Schenk et al., 1967), and biochemical studies (Krane et al., 1967; Mankin and Lippiello, 1969) are furthering knowledge about calcification. The most recent advance has been the discovery of membrane-bound vesicles, rich in alkaline phosphatase and sometimes containing hydroxyapatite crystals (Ali et al., 1970; Nichols and Wasserman, 1971; Anderson, 1973; Ali, 1976). In addition, there is a growing field of study in phosphate metabolism centered about the role of pyrophosphatase (Fleich et al., 1970; Nichols and Wasserman, 1971). Developments in these fields however, have not yet advanced to the point where they have become incorporated in diagnostic procedures. Histological sections only show the state of the growth plate at a moment in time, from which inferences may be drawn. The cumulative result of all the activities during growth are the bones, whose gross appearance are often helpful in diagnosis. There are excellent studies of skeletal abnormalities as revealed by radiography (i.e., Fairbank, 1951; Rubin, 1964). Disorders of the growth plate are discussed by Rang (1969).

IV. REMODELING AND TURNOVER

Once bone tissue has been formed, whether by endochondral growth or by apposition, it may be altered by the turnover or remodeling process.

This is but one process with two names. Since it may alter the mass and architecture of bone, remodeling seems an apposite term. But at the other end of the scale, there is only equal bone removal and replacement, a turnover of tissue. There is activity of some degree in some part of every skeleton throughout life. The two components of the process are resorption and formation. It has been established that the removal of bone matrix and mineral simultaneously is through the agency of osteoclasts (Hancox and Boothroyd, 1963). However, some still believe that osteoclasts do not occur in normal bone. As discussed in detail in Section V, the metabolic role of osteocytes is currently a matter of investigation. It is too early to know whether they participate in the turnover of the whole tissue or only in the turnover of mineral. Controversy has raged about bone formation (Löe, 1959), but there is no longer any doubt about the function of osteoblasts in producing osteoid nor about a delay before mineralization occurs (Kirby-Smith, 1933; Sandison, 1928; Frost, 1966). This is not to say that all aspects of both processes are known; far from it, but it does mean that the hypothesis of bone removal by osteoclasts and of osteoid formation by osteoblasts with subsequent mineralization is incontrovertibly founded. Most of the appearances of bone in metabolic bone disease can be seen as a manifestation of these three normal activities, modified by and coupled with other known phenomena, such as hormones, vitamin concentration, or electrolyte balance, and probably a host of other factors as yet unknown. Consequently, the diagnostic histologist in examining a bone biopsy is looking at the effects wrought by the remodeling process and is trying to decide how it has been modified and why.

All observations of bone indicate that resorption and formation are surface activities. Once a bone has been formed, it is modified in shape and structure by focal resorption and formation, and altered in mass through inequality between the amounts removed and formed. Normally, resorptive or formative activity take place over a small portion of the available surface at any given time. Several studies have indicated that they occur sequentially and move in a wave that is initiated by resorption and followed by formation (Frost, 1969; Dhem, 1966; Johnson, 1964). Because, in addition to being static, a histological section is only two-dimensional, the wave concept of resorption and formation is not readily apparent in it, and the sites of activity may seem widely separated.

V. RESORPTION (TABLE VI)

An excavation in the otherwise smooth bone surface is the hallmark of osteoclastic resorption. It has a clear-cut scalloped margin, along which osteoclasts may be found, but whose presence is not a prerequisite for recognition. The cavities range in length up to a few hundred micrometers with a depth of a few to tens of micrometers. The osteoclasts can be mononuclear (recognized by the cavity they lie in or by cytological features in good sections) or multinuclear cells. It has been evident from studies of bone in various metabolic states that as resorptive activity increases so does the number and size of osteoclasts, as well as the extent of surface upon which they have worked. The numbers of osteoclasts can be used as an index of resorption. During very active resorption, the cavities become deeper and often extend within bone, giving rise to an appearance of tunneling which, although regarded in the past as indicative of renal osteodystrophy, is nonspecific. Greatly increased resorption, such as seen in pathological states, is usually accompanied by some degree of marrow fibrosis; yet actual replacement of bone by fibrous tissue (osteitis fibrosa) seems to be more usual in hyperparathyroidism than in, e.g., Paget's disease or reactive bone (adjacent to osteomyelitis or fracture). Nevertheless, it has been described in acute disuse osteoporosis (Ball, 1960). Resorption cavities can readily be detected in microradiographs (Jowsey, 1966), where there is no possibility of seeing osteoclasts, or in undecalcified and decalcified sections, in which osteoclasts can be seen. The cavities are more difficult to recognize in decalcified sections, so undecalcified preparations are preferable. There can be problems in distinguishing cavities from artifacts and, although obvious, some quality control must be exercised in the preparation of sections.

Increasing attention has been paid to the role of the osteocyte (Table IX) in mineral physiology and bone destruction since 1963, when Bélanger *et al.* (1963) first produced additional evidence for this from observations on the bones of dogs intravenously injected with parathyroid hormone. Variation in osteocyte size had been recognized by von Recklinghansem soon after the turn of the century, and the possibility of a metabolic role for them had been argued (Vitali, 1968). It has long been at least inferred that osteocytes play a part in maintaining the integrity of bone, since their presence has been used as an indication of its vitality. But, as pointed out by Baud (1968), in 1956 the book on bone edited by Bourne contained no chapter on osteocytes; this is no longer the case (Bourne, 1971). The growth of knowledge about osteocytes has paralleled the growing understanding of lysosomes and mechanisms of tissue destruction, as may be seen from the review by Reynolds (1970). At the present time, the facts seem to be that osteocytes retain the cytological characteristics of osteoblasts for a time after their incorporation into matrix, but then their endoplasmic reticulum may (or does) become less prominent, with a less elaborate Golgi complex, and lysosomal structures appear. In association with these changes, the limiting sheath, an amorphous, dense, continuous lining of the lacunae, canaliculi, and vascular canals, disappears from the osteocyte lacuna, which increases in size through destruction of mineral and matrix. The subsequent events are at issue. Jande and Belanger (1971) suggested the ultimate death of the osteocyte, while others believe that a reversal of the process is possible (Vitali, 1968; Baud, 1968). Vitali and Baud support a more dynamic physiological role for the osteocyte in mineral homeostasis. This is compatible with the enormous surface area of the lacunocanalicular system [i.e., 250 mm^2/mm^3 of bone (Frost, 1963)]. The histological observations of Frost (1960a) and Arnold *et al.* (1971) in undecalcified stained section are also consistent with a functionally active lacunocanilicular system. In addition, many authors have demonstrated a similar perilacunar mineral reduction in osteomalacia by microradiography; this was first shown in vitamin D-resistant rickets, but is recognized in all types of osteomalacia including cases of chronic renal disease (Engfeldt *et al.*; 1956; Jowsey, 1964; Bohr, 1967).

Whatever major differences there may be between investigators in this field, there is a clear development of the evidence that osteocytes have an active role. Both onlookers and protagonists are divided into those seeing the function as a physiological mineral pump and those seeing it as a mechanism of tissue destruction comparable with osteoclastosis and as a manifest part of disease processes, such as hyperparathyroidism and osteomalacia. The pros and cons of this theory are reviewed by Bélanger (1969). Measurements of lacunar size are appearing in the literature (Meunier *et al.*, 1971b; Bordier and Tun Chot, 1972; Sissons *et al.*, 1975) as well as illustrations purporting to show osteocytic resorption (Jowsey, 1964; Robichon and Germain, 1968; Stewart *et al.*, 1972). My own position, based on a rather more modest experience than others claim, is that I have not seen perilacunar mineralization defects in cases other than osteomalacia of whatever type, nor am I aware of osteocytic bone removal in cases of hyperparathyroidism. However, I view small areas of resorption as compatible with or indistinguishable from osteoclastic activity extending from the surface. The actual appearances around which these arguments take place are not at issue, but only the definitions, criteria for recognition, and interpretations. It is extremely important for those uninitiated into the mysteries of microscopy to appreciate the distinction between seeing something and knowing what it means. Although not widely acknowledged, there is much evidence that one sees what one is looking for, a rule from which microscopists are not exempt. To enlarge on this thesis would be outside my present brief, but this cautionary tale, which has applications both for practice and research in medicine, can be further explored at various practical and philosophical levels (Feinstein, 1967; Harris, 1970; Byers, 1975).

VI. REVERSAL LINES

The limit of each resorptive wave is marked by a narrow line of modified matrix, the reversal line. It is not clear what the modification is, nor whether it is in the old or new matrix, or something between them, but it only becomes apparent when the cavity has been filled by bone. The line can be detected in most types of decalcified or undecalcified histological preparations but not necessarily in all decalcified paraffin sections. Despite the scalloped outline of resorptive cavities, the reversal lines in normal bone are smoother; Johnson (1964) refers to the planing effect of the osteoclasts at the end of the resorptive phase. On the other hand, Hattner *et al.* (1965) state that most reversal lines are scalloped, employing this as part of an interesting exercise in testing the hypothesis that resorption always precedes osteoblastic activity. One's difficulty lies in not knowing precisely what criteria are used for recognizing "scalloped" as opposed to "smooth" reversal lines. On the whole, it is only where turnover is rapid, as in Paget's disease or hyperparathyroidism, that reversal lines show the coarse scalloping of a resorption cavity. This coupled with their increased number, proximity, and disordered orientation results in the "mosaic pattern" of bone. Variations in the rate of turnover give rise to variations in the reversal line pattern; there are no quantitative values to indicate when the description "mosaic" is appropriate, and only judgment and experience can help.

VII. FORMATION (TABLES, II, III, and VIII)

The recognition of bone formation is fundamental. The usual criterion in undecalcified histological sections (only undecalcified preparations are reliable) is the presence of osteoid (unmineralized bone tissue or preosseous tissue) which indicates that osteoblasts have been active at some unspecified time and that the result of their labor has not yet been mineralized. In contrast with this, the criterion for formation in microradiographs is a surface layer of very low mineral content (Jowsey, 1966), which indicates that osteoid has been laid down at some unspecified time and is in the process of mineralization. Recognition depends, therefore, on active mineralization, since osteoid cannot be recognized in a microradiograph. Neither method of recognizing osteoid, each of which is a valid indicator that formation has occurred, tells anything about the rate of formation or exactly when the tissue was formed. Investigations with tetracycline labeling have established that in normal bone there is a measurable appositional rate which is about 1 μm/day (Lee, 1967). Estimates have been made of the time required to excavate and fill in an osteonal resorption cavity (Johnson, 1964). Frost (1969) gives a comprehensive table of his estimates of remodeling parameters for the sixth rib. The conclusion is that when an osteoid seam is begun there is steady progress to its completion, and following a pause of 10–21 days it is mineralized. Microradiographic studies (Amprino and Engstrom, 1952; Jowsey, 1966) have shown that initial osteoid mineralization reaches levels up to 75% of the maximum mineral content of bone in a few days, a difference easily distinguished in a microradiograph, and that mineralization is "completed" over a period of months or years. Initial mineralization of a seam occurs from below and proceeds upward; the end of this phase and the beginning of the phase of completion of mineralization, which moves in the reverse direction, is evident in microradiographs as a layer of denser mineralization on the inner edge of a surface band of low mineral density. This appearance indicates that initial mineralization is complete and that this low level band can no longer be classified as formation.

Osteoid is constructed of collagen and a mucopolysaccharide matrix. The latter is composed of both acid and neutral types, whose proportions and concentrations vary and are responsible for zones sometimes seen in osteoid (a superficial pale region of young tissue) and for a deeper staining older region adjacent to the bone (Löe, 1959). Both the periodic acid–Schiff reaction and metachromatic dyes can demonstrate these layers. A more detailed analysis of matrix can be had from chemical analysis (Herring, 1964). The collagen of bone is discussed at length by Miller and Martin (1968), and is reviewed in some detail in Chapter 1. Careful observation of very thin, stained, undecalcified sections by Raina (1972) showed all the internal surfaces, excluding resorption cavities are covered by osteoid, most of which is thin; however, there is a focally distributed portion that is thicker and constitutes the "osteoid seams." The thin layers, categorized as inert surfaces, are covered by inactive, flattened, sparse osteoblasts, whereas the thicker layers, the active formation sites, are covered by many, plump, active osteoblasts. This formative activity occurs, in the turnover process, at sites where bone has been resorbed. Osteoblasts become larger and more numerous when making osteoid and appear as a prominent single row of contiguous cells. Estimates of the number of osteoblasts can be used as an index of formation (Table VII).

The actual limits of the seams are often hard to fix, since they may narrow more or less gradually to the thickness of the inert layer. This can be a source of error in quantitation.

The collagen fibers of rapidly formed osteoid, and hence bone, are arranged in a criss-cross or woven pattern, in contrast to their lamellar arrangement when formed at slower rates. The rapid formation in infancy produces woven bone. From infancy onward, the modeling and turnover processes replace this woven bone with lamellar bone. In disease states, with rapid turnover, lamellar bone is replaced by woven bone, matters being reversed after the disease is arrested. Special mention should be made of two conditions in which collagen fiber arrangement is altered. One is osteomalacia, in which regions of osteoid are abnormally structured and often held accountable for some of the failure in mineralization. Support for this has been claimed from the second and more recently described condition, fibrogenesis imperfecta ossium (Baker, 1956; Baker et al., 1966), in which there is excess osteoid whose collagen content is greatly reduced and disordered (woven) in pattern, but in which there is no accompanying biochemical changes. The failure of mineralization in this latter case is therefore attributed to a matrix defect.

During the formation of osteoid, a portion of the osteoblasts are incorporated, giving rise to the osteocytic system with its enormous surface area and potential as a homeostatic system, already referred to in Section V in connection with osteocytic osteolysis. The distribution pattern of osteocytes together with information from tetracycline labeling has allowed Johnson (1964) to make a number of calculations about cellular dynamics and osteonal formation rates.

Löe (1959) reviewed, beginning with Virchow, the concept that an unmineralized matrix was formed first and later mineralized. This was supported by studies of Tomes and de Morgan (1853), Muller (1858), Pommer (1895), Wietland (1909), and Baker (1954). On the other hand, there was opposition from von Recklinghausan (1910) who believed, particularly in osteomalacia, that mineral withdrawal resulted in osteoid; a process he called "halisteresis." Maclean and Bloom (1940) and Bloom et al. (1941) were critical of the thesis that osteoid was a necessary stage in bone formation. The great many studies of bone since then, in association with clinical and biochemical observation, leave no doubt that osteoid is formed as a precursor of bone and, after an interval, is mineralized (Tables III and IV). The mineral appears in a narrow zone, the calcification front, parallel and adjacent to the bone, and progressively advances toward the surface. In disease states where mineralization is defective, the calcification front is deficient and disordered and can be used as confirmatory evidence of the defect. The usual evidence for deficient mineralization is excess osteoid, which continues to form despite the inadequate mineralization. For whatever reason, the calcification front has received scant attention from diagnostic pathologists. More recently, Bordier and his colleagues have quantitated the calcification front (Bordier and Tun Chot, 1972) as part of their assessment of metabolic bone disease, and have made others more conscious of it. Methods for its demonstration by the staining of histological sections have not been widely investigated so that their meaning and value are difficult to assess. On the other hand, the tetracyclines have been widely accepted and used for this purpose, and Bordier and Tun Chot (1972) can claim a high degree of correlation between identification by staining procedures and tetracycline labeling (Table VIII).

The tetracyclines are the latest in a long series of *in vivo* methods for marking bone. Madder was first observed as a marker by Belchier in 1736 and had a long history of use (Cameron, 1930), which has continued until at least 1960 (Hoyte, 1960) in the form of its synthetic and less toxic derivatives (e.g., alizarin). Lead acetate and a number of organic fluorescent compounds have also been used, but were hampered by the dangers of toxicity. The recognition by Harris (1960) and Frost (1960c) that the incorporation of tetracycline into the forming surfaces of lamellar bone described by Milch *et al.* (1958) could be used as a nontoxic *in vivo* marker for the microscopical study of appositional growth opened the way to a number of investigations of humans and animals. Tetracycline is deposited in bone at the sites where mineralization is taking place while the compound is in the blood; it remains as a permanent feature thereafter until the bone is resorbed. Some recent work indicates that there is a temporary inhibition of osteoblastic activity for 24–72 hours following intravenous administration of chlortetracycline into rabbits (Hong *et al.*, 1968).

One gram of tetracycline given as a single dose will appear after 48 hours as a fairly discrete line. Administered on a second occasion after an interval of a few weeks, a second line will appear where mineralization has not been completed, or a single line where mineralization has started in the interval after the first administration of tetracycline. Wider bands appear when administration has been continuous, either therapeutically or experimentally. Information can be gained about the mineralization process and also about appositional bone growth if one equates rates of mineralization to rates of osteoid apposition. The technique can be elaborated by taking advantage of the fluorescent color differences of various tetracyclines. The subject has been reviewed by Frost (1969). Tarn *et al.* (1974) have explored the use of single intravenous doses in animals and man with interesting results for bone growth kinetics (Swinson *et al.*, 1975).

VIII. TECHNICAL CONSIDERATIONS

A. The Biopsy Site

The iliac crest is the site most frequently used for biopsy because it is so accessible and because it is safe and easy to remove a portion of it. Even a percutaneous trephine can be used; an instrument and technique based on a method introduced by Bordier and his colleagues (1964) has been described by Byers and Smith (1967). Other techniques for obtaining iliac crest biopsies have been described [see, for example, Williams and Nicholson, (1963), and Velashy (1973)]. Rib is readily accessible, but the sample is taken by conventional surgical procedures (Sedlin et al., 1963). Opportunities to obtain bone often arise during surgical operations or at autopsy, and many sites can provide bone to meet the histologist's requirements of an abundance of surfaces for study. Ideally, a specimen should come from a site about which there is already a good deal of quantitative information. When interest centers on the growth plate, an open wedge biopsy of the iliac apophysis is very suitable. A biopsy specimen 1–2 cm long and 5–10 mm thick is easy to handle and provides adequate material for several types of histological preparations.

B. Techniques of Histology and Microradiography

Some histological features of metabolic bone disease can only be demonstrated with certainty by undecalcified sections. Decalcified sections are a useful adjunct, but should be sacrificed if there is a shortage of tissue. Descriptions of technical procedures have been given by Jowsey et al. (1965) and by Drury and Wallington (1967). Very satisfactory histological sections 15 to 25 μm thick can be prepared by a simple procedure of grinding slices, sawed by hand if necessary, from the face of a plastic block in the case of iliac crest or of unembedded whole rib. The lack of a microtome is the last thing that should impede the study of undecalcified sections. Plastic embedding is not difficult but requires some practice before it is mastered, usually because experience is required for good impregnation and for controlling the hardening process.

Undecalcified sections are needed for the reliable differentiation of osteoid and bone. A wide variety of staining procedures bring out the distinction (Löe, 1959; Frost, 1959; Matrajt and Hioco, 1966; Merz and Schenk, 1970), although even in unstained undecalcified sections, osteoid can be recognized. The techniques of impregnating the biopsy with silver and subsequently decalcifying and sectioning (Tripp and MacKay 1972) is quicker than plastic embedding and cutting or grinding but seriously limits the range of preparations from the biopsy. Osteoid may be seen in decalcified bone sections, particularly if embedded in celloidin, but this is inconsistent and therefore unreliable. Undecalcified sections have the additional advantage that the calcification process may be studied, especially through tetracycline labeling, and the mineral distribution examined by microradiography or, less reliably, by staining. No single histological preparation demonstrates all aspects of bone. Stained and unstained undecalcified sections, a microradiograph, and a decalcified paraffin section are ideal, combined with facilities for microscopy by ordinary light, polarized light, and ultraviolet light. Polarized light provides one of the simplest and most effective ways of detecting collagen fibers in histological material. They stand out brightly against the dark background, and, particularly with a rotating stage, their orientation is readily established. The method is applicable to decalcified and undecalcified sections; unstained undecalcified sections give the best results. Ultraviolet light, or at the least the short wavelengths just beyond the blue end of the spectrum, is necessary for fluorescence microscopy and the identification of tetracycline labels.

The technique of microradiography or, more accurately, contact microradiography as applied to bone, has an historical background going back to 1897 when it was used to examine alloys (Heycock and Neville, 1898). Lamarque (1938), with improved techniques, extended its use to biological studies. Both qualitative and quantitative assessments of the mineral distribution in bone were made over the ensuing years (Engstrom et al., 1960). Quantitative assessments showed a narrow range of mineral distribution which is altered in osteoporosis (Jowsey, 1964) and hyperparathyroidism (Smeenk, 1961); however, the technique of quantitative densitometry is sufficiently exacting for it not to provide a useful diagnostic procedure. The original qualitative assessments were mainly of value in studying osteoid mineralization (Amprino and Engstrom, 1952) but have lately been useful in the demonstration of periosteocytic (perilacunar) deficiencies of mineral. Jowsey (1963, 1966) developed the use of the contact microradiograph for surface and the area measurements of bone. It is these measurements that are now commonly referred to in discussions of quantitative microradiography. It is essentially the same as other methods in which undecalcified sections are used as a sample of patients who are drawn in turn from populations with wide natural variations, and characterizes their surface activities in proportional or absolute terms.

C. Quantitative Methods

Whatever bone is quantitated, the methods are the same. The following, based on histological sections, are those generally employed. These are all manual methods using the human eye as the sensing device. There are some machines in use (Lloyd and Hodges, 1971; Williams, 1972), and these will no doubt revolutionize quantitative procedures. Unfortunately they will not overcome the variations within and between skeletons, and it may be some time before they can record all parameters. The use of sections depends wholly or in part upon microscopy, which of itself can introduce an element of error into the methods, but I do not propose to discuss these. However, this subject has been studied by Frost (1962) in some detail. There are, of course, other sources of error arising from both technical factors and the observer. Error analysis will not be dealt with further, except to emphasize again its importance. There are many ways to express quantitative values, the choice often being determined by techniques or by some more obscure reason. The most satisfactory analysis would be of volumes of bone, surface areas per unit of volume, and rates of formation and resorption per unit of surface per unit of volume per unit of time. Frost (1966) and his co-workers have elaborated quantitative analytical methods that give a dynamic portrayal of bone metabolic activity, but which nevertheless do not overcome the difficulty of a broad no man's land between normal and abnormal activity and the element of uncertainty that sometimes exists about the significance of the result from a single site for the remainder of the skeleton.

1. Areas and Volumes (Tables I–V)

The whole of a bone section may be quantitated by using camera lucida drawings or enlarged photographs from which the proportional areas of the components of interest may be determined by such means as counting squares in a superimposed grid (Popowitz and Johnston, 1971), cutting out and weighing (Jee et al., 1966), and planimeter measurement (Jowsey et al., 1965). Absolute values are established from the original dimensions of the section and the magnification. On the other hand, a sampling procedure may be used, generally an eyepiece graticule with points that appear superimposed on the section. Random sampling methods have been reviewed by Weibel (1963) and Underwood (1970). The work of Hennig (1967) is most often referred to since he was responsible for the design of the Zeiss (1960) integrating eyepiece graticules. Although there were originally two eyepieces, they have now been combined into one pattern, suitable for both point and linear sampling. Most workers use the Zeiss eyepiece, although others have been described (van der Heul et al., 1964; Merz and Schenk, 1970).

The graticule contains an array of points within a perimeter line. The whole section is covered by overlapping or contiguous fields. Additional sampling may be achieved by rotating the graticule. The number of points falling on each component of interest are counted; their number is propor-

TABLE I

Bone Area in Sections of Normal Anterior Iliac Crest

Age	1[a]	2[a]	3[a]	4[a]	5[a]
0–9				18.5 (4.0)	20.8 (3.4)
10–19				20.5 (4.0)	17.8 (3.4)
20–29	22.8 (4.3)	21.7 (4.4)	23.5 (2.3)	21.6 (4.0)	17.7 (3.4)
30–39	22.1 (4.1)	19.8 (4.8)	21.2 (3.1)	21.7 (4.0)	19.1 (3.4)
40–49	21.0 (4.0)	19.9 (3.9)	18.3 (3.4)	19.2 (4.0)	17.7 (3.4)
50–59	19.6 (4.2)	18.5 (4.8)	17.8 (3.0)	18.1 (4.0)	15.5 (3.4)
60–69	19.1 (4.9)	15.3 (5.2)	16.4 (1.9)	16.7 (4.0)	13.7 (3.4)
70–79	17.1 (3.1)	15.0 (3.2)		14.0 (4.0)	11.2 (3.4)
80–89		15.4 (4.6)		14.4 (4.0)	7.1 (3.4)

[a] Columns 1–5: percentage area of cancellous space occupied by bone in sections of normal anterior iliac crest as determined by various authors (one standard deviation in parentheses). Column 1, 113 cases, Merz and Schenk (1969). Column 2, 132 cases, P. Meunier et al. (unpublished) from Bordier and Tun Chot (1972). Column 3, 54 cases, P. J. Bordier et al. (unpublished from Bordier and Tun Chot (1972). Column 4, 93 cases, Holley (1969) S.D. for whole series calculated by Byers. Column 5, 41 cases, Garner and Ball (1966) means and S.D. for whole series calculated by Byers.

TABLE II

Osteoid Areas in Normal Anterior Iliac Crest

	Area expressed as		
No of cases	% Bone + osteoid	% Bone + osteoid + marrow	Reference
41, all ages (range)	0–3.2	0–0.47	Garner and Ball (1966)
50, over 50 years of age		0–0.47	Jenkins et al. (1973)
41, adults (range)	0–5.0		Woods et al. (1968)
"Adults"	3.8 ± 1.6		⎫
"Older people"	9.7 ± 2.3		⎬ Bordier and Tun Chot (1972)
28, normals	5.7 ± 2		⎭
113, all ages (range)	0–6.85		Merz and Schenk (1969)

No of cases	Expressed as surface area/unit volume (mm^2/mm^3)	Reference
78 normal cases, range of mean values for 3rd to 9th decade	0.29–0.49	Sissons et al. (1967)

TABLE III

Some Mean Values (Standard Deviation) for Normal Sixth Rib[a,b]

Parameter[c]	Age (years)								
	0–0.9	1–9	10–19	20–29	30–39	40–49	50–59	60–69	70–89
1. Osteoid seams (No./mm²)	6.2 (3.2)	2.7 (1.0)	1.4 (1.3)	0.5 (0.4)	0.2 (0.5)	0.4 (0.4)	0.4 (0.2)	0.5 (0.4)	0.7 (0.5)
2. Resorption spaces (No./mm²)	3.3 (1.8)	2.0 (0.6)	0.6 (0.5)	0.3 (0.2)	0.3 (0.3)	0.5 (0.3)	0.5 (0.3)	0.6 (0.2)	0.8 (0.5)
3. Osteoid seam circumference (mm)	0.3 (0.1)	0.3 (0.04)	0.3 (0.1)	0.3 (0.1)	0.3 (0.1)	0.3 (0.1)	0.3 (0.1)	0.3 (0.1)	0.3 (0.1)
4. Labeled seams (% total)	95–100	95–100	95–100	90–95	90–95	90–95	90–95	90–95	90–95
5. Cortical to total area[d]	0.7 (0.2)	0.6 (0.2)	0.5 (0.2)	0.5 (0.2)	0.4 (0.2)	0.4 (0.2)	0.4 (0.2)	0.3 (0.1)	0.3 (0.1)
6. Cortical cross section area (mm²)		16 (4)	25 (6)	22 (7)	20 (5)	20 (3)	20 (3)	22 (4)	
7. Periosteal perimeter (mm)		20 (4)	29 (6)	31 (5)	31 (7)	29 (4)	31 (6)	32 (6)	
8. Endosteal perimeter (mm)		14 (3)	22 (3)	24 (5)	25 (6)	25 (6)	26 (5)	26 (6)	
9. Seams/unit endosteal perimeter (No./mm)		0.29 (0.15)	0.16 (0.08)	0.12 (0.09)	0.07 (0.0)	0.11 (0.07)	0.08 (0.05)	0.07 (0.04)	

[a] From Frost (1969).

[b] This table does not contain any of the dynamic values, e.g. appositional rate, radial closure rate, osteon formation time, activation frequency that form part of the original tables and are an important part of Frost's evaluation of bone.

[c] Parameters 1–5, determined in 356 cases; parameters 6–9 for 70 cases.

[d] Sex dependent.

TABLE IV

Some Quantitative Assessments of Iliac Crest in Metabolic Bone Disease

	Vitamin D deficiency[a]		Malabsorption[b] 27 cases	Renal osteodystrophy[b] 18 cases	Osteomalacia[c] 27 cases	Osteomalacia[d] (p)	HPT[e] 23 cases	Paget's disease 10 cases
	Mild 10 cases	Severe 30 cases						
Bone + osteoid (% total area)	21.7 ± 3.4	27.8 ± 3.8	6.7–30.7	13.6–67.3				31.6–65, woven bone 13–14
Osteoid (% bone + osteoid)	8.2 ± 3.4	20.9 ± 7.7	0–55	3.5–61	8–62	–90		
Osteoid (% total surface)	36.3 ± 8.9	67.6 ± 13.7			70–100		12–78	27.6–67.2
Osteoid with active 'blasts (% total surface)						3		12.9–97.8
Calcification front (% total surface)	35.8 ± 6.4	33.8 ± 5.6						61 in 6 patients (normal) 7.5–50 in 4
Resorption (% total surface)	21.9 ± 4.1	19.2 ± 18.3					13–47	
Osteoclasts (No/mm² section)								1.6–6.7

[a] Bordier and Tun Chot, 1972.
[b] Ball and Garner, 1966 (see also Table V).
[c] Paterson et al., 1968.
[d] Merz and Schenk, 1970.
[e] Byers and Smith, 1971.
[f] Bordier et al., 1972.

TABLE V

Quantitative Assessment of Iliac Crest in Malabsorption and Renal Disease[a,b]

Bone disorder[c]	Malabsorption				Renal failure			
	No. of cases	Bone + osteoid % section area	Bone	Osteoid	No. of cases	Bone + osteoid % section area	Bone	Osteoid
			% bone + osteoid				% bone + osteoid	
OP	7	6.7–11.6	100–99	0–1				
OP + OM	6	7.3–11.9	84–68	16–32				
Normal	2	13.1–13.2	97.7–97.0	2.3–3.0				
OM	10	13.0–23.4	90–34	10–66	5	13.6–22.3	90–71	10–29
OS + OM	2	28.8–30.7	68–45	32–55	13	26.8–67.3	89–39	11–61

[a] From Garner and Ball (1966).
[b] "Bone" and "osteoid" converted to % bone + osteoid; cases divided into "bone disorders" by their criteria; see Table I.
[c] OP, osteoporosis; OM, osteomalacia; OS, osteosclerosis.

tional to the area the component occupies in the section and to its volume in the bone. Assumptions have to be made concerning random distribution, and, in order to convert to volumes, section thickness; these can of course be tested. The accuracy of point sampling is related to the number of points falling on the component of interest in proportion to the total points; thus to attain a given degree of accuracy, many more points must be counted when it occupies a smaller proportion of the section. On the other hand, it may not be necessary to count many points if all that is required is the confirmation that the component is above or below a particular level. Curtis (1960) gives the Gauss equation for standard error, expressed as a percentage of the component of interest:

$$\frac{S}{x} = 67.45 \frac{100 - c}{nc}$$

where n is the number of points falling on it and c is its percentage of the whole area. He also provides a tabulation, given below for values of S/x for various values of c and n:

n \ c	5	15	20	30
100	29.3	16.0	13.4	10.0
500	13.1	7.0	6.0	4.3
1000	9.2	5.0	4.2	3.2
10,000	2.9	1.6	1.3	1.0

2. Surfaces (Tables VI–VIII)

The extent of the bone surface occupied by any component can be measured directly from photographs by using a planimeter (Jowsey, 1966). However, it is more usual to use eyepiece graticules for linear random sampling. The theory is discussed by Weibel (1963) and by Underwood (1970). A number of parallel lines are marked on the graticule, and intercepts can be achieved by moving the section and rotating the graticule. The character of the surface at each intercept is recorded. The number of intercepts with any given type of surface, for example, osteoid, in relation to the total intercepts is proportional to the bone surface covered by osteoid relative to the total surface. The graticule area and the line length can be determined for any given microscopical conditions, and hence absolute values (surface areas/unit volume) can be calculated on the assumption that the section is infinitely thin. In most graticule designs, the lines are straight, but in that of Merz (1967; Merz and Schenk,

TABLE VI

Percentage of Trabecular Surface in the Normal Anterior Iliac Crest Undergoing Resorption and Resorption Indices[a,b]

Age	1	2	3	4	5 Total resorption	6 % with osteo- clasts	7 Osteoclast lacunar ratio
0–9	20.0 (4)						
10–19	12.4 (4)	10.5 (1)					
20–29	8.4 (4)	4 (1)			5.3 (1.7)	0.5 (0.4)	13.0 (10.8)
30–39	12.0 (4)	6 (1.5)			6.3 (2.5)	0.5 (0.5)	8.1 (4.9)
40–49	9.3 (4)	7 (2)	15.4 (4)	2.4 (0.4)	7.5 (4.3)	0.6 (0.7)	8.7 (7.9)
50–59	12.1 (4)	7.5 (2)			6.1 (2.7)	0.5 (0.4)	8.5 (7.9)
60–69	12.7 (4)	8 (2)			8.0 (4.0)	0.5 (0.5)	7.7 (6.8)
70–79	10.2 (4)	11 (2.5)			5.8 (2.9)	0.6 (0.5)	8.7 (6.4)
80 +	12.6 (4)	12 (2.5)					

[a] One standard deviation (in parentheses) as determined by various authors. Lowest and highest values given (mean ± 2 S.D.).

[b] Column 1, 93 cases, Holley (1969) S.D. for whole series calculated by Byers. Column 2, Jowsey (1966) read from graph. Number of cases not specified. Column 3, 28 cases, Bordier and Tun Chot (1972). Column 4, 31 cases, Meunier *et al.* (1971d). Column 5–7, 113 cases, Schenk and Merz (1969); this does not include their values for empty resorption cavities nor their osteoclast index.

TABLE VII

Percentage of Trabecular Surface in the Normal Anterior Iliac Crest Covered by Osteoid[a,b]

Age	1 Total osteoid (% bone surface)	With active 'blasts (% osteoid)	2	3	4
0–9			14.2 (7.5)		
10–19			14.7 (7.5)	10 (3)	
20–29	13.8 (6)	5 (3)	11.1 (7.5)	3.5 (1)	12 (6)
30–39	11.6 (6)	5 (3)	13.8 (7.5)	4.5 (2)	
40–49	13.1 (5)	3.8 (2)	9.3 (7.5)	2 (2)	16.6 (4)
50–59	17.1 (9)	5.2 (5)	8.3 (7.5)	3.0 (2)	
60–69	17.5 (10)	5 (5)	11.8 (7.5)	3.5 (2)	19 (4.7)
70–79	20.5 (14)	3.5 (4)	14.4 (7.5)	3 (2)	
80+			12.1 (7.5)	3.5 (2)	

[a] One standard deviation (in parentheses) as determined by various authors.

[b] Column 1, 113 cases, Merz and Schenk (1970). Column 2, 93 cases, Holley (1969). S.D. for whole series calculated by Byers. Column 3, Jowsey (1966). Values read from graph (number of cases not specified). Column 4, 28 cases, Bordier and Tun Chot (1972).

TABLE VIII

Calcification Front in Normal Anterior
Iliac Crest[a]

Age	1	2
0–9		
10–19	16 (4.5)	
20–29		84.6 (7.5)
30–39	11.5 (4.5)	
40–49	14.5 (4.5)	
50–59	10.5 (4.5)	83 (±7)
60–69	13.3 (4.5)	
70–79	12 (4.5)	76 (±4)
80+		

[a] Column 1, percent bone surface
showing tetracycline uptake. 16 cases,
van der Sluys Veer *et al.* (1964). Column 2, percent osteoid with calcification front. 28 cases, Bordier and Tun
Chot (1972).

1970), they are composed of alternate halves of semicircles joined at their
ends. This graticule allows trabecular width to be calculated in addition to
the surface estimates (Whitehouse, 1974a,b). The accuracy of the method
is proportional to the number of intercepts counted. Its precision is a
reflection of the ability to recognize the various surface characteristics, a
problem to be dealt with later. At least theoretically, one can determine
the proportion (or absolute value) of bone surface that shows any of the
following features: (1) osteoid with active osteoblasts, (2) osteoid without
active osteoblasts, (3) osteoid with calcification front, (4) osteoid without
calcification front, (5) resorption with osteoclasts, (6) resorption without
osteoclasts, and (7) inert surface. Clearly, some of these values can be
derived by calculation from basic observations. As has more than once
been stated, the main requirements are good definitions and good criteria
for surface activities.

3. Linear Measurements (Osteoid Thickness, Tetracycline Labels, Osteocyte Lacunae)

Thickness of osteoid seams has been the most used expression for quantitative descriptions of osteoid, and yet it was only in recent years that
actual values for normal seam thickness were available. Technically the
measurement is made by an eyepiece graticule marked with gradations
that can be quantified for any given set of circumstances, and the values
are thus determined as with a ruler. Here, as in the other microscopic

methods, appropriate optical conditions must be used (Frost, 1962). A more refined method is to use an eyepiece with a mobile point activated by a spindle that records the distance traversed when the spindle is turned. Since the slide can be moved, and either the eyepiece or stage rotated, successive sites for measurement can be brought into position and their values accumulated on the spindle. For example, several measurements of the thickness of an osteoid seam or of the distance between tetracycline labels can be accumulated and mean values calculated. In practice, this apparatus is much more refined than described here (Weibel, 1963; Lee, 1967). With growing interest in osteocytic activity, the size of their lacunae is of growing importance. Measurements of the longest and shortest axes are adequate to establish differences from normal lacunar size in disease, i.e., hyperparathyroidism (Meunier *et al.*, 1971b; Rasmussen and Bordier, 1974). Absolute values for cell size in ordinary sections are difficult to obtain (Sissons *et al.*, 1975) because accurate information on section thickness is lacking. The measurements are made either with an eyepiece micrometer or from enlarged photographs. The width of trabeculae is of interest, and some estimates have been made by Wakamatsu and Sissons (1969) and Whitehouse (1974a). Whitehouse emphasizes the ease with which this data, together with a mathematical expression of trabecular orientation and surface values can be obtained with the Merz (1967) graticule.

4. *Numeration (Osteoid Lamellae, Formation Foci, Osteoid Seam, Resorption Foci, Numbers of Osteoclasts, Periosteocytic Mineral Defect) (Tables III, IV, IX)*

Woods *et al.* (1968) have measured osteoid in normal bone and used the number of lamellae as an index of thickness. When undecalcified sections are stained for calcium (Von Kossa's stain), the mineralized portion becomes black and the birefringence of its collagen is obscured, but the osteoid is unstained and the birefringence of its collagen is undisturbed. Successive layers of collagen fibers in the osteoid (lamellae) have different axes of orientation, so that in a field of polarized light only alternate bands of collagen are bright for any orientation, the number of bright lines therefore represent half the lamellae. These authors never found more than 6 lamellae (3 bright lines) in any of 48 normals. A review of the material studied by Byers (1962, 1963) revealed that this limit could be exceeded on occasion (P. D. Byers, unpublished results). The actual number of seams can be counted as an index of formation. This forms part of Frost's basis for quantitating bone (see below) using cross sections of ribs; he counts all the seams. In addition, he identifies those that incorporate tetracycline, which gives an index of mineralization or active formation sites.

TABLE IX

Osteocytic Alterations in Iliac Crest

| | Normal 35 cases | Hyperparathyroidism | |
		Primary 24 cases	Secondary 20 cases
Mean lacunar[a] size (S.D.)	48.3 (4.8)	68.3 (9.5)	67 (8.1)

	Mean of 11 normal cases
% Total cortical and cancellous lacunae showing osteocytic osteolysis[b,c]	3.9 ± 0.6

[a] From Meunier et al. (1971).
[b] From Bordier and Tun Chot (1972).
[c] See also Baud and Anil (1971) for differential osteocyte count in alveolar bone.

Similarly, Frost uses the number of resorption cavities. In both instances this histological data is coupled with other information. Osteoclasts and resorption cavities are counted as an index of resorptive activity (Schenk et al., 1973; Woodhouse et al., 1971); this means that all the osteoclasts in a biopsy should be recorded. An estimate of osteocytic activity can be made by counting loci of periosteocytic mineral deficiency (Bordier and Tun Chot, 1972).

IX. SKELETAL VARIABILITY AND THE VALUE OF BONE BIOPSY

A bone biopsy is a sample of the skeleton from which to judge its qualities. This assumes a degree of uniformity both within an individual and between individuals for any given condition. This could be tested by measuring the reliability of a histological section as a sample of a comparatively huge volume of bone by assessing variability between people and the precision with which the features can be measured by many observers and by critically evaluating the basis of the methods. To date, one does not feel that any adequate assessment of all these facets has been made. Notwithstanding this it is possible to piece together a number of studies that let one formulate an opinion. "Bone biopsy" makes no statement about the site, many of which can be (and are) biopsied during operations or in the investigation of a focal disturbance. Nevertheless, it is now the practice nearly everywhere to sample either iliac crest or rib in investigating metabolic bone disorders. This is primarily because these are the sites safely and easily approached which give an abundance of bone surfaces for study.

The range of surface lengths in sections from the anterior half of rib and in, perhaps, larger sections of iliac crest cancellous space from Lloyd and Hodges (1971) study are shown in the following tabulation (surface to volume ratio in parenthesis). The criterion of available surface weighs

	Anterior rib (cm)	Iliac crest (cm)
Maximum	29.3 (219)	37 (284)
Minimum	12.9 (91)	10 (139)

slightly in favor of iliac crest. However, the study of rib cortex cut at right angles to the osteons with their systematic organization that permits their identification as units of structure, each with an isolated surface on which loci of activity can be visualized (Frost's 1966 "bone modeling unit"), presents many advantages over iliac crest, particularly in tetracycline-labeling measurements. However, if the growth plate is to be studied, then the iliac crest is an excellent site, since the apophyseal growth plate is easily accessible and remains active late in childhood. Irregardless of the merits of these two sites, skeletal variability and the diagnostic value of bone biopsy must be considered in the light of the probability that one or other site will be used as the sample of the skeleton.

Amprino and Bairati (1936), in a study of bones from 94 humans, remarked on a wide range of activities between individuals, but noted that they were similar in the bones of one individual. However, in 1947, Amprino and Sisto, noting that the appearances in a pair of femurs were similar, found wide variations at different levels. Nevertheless, studies by Jowsey et al. (1965) showed a good correlation between measurements of surface activities and bone volume at several sites and concluded that it was valid to use bone from one site as representative of the whole skeleton. Other studies of the correlation between bone mass at two sites (Meema, 1963; Saville, 1965; Chalmers and Weaver, 1966; Dequeker et al., 1971) indicate that they parallel one another. This hypothesis is widely accepted, and there are many measurements of bone density in health and osteoporosis where single bones are used as indicators of skeletal mass. On the other hand, a study by Arnold and Bartley (1965) showed that the weight per cubic centimeter of a lumbar vertebra and the midshaft of femur from each of 150 autopsies gave three categories of relationship: (1) reduced cortical and vertebral ash, (2) normal cortical but reduced vertebral ash, and (3) reduced cortical ash with a normal vertebra. Trotter *et al.* (1959) examined the densities of a cervical and a lumbar vertebrae, a humerus and femur from every one of 80 cadavers of mixed race and sex (Caucasians and Negros, males and females). Their objective was to study differences between classes of bone (i.e., vertebrae, humeri, and femurs) and sex–race groups. They did not analyze correlations between densities of the bones of individuals, but it is apparent from the display of their data that the density of any one bone would not predict that of another bone of the same individual with great reliability. On the other hand, Doyle (1972) reviewed the value of knowledge of bone mass in one part of the skeleton in predicting that of another part and of bone strength in other parts. His own work and that of Mazess (1971), Cameron and Sorensen (1963), Horsman *et al.* (1970), Dunnill *et al.* (1967), and Chalmers and Weaver (1966) lead to the conclusion that weights and densities of one normal long bone will predict that of another from the same skeleton within 5 to 10%; however, the vertebral density will not be accurately predicted by long bone values nor by those obtained from iliac crest samples (see Chapter 6). Regional inequalities in bones are clearly evident in many disorders, for example, the juxtacortical osteoporosis associated with many diseases, the localized manifestations of hyperparathyroidism, the regionalized bone density of renal osteodystrophy ("rugger-jersey spine"), and the regional nature of Paget's disease.

The variability of formation, both within and between individuals with time, has been assessed in dogs by Harris *et al.* (1968). Porosity of bone was also measured at the end of the experiment. Using two tetracycline labels in three dogs, each administered continuously for 12 weeks with a 12-week interval, they examined four sections from four sites of five paired long bones (femur, tibia, ulna, radius, humerus), and three sections from three sites of three pairs of ribs (fourth, seventh, eleventh). They found that for two test periods, bone formation in the same section in the same region and in different regions were variable, in some instances by as much as a factor of 10, the differences being significant on *t* tests of covariance. One section was not representative of its own bone or all long bones of the same animal, any more than was one region; one bone was not representative of all bones in one dog. It was not until all the data from every bone of each dog was considered that the difference in cortical bone formation between dogs in the two labeling periods ceased to be significant. When the data for only one labeling period was considered, differences were significant. Studies of porosity of the bones showed highly significant differences between dogs, between the sites, and between long bones, but not between sides or ribs. In assessing this work, it must be remembered that there is some evidence of inhibition of osteoblasts by tetracyclines (Hong *et al.,* 1968). However, even so, the demonstration of variability throughout the skeleton is not invalidated. Variations such as these clearly indicate the need for a larger sample not only of an individual but also of the population before one can feel sure that it is adequately described.

Information about variation within the iliac crest of "normal" individuals was obtained in a study carried out by Sissons *et al.* (1967) and Holley (1969) working with 2–4 cm blocks cut from its anterior portion. In repeat measurements of single sections using point and linear sampling, Sissons *et al.* (1967) found a theoretical standard error of up to 1% for area, and 6–7% for resorption and osteoid. When sections were taken from blocks over a distance of 7 cm, these errors rose to 9.8, 15.1, and 11.1%, respectively. Equally important for the diagnostic pathologist were significant differences between the center and periphery of the blocks and between areas at different depths, which emphasizes the additional hazards of using small or fragmented biopsies for quantitation.

The variations that can occur throughout individual bones were shown in great detail by Lloyd and Hodges (1971) using a computerized automatic scanner in an examination of femoral cortex, femoral head, seventh thoracic vertebra, a lumbar vertebra, sixth rib, iliac crest, and cranium of a human. From each specimen up to 40 sections (rib) were prepared and microradiographed. The latter were scanned and bone area and perimeter measured. The maximum and minimum surface volume ratios are shown in the following tabulation (numbers in parentheses are the number of sections).

| | Femur | | Vertebra | | Rib | | Ilium | |
| | Cortex | Head | T | L | All | Ant. half | trabecular | Cranium |
	(4)	(8)	(8)	(10)	(35)	(18)	(12)	(9)
Maximum	34	103	160	143	218	218	284	53
Minimum	27	89	84	79	43	91	139	32

The difference that may occur between observers appear in Byers and Smith (1972) where the results of two observers (Byers and Holley) are recorded when assessing surface activities by line sampling of the same sections, although not of precisely the same areas. No significant difference was found between them when the group of cases was considered, but some individual results differed by a factor of two or more.

The greatest source of variance in Holley's (1969) study was between individual cases. He calculated a normal range of bone area in the iliac crest of 10–26% at birth, rising to 14–29% at 35 years, and declining to 6–22% at 75 years. His surface activity values were comparable in range to those independently determined by Byers and Smith (1971) for a smaller number of normals selected from his cases. The percent surface covered by osteoid was 8.6%, 95% confidence limits 3–28%; the resorption surface was 10.9%, 95% limits 6–19%. The wide skeletal variations suggest that a broad overlap of values in health and disease is possible. This is confirmed by most quantitative studies. Byers and Smith (1971) found a statistically significant difference for formation and resorption between groups of normal and hyperparathyroid patients. It is apparent that abnormality in the bone of an appreciable number of individuals in the hyperparathyroid group could not be recognized by quantitation of the surface activities. The same holds true in the case of osteoporosis [see, for example, Jowsey et al. (1965) (Fig. A-9)].

It seems reasonable to conclude that, as in many laboratory examinations, a result in the normal range does not assure one of a healthy state, either because the biopsy is unrepresentative, or because the skeleton has not yet responded or has responded in a way we do not yet know about, or because there are known changes present that are significant for the patient but still lie within the statistical range of normal. On the other hand, abnormal values must be significant for at least the site of the biopsy; however, in how far they are generalized is a matter of judgement and of assessment in other ways. This means that one is looking for levels that show whether the values must be regarded as abnormal, must be considered in the normal/abnormal range, or can with certainty be regarded as normal. Some might feel that, in consequence of the foregoing discussion, qualitative examination of a diagnostic biopsy would be adequate. However, the fact is that in asking himself whether resorption, osteoid and its mineralization, and the bone mass are pathological, the pathologist is seeking to estimate their quantities. He should use quantitative methods because vision is a method of perception subject to many deceptions; Byers and Smith (1972) give an example of the value of quantitative methods in correcting visual impressions. Quantitative values convey information that can be checked and give values that can be set against inclusion and exclusion levels which indicate the categories in which a case must be considered.

X. QUANTITATIVE VALUES IN BIOPSY DIAGNOSIS

This section draws together a few threads for the convenience of the diagnostician. This is done with iliac crest biopsy in mind, not because it is the only, or even the best, site but because it is most generally used and is the basis of my exerpience. Frost's methods, based on rib, overcome the difficulty that osteoid areas and surface coverage do not indicate anything about rates of formation, and that extent of resorption cavities only indicate that an event has occurred and not at what rate nor how much was removed (Frost, 1973). In rib, the number of forming foci, their surface area, and the appositional rate (from double tetracycline labels) give bone accretion in unit time. The volume of tissue in which this is taking place can be determined, so that we can determine rates in unit time per unit mass. Less easily determined are comparable values for resorption, or perhaps one should say that greater assumptions have to be made in doing so. Nevertheless the number of resorption foci, the specific resorption surface per focus, and the mean linear rate of destruction are used by Frost to calculate resorption rates that form the companion piece to the rates of formation just described (Frost, 1963). With these parameters Frost and his colleagues have given a dynamic picture of bone (Table III) and of its metabolic disorders that no one else has done. The mathematical basis for his parameters and their development in physiological terms has brought much criticism from those who understand such things, and has baffled those not so trained. One of the latter group, I find his basic concepts and methods attractive. The work of Schenk (1969), Merz and Schenk (1970), and Schenk *et al.* (1972) adds a dynamic element to iliac crest biopsies. Quantitative measurements of surfaces, areas, and volumes can be used to decide if a parameter exceeds a critical level for admission into a category without going to the length of determining its actual value. Whatever the precision of quantitation, the critical levels must be established, and for this purpose use can be made of those currently available values listed in Tables I, III, VI, and IX. Quantitative data are not numerous, and consequently figures can be conservatively suggested only for bone and osteoid volume and for surface activities.

The use that has been made of quantitation techniques in the study of bone disease can be seen in Tables IV and V. These tables are by no means comprehensive. They are based on groups of cases defined by nonhistological parameters; the range of disorders that the bone undergoes are determined by histological quantitation. The diagnostician's problem, of course, is to know when a case can be admitted to a group using the bone parameters. There is no doubt that this decision is best taken using all the information about the patient. The ideal is a close liasion between the interested parties.

A. Iliac Crest Bone Volume

An examination of published values shows that there is a fairly good agreement as to bone area values for normal iliac crests (Table I). Using these figures to obtain highest and lowest levels per decade can provide part of the information required. A review of the literature for a level of bone volume in the iliac crest cancellous space below which osteoporosis occurs does not give a very satisfactory answer. Bordier and Tun Chot (1972) state that a histological diagnosis requires a significant reduction in cancellous bone without defining this reduction. Clearly, the matter is a difficult one, since osteoporosis must first be defined and recognized before the iliac crest values can be obtained. The clearest statement is by Meunier *et al.* (1971) who found that in 54 clinically diagnosed osteoporotics, none had more than 16% bone in the cancellous space of the iliac crest. Until more work is done, this is the most reliable value for a critical level at which osteoporosis must be considered. The paper of Garner and Ball (1966) contributes to ideas on critical levels for both bone volume and osteoid (Table V); they studied iliac crest bone biopsies from 27 patients with intestinal malabsorption and from 18 patients with renal azotemia and compared these with 41 control cases from which they determined ''normal ranges.'' Osteoporosis and osteosclerosis were recognized when levels above (24.7%) or below (12.3%) the normal range of bone (mineralized and unmineralized tissue) were present. Osteomalacia was present when osteoid area was greater than 1% of section area, and bone (mineralized tissue) area was less than 90% of the combined area of mineralized tissue and osteoid. Perhaps the striking finding in this study are cases of malabsorption with reduced bone volume, with and without excess osteoid, and others with a normal bone complement. The authors make no reference to the calcification front; one wonders what tetracycline labeling would have shown in the cases without excess osteoid. In the two malabsorption cases that can be classified as osteosclerotic from their data (Table V), mineralized bone was only 68 and 45% of bone and osteoid, whereas the 13 renal failure cases with increase in bone and osteoid had mineralized tissue ranging from 89 to 39%.

B. Iliac Crest Osteoid and Calcification Front

Parameters that can be used for osteoid quantitation are osteoid area, bone surface covered by osteoid, proportion of osteoid with active osteoblasts, and proportion of osteoid with calcification front. Notwithstanding that the popular reference to excess osteoid is ''wide osteoid seams,'' this list does not include that parameter, since it is not a sensitive index to excess osteoid, as the extensive studies of Wilson *et al.* (1968) show. Critical levels can be determined for each listed item from currently available figures, which could well be augmented by further studies.

Area values for osteoid have been reported by not only Garner and Ball (1966) but also by Woods *et al.* (1968) and Bordier and Tun Chot (1972)

(Table II). The higher normal values for osteoid content reported by Bordier and Tun Chot, particularly for "older people," suggests that they have some cases with abundant osteoid in their normal group as suggested by Sissons *et al.* (1967), (see also Merz and Schenk, 1970; Jenkins *et al.*, 1973). Garner and Ball and Woods diagnosed osteomalacia in vitamin D deficiency when osteoid exceeds normal values. Bordier and Tun Chot stated that they diagnose osteomalacia in the presence of excess osteoid and a reduction in calcification fronts, although they did not state at what point osteoid is in excess or calcification front reduced. Their data suggest that they must on occasion make a diagnosis in the range of normal osteoid, presumably on the basis of a reduction in calcification front. Since this is in contradiction with the usual definition of "osteomalacia," it suggests the need to modify the definition or to coin a new term for this class of disease. Because of the different criteria, it is not possible to know if osteomalacia actually occurred in case reports of "malabsorption and osteoporosis." On the basis of osteoid area as a percent of total bone (mineralized and unmineralized areas), one can assume that definite osteomalacia occurs with osteoid areas above 14%, possible osteomalacia above 3.2%, and exclusion of osteomalacia with values below 1.4%. The proportional surface values for osteoid are given in Table VII; a critical level of 30% above which osteomalacia is certain can be established from these data. From data of Bordier and Tun Chot (1972) a level below 18% would exclude osteomalacia, but perhaps with the proviso that the calcification front is normal. These authors find surface coverage a more sensitive index of osteomalacia than osteoid area.

The proportion of surface with active osteoblasts offers a semidynamic parameter. The criteria for recognizing an active osteoblast are difficult to standardize, however. This is not a popular parameter with only one set of normal standards available for comparison (Table VII) as published. Bordier and Tun Chot (1972) indicate that 60% is a critical level for definite osteomalacia. The reader's attention is drawn to the earlier reservations about staining procedures for detecting calcification and to the desirability of using tetracycline. But even in the case of the latter view, information about its incorporation is accumulating which could in turn lead to modifications in the technique of its use (Swinson *et al.*, 1975).

C. Iliac Crest Resorption

Proportional surface values for resorption cavities with or without using osteoclasts as an index of resorption are available (Table VI). The critical level for abnormal resorption seems to be above 25%. The use of osteoclasts in a dynamic index is desirable, but must have great problems in observation error, which need be assessed before the index can inspire confidence. As indicated by the data of Byers and Smith (1971), there is no critical level for excluding hyperparathyroidism. Normal parameters of bone remodeling and bone turnover obtained from rib biopsies are illustrated in Table III.

XI. BONE CHANGES IN METABOLIC BONE DISEASE

A. Osteoporosis

Osteoporosis has been defined as a decrease in the mass per unit volume of tissue (Tables I, III, and VII) (Nordin, 1964) and as a decrease in absolute skeletal volume below a defined limit (Frost, 1964). Because of the great variation in bone mass in older groups, the increased incidence of osteomalacia in the elderly, and the relative insensitivity of ordinary radiological techniques as discussed in Chapter 6, the diagnosis of osteoporosis is more than the recognition of "skeletal demineralization" or of "reduced bone volume," now commonly referred to as "osteopenia." It is for the diagnostic pathologist to set bone mass, determined quantitatively, in the perspective of other histological parameters and for the clinician to interpret its meaning for his patient. Normal values for iliac crest are given in Table I, and for rib in Table III. In osteoporosis, bone architecture is altered in several ways. The diameter is increased, a normal change with age, shown in the femur by Trotter and Peterson (1967) and by Takahashi and Frost (1966) in the rib, through periosteal new bone formation. The porosity of the cortex is increased by enlargement of osteonal canals (a sign of resorption without equal formation). The thickness of the cortex is reduced by removal from the endosteal surface (further evidence of unequal turnover activites). These three sites (endosteal, osteoneal, and periosteal) are treated separately by Frost (1966) in his quantitative procedures. Bone trabeculae are reduced in number and more widely separated, but the thickness of residual trabeculae is only slightly reduced (Wakamatsu and Sissons, 1969). The structure of bone remains normal. Although mineral density is altered with age (Jowsey, 1964), this is not detectable by visual inspection of microradiographs. However, the occlusion by mineral of Haversian canals and of osteocyte lacunae is readily seen (Jowsey, 1960). Periosteocytic mineral reduction is not evident (a statement made with reservations and discussed in Section V). Despite at least one paper to the contrary (Stewart et al., 1972; see Section V), osteocyte bone resorption seems a most improbable mechanism for the production of osteoporosis and cannot be accepted without better definitions and criteria for recognition, and above all without a better knowledge of its dynamics.

Cell populations at surfaces will be altered in keeping with whatever changes there may be in the turnover. In addition, the marrow becomes less cellular and more adipose; a quantitative assessment of this has been made by Meunier *et al.* (1971a). Although not widely explored, there is an interest in marrow factors in relation to osteoporosis (Frame and Nixon, 1970) which arises partly out of the osteoporosis of mast cell disease and of high heparin dosage. However, the report of osteosclerosis in a case of systemic mast cell disease reported by Sirois (1963) should be kept in mind. Reduction in bone mass may be a secondary phenomenon, as in immobilization, rheumatoid arthritis, or even hyperparathyroidism (Chapter 6). In many of these there is a high turnover rate. Ball (1960) reviewed evidence for this in hyperthyroidism and quoted both Askenazy and Rutishauser (1933) and Follis (1953) who noted patterns that resembled osteitis fibrosa. Ball (1960) also investigated the increased resorptive activity in immobilization osteoporosis and was able to show both tunneling resorption and fibrous replacement, features that are not, therefore, specific for any disease.

B. Osteopetrosis

Osteopetrosis (Albers–Schonberg disease or marble bone disease) is an unusual type of osteosclerosis. The latter is a group of disorders, usually arising as the result of an imbalance between formation and resorption, which has many causes. The fact of sclerosis may be ascertained in a biopsy, the problem being similar to but at the opposite end of the scale from osteoporosis. As noted in detail in Volume II, Chapter 7, severe cases die in childhood from anemia presumably because of the failure to produce a marrow cavity. Mild cases survive and are generally recognized incidentally in adult life when radiographs show zones of density in otherwise normal bones (Dent *et al.,* 1965). A biopsy of an affected area shows bone architecture affected by the increased volume of bone. The structure is lamellar bone, with possibly some woven bone, encasing cores of calcified cartilage. This pattern is diagnostic. If it is not found, the problem is of a differential diagnosis of osteosclerosis and must be made from other features, such as the gross skeletal changes and their distribution. Acquired forms of osteosclerosis are readily studied in radiological literature (Murray and Jacobson, 1971).

C. Rickets and Osteomalacia

The iliac apophysis is a very accessible and suitable site in which to study the growth plate. Biochemical and radiological features of rickets are described in detail in Volume II, Chapter 7 and need little elaboration. The failure to calcify the cartilage matrix adequately interferes with growth and ossification, which is most readily seen in sections as a failure of the cartilage cells to form orderly columns and an increased thickness of the cartilage plate. The osteoid that is formed is not mineralized, and this in turn affects the remodeling process and results in osteomalacic bone. In the minimally affected cases, characteristically seen by present day clinicians, the changes may not strike the eye unaccustomed to looking at growth plates, and it is therefore useful to have some normal preparations covering the growth period available for comparison.

It is generally accepted that the ultimate diagnostic criterion for osteomalacia is an excess of osteoid. However, this can be found in a large number of disorders affecting bone, so that this unqualified criterion is useless. Qualifications can come from clinical, radiological, and biochemical sources as described in Chapter 5 and histologically. A number of diseases, such as hyperparathyroidism, thyrotoxicosis, and Paget's disease of bone, have a high bone turnover rate that of itself is responsible for increased osteoid. Nevertheless, exceptional circumstances may arise in which vitamin D deficiency or hypophosphatemia occur so that osteomalacia is also present (Arnstein et al., 1967). Stanbury (1972) concludes that primary hyperparathyroidism should also be included in the differential diagnosis of osteomalacia. This and the findings of a wide range of appearances in osteomalacic bone leads to the general conclusion that the pathogenesis of this disorder may not be simple and that a variety of disease patterns may exist.

It has been widely accepted that the basic pathogenetic mechanism in osteomalacia is a failure to mineralize osteoid. The calcification front can be detected histologically. That it has not formed part of the criteria in histological diagnosis must be partly due to the uncertainty about the reliability of staining methods for demonstrating calcification fronts (Stanbury, 1972). Despite the interference with mineralization in osteomalacia, the reduction in calcification front is not complete and tetracycline deposition can be found in some part of the osteoid (Frost, 1969; Bordier and Tun Chot, 1972). The mineral deposition is often irregular, extending up toward the surface in an abnormal fashion; microradiographs and staining procedures have also been used to demonstrate this (Bordier and Tun Chot, 1972; Haas et al., 1967).

The bone architecture is not altered in osteomalacia, and both cortical and trabecular elements are readily recognized in their usual relationships. The total amount of tissue, that is bone plus osteoid, may be slightly increased (Ball and Garner, 1966; Bordier and Tun Chot, 1972) (Tables IV and V). This increment may be much greater than indicated in Table IV and V and leads to a dense skeleton when the osteoid mineralizes as the result of treatment. The skeletal density will be reduced subsequently by remodeling processes (Perry *et al.,* 1976).

In the bulk of osteomalacic bone, the lamellar collagen is unaltered but abnormal osteoid does occur. Ball and Garner (1966) found this in 14 out of 16 osteomalacic biopsies from cases of renal failure, but not in those from 18 cases of malabsorption, with one doubtful exception. My own experience in the latter type of case is that foci of woven osteoid are not unusual. This may be confused with osteitis fibrosa of secondary hyperparathyroidism which superimposes the changes of that condition on those already present. Treatment increases mineralization and reduces the amount of osteoid; some details are reported by Melvin *et al.* (1970) and Haas *et al.* (1967). A well-recognized phenomenon is the failure to mineralize (some) osteoid, which persists buried beneath normally mineralized tissue. Ball and Garner (1966) studied this and concluded that this abnormality is due to something more than the woven pattern of collagen, since fracture callus in osteomalacia mineralizes normally.

In osteomalacia, as in other conditions, the number and size of cells can be used as an indication of activity in terms of both formation and resorption. Large osteoblasts indicate recently formed osteoid, and osteoclasts show where resorption is taking place. Haas *et al.* (1967) and Schenk and Merz (Schenk *et al.,* 1972) have used this to demonstrate the dynamics of osteomalacia. A perilacunar mineral deficiency is found in many biopsies of osteomalacia, affecting a variable number of cell sites (Table IX). It has been said that this mineral defect is peculiar to vitamin D-resistant rickets (Arnstein *et al.,* 1967). However, additional experience has shown that the perilacunar mineral defect is present in all types of osteomalacia (Bohr, 1967). Bordier and Tun Chot (1972) (Table IX) even go so far as to say it is found in microradiographs of normal bone. If this is confirmed, it is an observation that provides further support for this as a normal physiological mechanism or "bone mineral pump" which is accentuated in osteomalacia.

Even though conventional considerations of bone in osteomalacia do not give much attention to resorption, this is a very important aspect, since it is through assessment of this that the histologist must hope to recognize secondary or tertiary (autonomous) hyperparathyroidism in osteomalacia. Both surface resorption and tunneling resorption may be seen. There are at present only limited quantitative assessments of these (Ramser *et al.,* 1966; Haas *et al.,* 1967; Bordier and Tun Chot, 1972). It seems to be the case that a significant increment in bone resorption is seen in uncomplicated osteomalacia, but by what criteria is the presence of complicating hyperparathyroidism to be detected? The histological distinction between primary hyperparathyroidism with abundant osteoid and hyperparathyroidism secondary to osteomalacia could be made on the basis of the degree of osteoid mineralization. When hyperparathyroidism complicates osteomalacia, one would anticipate a greater degree of resorption, a different pattern of resorption, and fibrous replacement of bone. In the first instance, we have few quantitative values for resorption in uncomplicated cases. In the second, there are no good studies of resorption patterns with this problem in mind. The third is the most useful one, with the reservation that in my own experience it can be difficult to decide between abnormal osteoid and fibrous replacement. This dilemma leads to uncertainty in histological confirmation of osteomalacia with secondary hyperparathyroidism.

A description of the bone in osteomalacia would not be complete without reference to Looser's zones. Their histopathology was described by Ball (1960). They are regions of fibrous tissue in which trabeculae of immature (woven) bone appear. The general pattern is that of reactive tissue. This immature bone is capable of mineralization, as is other reactive bone tissue in osteomalacia of both malabsorption and azotemic cause (Ball and Garner, 1966).

D. Hyperparathyroidism

The effect of parathyroid hormone (PTH) on bone has been reviewed by Vaughan (1975) with emphasis on osteoclastic resorption, osteocytic osteolysis, and osteoblastic activity. PTH injection in animals increases the number of osteoclasts (Bingham *et al.*, 1969). Increased bone removal by osteoclasts is due not only to an increase in number of cells but also to their increased metabolic activity (Vaughan, 1975). An active role for PTH activating the osteocyte of bone seems indisputable, but whether this response leads to significant bone resorption is less certain. Meunier *et al.* (1971) (Table IX) showed a 50% increase in mean size of osteocyte lacunae, which, considering their number [Frost (1964) gives 20,000/mm^3], could well mean the removal of a significant amount of tissue. The tissue culture work of Gaillard (1965), Vaes and Nichols (1962), Flanagan and Nichols (1964), and Bingham *et al.* (1969) is cited by Vaughan (1975) to show that PTH affects osteoblasts. The first action may be inhibitory, although stimulation ultimately follows. There is a general agreement that PTH in humans increases bone turnover (Volume II, Chapter I). Byers and Smith (1972) concluded from their studies and those of others that probably all the bones in every case of hyperparathyroidism are affected, but because the changes may be within the broad range of normal, they are not always recognizable on radiographs or by quantitation of biopsies (Fig. 1). In addition, the changes may be unevenly distributed throughout the skeleton, so that only local lesions may be found.

The features to be looked for in a bone biopsy specimen are increased

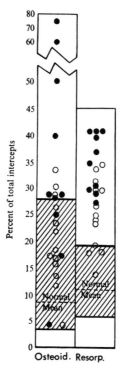

Fig. 1. Quantitative values for osteoid and resorption in bone biopsies from the iliac crest of 23 patients with hyperparathyroidism. X-Ray evidence of osteitis fibrosa is represented by closed circles. The shaded areas represent the 95% confidence limits of the normal means. [Adapted from Byers and Smith (1972) with permission of authors and publishers.]

resorption and formation, normal mineralizing activity, fibrous replacement of bone ("osteitis fibrosa"), accentuated reversal lines, and abnormal ("woven") bone. These histological appearances are nonspecific. They may be taken as evidence of hyperparathyroid bone disease, but other evidence is necessary for confirmation. Conventional clinical (Dent and Watson, 1968) and radiological criteria (Dent and Hodson, 1954) are most used, since PTH assays are still not widely available and may prove normal despite active disease (see Volume II, Chapter 1). A good correlation can be found between bone resorption and formation, plasma alkaline phosphatase, and urinary hydroxyproline (Byers and Smith, 1972). The local skeletal lesions of hyperparathyroidism take the form of so-called "brown tumor." This is a term descriptive of the gross appearance, which is often light or dark brown in color, and in small bones frequently appears as a swelling. Larger bones mainly show an osteolytic focus, usually in the metaphysis and/or epiphysis. It is not uncommon for these to be the presenting lesion, particularly when the jaw, one of the commonest sites, hands, or feet are affected. They are a mixture of fibrous tissue and multinucleated giant cells in varying proportions, a picture that is often difficult or impossible to distinguish from giant cell tumor of bone (osteoclastoma). It is now recognized by bone tumor pathologists that in every case diagnosed as giant cell tumor, serious consideration must be given to the possibility that it is a manifestation of hyperparathyroidism and that the only sure way to do this is biochemically. Enlarged intratrabecular spaces are evident in some cases of hyperparathyroidism, spaces which are, nevertheless, still relatively small, such as would accommodate a few large cells (see, for example, Jowsey *et al.*, 1964). Protagonists of the "osteocytic osteolysis" theory regard these changes as manifestations of osteocytic bone resorption; whereas those who question this role for osteocytes feel that these cavities were caused by osteoclasts penetrating from the surface. Meunier *et al.* (1973) have published data for size of osteocyte lacunae (Table IX) indicating they are significantly larger in hyperparathyroidism, an observation that needs confirmation. Apart from exceptional cases referred to in Section V,D on osteomalacia, mineralization of osteoid is not at fault in primary hyperparathyroidism. There is evidence (Smeenk, 1961) that the mineral distribution of bone is abnormal, but this is not detectable by visual inspection of microradiographs.

E. Renal Osteodystrophy and Dialysis Bone Disease

Segregating the bone changes of renal failure under the heading renal (or azotemic) osteodystrophy facilitates discussion and investigation. The response of bone is limited, and renal failure can only invoke alterations in bone turnover and mineralization as in other metabolic bone diseases, with the consequence that nonspecific osteomalacic or hyperparathyroid bone changes may occur. However, there is a complex and not completely understood concatenation of factors acting on the bone in renal failure which can effect a range of changes from osteoporosis to osteosclerosis, embracing osteomalacia and hyperparathyroid bone changes in their full panoply (Fig. 2). This complex state of affairs is futher compounded by the effects of dialysis. These influences are discussed in detail in Volume II, Chapter 2. Nevertheless, accumulated observations indicate that glomerular disease leads primarily to hyperparathyroid changes and tubular disease to osteomalacia. Combinations of glomerular and tubular disease induce both histological patterns in varying proportions. It hardly needs

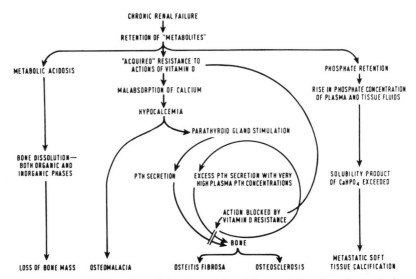

Fig. 2. Schematic illustration of the changes in calcium and phosphate homeostasis and vitamin D metabolism in chronic renal failure and of their roles in the etiology of the types of bone disease found in that condition. [Reproduced from Wills (1971) with permission of author and publishers.]

mentioning that bone biopsy is unlikely to be used for diagnostic purposes in renal failure. However, it is useful in the cause of elucidating the pathogenesis of bone changes. It may be that in the future it could be used to follow and control therapy, but this would depend on the accumulation of much more adequate information than we now have. Stanbury (1972) emphasized the lack of appropriate histological documentation of osteodystrophy which makes it difficult to assess and compare findings obtained by different individuals in patients from varying geographical locations.

There have been recent studies of bone in cases of renal failure, both with and without overt bone disease (Cochran and Nordin, 1969; Barzel and Jowsey, 1969; Kaye *et al.,* 1970; Kerr *et al.,* 1969; Katz *et al.,* 1969; Kim *et al.,* 1968; Jowsey *et al.,* 1969). These studies impart a better understanding of renal osteodystrophy than of hemodialysis bone disease, but raise many questions about both, even, are they appreciably different. There is still a need for more knowledge about the range of bone changes; indeed, about whether they occur at all in some circumstances (Wills, 1971). Not only is accurate documentation required but there should also be some uniformity of methods and criteria.

To describe in detail the bone in renal disease would be a repetition of previous comments made regarding osteomalacia and hyperparathyroidism. If dissolution of bone substance really occurs in acidosis, and the evidence is summarized by Wills (1971), then presumably osteoporosis would ensue. In addition, a not uncommon feature of renal osteodystrophy is osteosclerosis. There may be a general increase in bone and osteoid (often not easily detectable) or a striking, and perhaps regional, one. Osteosclerosis is manifested by an increase in the bulk of the trabecular bone and the consequent reduction in marrow space. There is little information about what happens to the cortex; any increase in the bulk would have to be periosteal or endosteal.

The structure of the bone may, in places, be woven collagen because of past increases in turnover. Equally, there may be some disorder of reversal lines. Bone surfaces can have varying amounts of osteoid, and as was evident from Garner and Ball's (1966) work, it may be that the increased bulk of tissue is due to osteoid, whereas the bone is normal or even reduced in amount (Table V). This is an important point to bear in mind when considering the interpretation and value of radiographs in assessing metabolic bone disease. Defective mineralization of osteoid will be manifested in the calcification front, and altered periosteocytic mineral concentrations can be observed.

F. Paget's Disease of Bone (Osteitis Deformans)

This disease is a localized disorder of the skeleton due to extremely active bone remodeling, in Caucasians in Europe, North America, and Australia over 40 years of age. Many individuals suffer from very restricted skeletal involvement, perhaps one or two vertebrae, without the disease coming to notice (Collins, 1966). On the other hand, more widespread involvement can give rise to pain, circulatory disorders (Barry, 1969), and deformity that may be very bizarre (Byers and Jones, 1969). Bone sarcoma is a well-recognized complication (Price, 1962). Further details of the clinical and epidemiological aspects of the disease are to be found in Volume II, Chapter 5. Because it is a localized disease, diagnostic information can be gleaned only from the affected sites.

The initial manifestation of Paget's disease is a wave of predominantly osteoclastic activity leading to regional osteoporosis. Radiographically, this appears as a sharply circumscribed area of reduced density, designated as "osteoporosis circumscripta" in the skull. In long bone, where the "flame shape" is often alluded to, it may be biopsied as a bone cyst of an osteolytic neoplastic lesion. After an interval of time, osteoblastic activity is more dominant, and an abnormally large amount of bone is produced at the site; not only does the cancellous space contain more bone but the diameter of the bone is increased as well. At both stages, histological sections show an increase in resorption and formation, and from early in the disease the mosaic pattern of reversal lines is evident. Fibrosis of the marrow is an associated aspect of the process, appearing at a fairly early stage. The alteration in the vascular network responsible for the change in the dynamics of blood flow may or may not be apparent as dilated capillaries and engorged blood vessels. The increased turnover is, as in other bone disease, the result of increased cellular activity, and both osteoblasts and osteoclasts are prominent at bone surfaces (Table IV). The disease runs a course at any given site and eventually becomes quiescent, at which point the cells become greatly diminished in number and size to the point of disappearing.

There is no doubt that the more florid patterns of increased bone turnover are usually seen in Paget's disease, and that the most profound effects are found in this disease and indeed may be pathognomonic, as Sissons (1966) suggests. Unfortunately, these comparative terms have no absolute values; each pathologist formulates his own standards out of his experience, which are not readily expressed as means and standard deviations and expected ranges.

A further use for the bone biopsy in Paget's disease has been occasioned by the discovery of compounds that reduce bone turnover; fluoride, cytotoxic antibiotics (mithramycin and actinomycin D), calcitonin, and diphosphonates seem to offer new means of therapy. These compounds have been employed with varying success to relieve symptoms. Various objective assessments have been used to demonstrate reduction in turnover, viz., hydroxyproline levels, calcium kinetics, alkaline phosphatase, and quantitative histology. Woodhouse (1972) reviews the disease and its treatment. (Further details may also be found in Volume II, Chapter 5.) The effect of treatment must be assessed by biopsies before and after use, since there are no "standard" values for the disease, and, in fact, quantitative values are few (Table VII).

G. Fibrogenesis Imperfecta Ossium and Axial Osteomalacia

Only five cases of "fibrogenesis imperfecta ossium" have been published (Baker, 1956; Baker et al., 1966; Thomas and Moore, 1968; Frame et al., 1971). This may be because, as Baker has pointed out in his meticulously detailed studies, such cases may often be mistakenly diagnosed as simply osteomalacia. On the other hand, the specific radiological changes might well lead to more cases being examined histologically with this diagnosis specifically in mind—verbum sapienti. This eventuality having occurred in at least one instance, the result was a surprise in that no evidence of fibrogenesis imperfecta ossium was discovered, and the conclusion was reached, among others, that the radiographical findings are nonspecific (Stanley *et al.*, 1971). In the bones of all five reported cases, there was an abundance of matrix, sufficient to suggest a diagnosis of osteomalacia, but the matrix and some of the bone was greatly deficient in collagen, a fact discovered only during examination of the sections under polarized light. Two of the patients died, and bone was first examined histologically following autopsy. Both had had fractures, and the callus was mineralizing normally. This led to the conclusion that there was no abnormality of mineralization but that there must be a defect in the osteoid associated with its reduced collagen content which prevented it. This conclusion is now quoted in support of the hypothesis that an abnormality in the osteoid of osteomalacia interferes with its mineralization, as already discussed. Perhaps it is worth recalling that Garner and Ball (1966) found that fracture callus mineralization is normal in patients with renal failure and osteomalacia. Nothing is known of the biochemical or biophysical properties in fibrogenesis imperfecta ossium, the histological studies having only demonstrated that the number of collagen fibers is reduced. So far as can be judged, each individual fiber in such a case is as strongly birefringent as in a normal individual; but since there are fewer of them, the total amount of visible light in the dark polarized field is reduced. This finding is quite striking and distinctive.

In discussing their case, Frame *et al.* (1971) reviewed the relationship of these cases to the unusual examples of osteomalacia that they had reported earlier under the name of "axial osteomalacia." Thomas and Moore (1968) suggested they are one and the same disease. Radiological patterns in vertebrae are similar, but the lack of severe pain and tenderness, the normal alkaline phosphatase, and the normal collagen content of the osteoid in the axial osteomalacia patients are against this conclusion. These cases came to light because of mild discomfort in the spine. The radiographs revealed coarse trabeculation of vertebrae and, in one case, of the ribs and pubis. The bone examined in each case was a biopsy of the iliac crest, thus none of the grossly affected bone was studied, and one can only speculate that in those parts some different pattern in the tissue was present. One should always consider this rare disorder of skeletal metabolism in the differential diagnosis of osteomalacia.

XII. APPENDIX

Definitions and criteria have been given in the text for the recognition of those elements of bone that are of value in histological diagnosis. Something of their range of variation, means of quantitating them, and possible interpretations have been discussed. This section is a summary of what to look for and how to look for it (Table A-1) and illustrates what one might expect to see. It is not an attempt to illustrate the histological appearances of the bone diseases that have been considered.

Every histological section contains all the components of the tissue unless removed by solvents either purposively, as in decalcification, or incidentally, as in defatting paraffin embedded sections, but not all necessarily will be rendered clearly or even at all visible by any given method of preparing the section. Moreover, the procedures themselves introduce variations which compound the natural variations of the tissue. All the

TABLE A-1

Diagnostic Features (Numbered List), Histological Conditions, and Illustration Guide

1. Osteoblasts
2. Osteoid
3. Calcification front or calcifying osteoid
4. Bone (as a tissue without specification of what part is visualized)
5. Collagen fibers
6. Bone mineral density
7. Osteocytes and/or lacunae
8. Osteoclasts
9. Resorption
10. Reversal lines
11. Fibrous tissue
12. Marrow

Section preparation	Microscopical light conditions[a]		
	Plain	Polarized	UV
Undecalcified			
Ground or microtome stained	1,2,3,4,7,8,9,10,11,12 ground Fig. A-2, microtome Figs. A-3, A-5, A-11, A-12	5, Fig. A-4	
Ground or microtome silver impregnated	2,4, Fig. A-1	2,5	
Ground microradiograph	3,4,6,7,9,10, Figs. A-7– A-9		
Ground or microtome unstained, labeled		5	3, Fig. A-14
Decalcified			
Stained	1,4,7,8,9,10,11,12, Figs. A-6, A-10	5, Fig. A-13	

[a] Numbers refer to histological features.

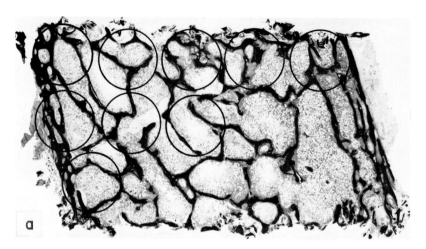

Fig. A-1a

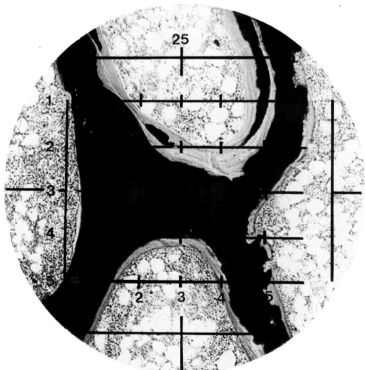

Fig. A-1b

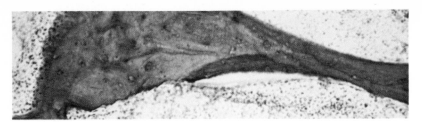

Fig. A-2

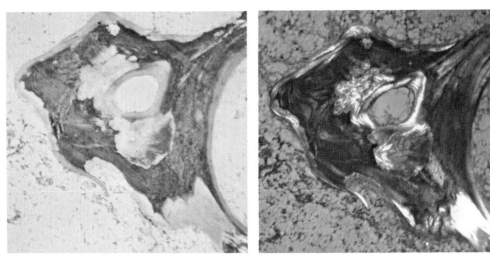

Fig. A-3

Fig. A-4

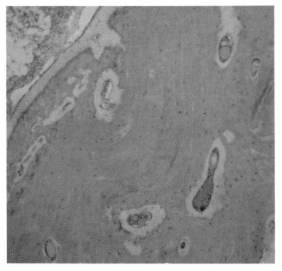

Fig. A-5

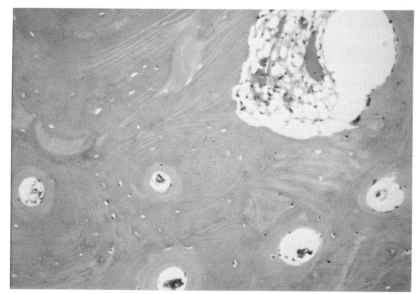

Fig. A-6

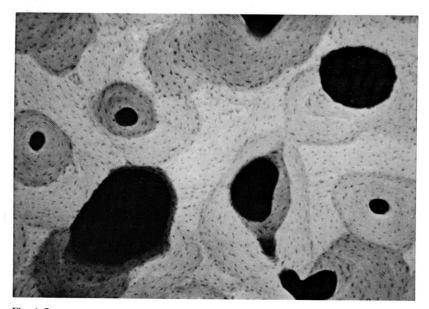

Fig. A-7

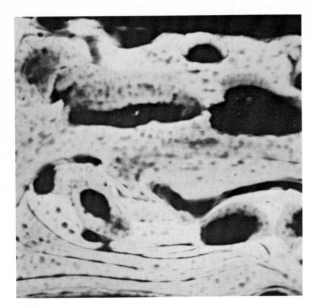

Fig. A-8

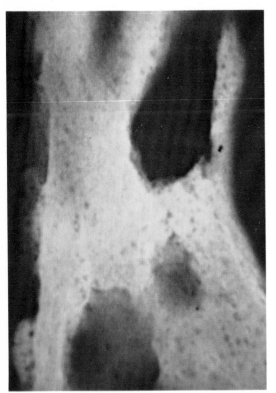

Fig. A-9

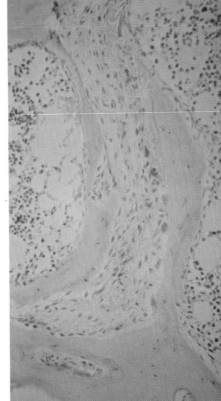

Fig. A-10

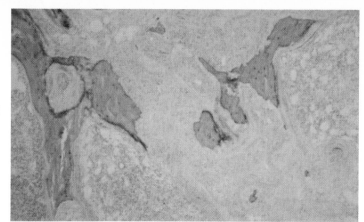

Fig. A-11

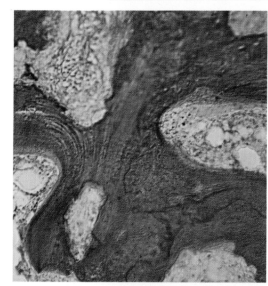

Fig. A-12

Fig. A-13

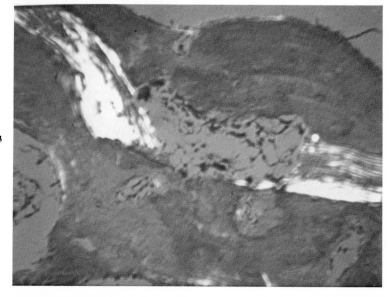

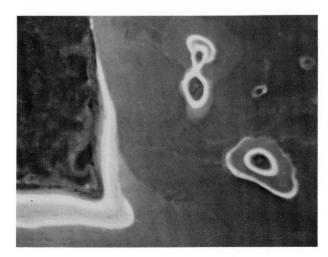

Fig. A-14

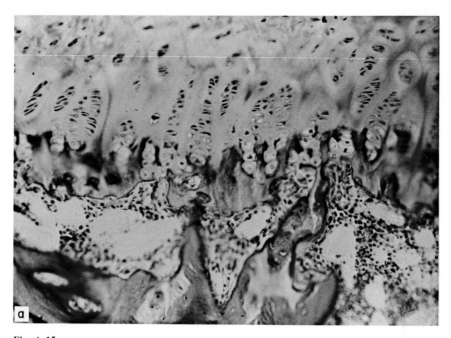

Fig. A-15a

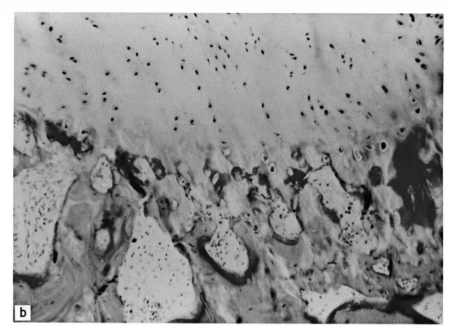

Fig. A-15b

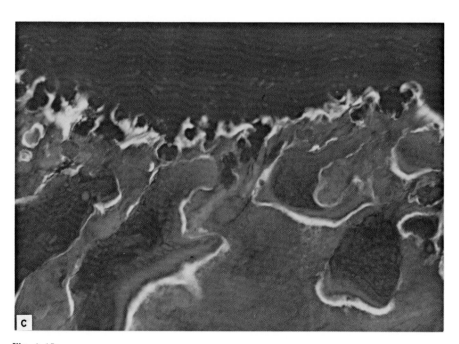

Fig. A-15c

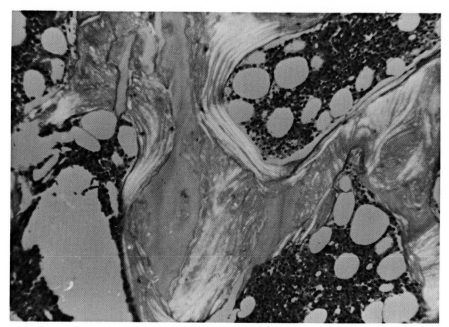

Fig. A-16

important diagnostic features available in histological preparations are listed in Table A-1 together with the type of section and microscopical lighting conditions in which they can be seen to advantage. The photomicrographs in which these features are illustrated are included in Table A-1.

However, a brief comment might be useful. In histological preparations the distinction between bone and osteoid is only reliably demonstrated when the mineral is present. In an undecalcified section hematoxylin stains the mineralized tissue, and osteoid is stained by eosin; when the mineral is removed all the tissue then stains with eosin. The decalcified bone and osteoid may or may not stain with a different intensity, but this cannot be controlled. Hence a positive finding is meaningful but a negative one is not. Most stains will give a distinction between bone and osteoid in undecalcified sections, some being more satisfactory than others. Solochrome cyanin of itself stains them differentially. It has been popular because of claims for the staining of the calcification front; but it is only one of a number of dyes that will do this. As has been pointed out in the text, the reliability of stains is questionable in demonstrating the front. Stained, undecalcified sections show where the mineral is, but they do not generally demonstrate variations in its density. Stains that do show variations in density have been described (Villaneuva, 1967) and may be used diagnostically instead of microradiography. However, the latter shows in great detail the aberrations of mineral density described in this chapter as a periosteocytic mineral defect. When the mineral is completely absent from these defects they can be seen in stained undecalcified sections. The microradiograph may be used to characterize surface activity. It is a good preparation in which to measure osteocyte lacunae; however, it cannot be used as an index of cellular activity without benefit of other stained preparations. Cytological details are good in most decalcified or undecalcified stained sections. The features do appear differently in the two types of section, and one may be preferred over another, but given adequate preparation the undecalcified may well be superior. Nevertheless there can be difficulties in determining cell types which should not be underestimated. There are special stains for collagen, but they are unnecessary because collagen can be visualized simply by polarized light. The birefringence of the fibers is obscured by some stains, and maximum resolution is achieved with unstained sections, but the recognition of lamellar or woven patterns or the reduction or absence of the fibers can be adequately assessed in stained section. The demonstration of resorption is very much a matter of being able to recognize surfaces where osteoclasts have been active. (It is an obvious bit of pedantry to say that nothing is happening in a histological section since the tissue is dead, and every attribution of current activity is an interpretation). Multinucleated osteoclasts are readily recognized but mononuclear osteoclasts are more problematical; nevertheless both almost certainly mean active resorption and may be used for a resorption index. Reversal lines do not always stain well in histological sections, whether decalcified or undecalcified, but one can frequently get a good indication of their pattern from the pattern of the tissue, particularly that of the collagen fibers.

Fig. A-1. Illustrating a quantitative method for areas and surfaces applicable to bone and osteoid. Iliac crest biopsy in osteomalacia. Undecalcified, plastic embedded, ground section; impregnated by silver after the Von Kossa method. (a) ×10 and (b) ×53.

Circles on the Fig. A-1a of the whole section indicate how successive fields are examined with a graticule eyepiece until the whole section has been covered. Strictly speaking, there should be a distinction between cortex and cancellous bone, because of their different volumes and surface areas. The size of the sample can be increased by overlapping the fields and by rotating the graticule within a field. Figure A-1b shows an enlargement of one field with the Zeiss integrating disc 1 in the eyepiece (Gahm, 1968).

The size of the field is determined by the magnification used. Most details can be resolved at 80 to 100 times, but the resolution of cellular detail may require magnification up to 300 or 400 times. The graticule is constituted of five lines within a square, the boundaries of which can be used to determine field limits, but also absolute field size for given magnifications. Each of the five lines has five crossbars that locate the counting points. Surface values are obtained by recording the characteristic of the surface where it is intercepted by the lines. Thus, inert bone, resorption, osteoid with and without active osteoblasts, and/or calcification front can be determined as a proportion of total intercepts or in absolute values by using the total line length and field size for the magnification. Osteoclasts do not form continuous layers and they must be counted individually to calculate a resorption index. The graticule points may be used for area measurements; the tissue under each is recorded (bone, osteoid, marrow space), and their values are calculated in relative or absolute terms.

In the photomicrographs of this figure the bone is black, and the osteoid is a pale layer overlying it. Osteoid is excessively abundant both in terms of surface covered and area occupied. Irregular mineralization of the osteoid is shown by isolated tongues of mineral. The staining procedure does not distinguish between actively occurring (a calcification front) or established mineralization. If this section is viewed in polarized light, only the osteoid collagen is visible, and only its collagen structure can be studied.

Fig. A-2. Illustrating bone, osteoid, active osteoblasts, calcification front, reversal lines, resorption, osteoclasts, inert surface. Normal iliac crest. Undecalcified, plastic embedded, ground section, stained with hematoxylin and eosin. ×154.

The bone is purplish blue. One surface is partially covered by virtually colorless osteoid (an osteoid seam). This is covered in turn by a single layer of plump, dark cells—active osteoblasts. The bone rests on a crescent of bone more darkly stained, which may be the effect of recent mineralizing activity. This area is demarcated by a reversal line; several other lines are visible. The interface between bone and osteoid is clouded by a fine granularity that is the calcification front. In one direction the osteoid narrows gradually to the point of disappearance; in the other it narrows more abruptly and ends at a scalloped resorption surface. The latter extends to the top of the hump in the surface. The osteoclasts are obscure at this magnification because they are mononuclear and pale. The other surfaces are smooth and without active cells and are classed as inert.

Fig. A-3 and A-4. Illustrating bone, collagen, osteoid (normal and abnormal, with abnormal mineralization) and resorption. Iliac crest biopsy in osteomalacia. Undecalcified, plastic embedded, microtome section stained with hematoxylin and eosin. Figure A-3 photographed in plain light, Fig. A-4 in polarized light. $\times 45$.

The bone is bluish red and darker than the osteoid. Polarized light shows a lamellar collagen structure. (The background can be much darker but has been lightened for purposes of illustration; the inequality of birefringence is due to the variable orientation of the fibers with respect to the plane of the light, which can be overcome in practice by using a rotating microscope stage.) There is osteoid on all the surfaces and a large portion of the central area, but no osteoblastic activity nor evidence of calcification fronts. The interface between the osteoid and bone is scalloped in many places but smooth in others. Much of the osteoid is of a lamellar collagen structure, including that of the surface within the bone; but much osteoid deep to the latter has a woven collagen pattern that is abnormal in the adult. The poor staining quality of this osteoid in Fig. A-3 is indicative of its abnormal structure; the smudgy purple patch within it is the site of mineralization. A resorption cavity is being tunneled under the osteoid on the lower left surface; the polarized picture shows a thin layer of short, bright collagen fibers at this surface. Is this immature osteoid or fibrous replacement? At the top within the bony prominence there is a small intraosseous resorption cavity. (The single osteoclast within it is not clear in the photograph.) At some distance to right and left are a few pale areas within the bone suggesting a defect in mineralization (see also Fig. A-5, A-6, and A-8).

Fig. A-5. Illustrating bone, osteoid, active osteoblasts, osteocytes, perilacunar mineral defect ("halo volume"). Rib in osteomalacia. Undecalcified, plastic embedded, microtome section stained with solochrome cyanin. $\times 67$.

The bone is pale blue, and covered by a gray band on all surfaces, both osteonal and endosteal. The latter is covered by a layer of active osteoblasts. The osteoid bone interfaces are smooth and at the endosteal surface stains darkly and might be characterized as a calcification front. Nuclei of osteocytes are just discernible as pinpoint dark blue dots; some of these are surrounded by pale pinkish gray zones of various shapes, the sites from which mineral has been lost through osteocytic activity; the lacunae are not enlarged (see Figs. A-6 and A-8 for other preparations from this case).

Fig. A-6. Illustrating decalcified bone, lamellar collagen, resorption, osteoclasts, osteoid, osteoblasts, osteocytes, and lacunae. Rib in osteomalacia. Decalcified, paraffin section of rib stained with hematoxylin and eosin, same case as Fig. A-5 and A-8. ×154.

The bone is stained red and shows the details of cortical architecture rather more clearly than the previous photomicrograph. This consists of osteons whose limits can be recognized by their just discernible lamellar pattern; the reversal lines that bound them are not stained. The bone tissue between osteons, also of lamellar structure, is classed as interstitial. Five osteonal canals are small and are surrounded by a zone that is paler staining than the rest. This zone is osteoid and is unexpectedly differentiated in this decalcified preparation. Sparse, flattened, inactive osteoblasts lie on these osteonal surfaces. The larger cavity has been resorbed, and a few small osteoclasts are present in Howships lacunae that cover much of its surface. The remainder of the surface in this cavity is smooth, covered by a single layer of as yet inactive osteoblasts. The osteocyte lacunae are clearly evident and slightly variable in outline and in size; the osteocytes are visible in only a proportion of them. This is not unusual in paraffin sections. The crescentic pale red zones in interstitial bone suggest deficient mineralization that is confirmed by the undecalcified section (Fig. A-5) and the microradiograph (Fig. A-8). The tissue within the osteonal cavities has been distorted in the process of preparing the sections.

Fig. A-7. Illustrating the microradiographic appearances of normal cortical bone: resorption, formation, mineral density, osteocytes, and lacunae. Femoral cortex from normal 17-year-old male. Undecalcified, plastic embedded, ground section microradiographed at a thickness of 70 nm. ×109.

The osteonal architecture is evident; the orientation of the ovoid osteocyte lacunae indicates the orientation of the lamellar structure. The bone between osteons is interstitial and the most densely mineralized; it can be used as a standard for 100% mineralization. The osteons are of several generations and show a range of mineral density, generally less than the interstitial bone. Resorption on the surface of the osteonal canal in the bottom left-hand corner has transgressed the original osteonal boundaries; eventually a new region of interstitial bone will result. At the opposite corner a small portion of the large osteonal canal has a resorption surface, whereas the remainder, a dark gray band, is the mineralizing portion of a forming surface (see Fig. A-2). The cessation of mineralization, and hence of formation, is recognized when a thin white line appears on the surface, as is present in the remaining osteons. The magnitude of the range in size of osteocyte lacunae is evident, as is the absence of any perilacunar reduction of mineral.

Fig. A-8. Illustrating the microradiographic appearances of abnormal cortical bone: resorption, formation, osteocyte lacunae, and perilacunar defect. Rib in osteomalacia. Undecalcified, plastic embedded, ground section microradiographed at a thickness of 70 μm. The same case as Figs. A-5 and A-6. ×67.

At several points the surfaces are scalloped, indicative of resorption. A few low density surfaces indicate that some mineralization, and hence formation, is occurring. The striking feature is the extensive perilacunar mineral reduction, giving a smudgy quality to much of the microradiograph. The appearances suggest large osteocyte lacunae, but the stained sections in Figs. A-5 and A-6 show that bone matrix surrounds the lacunae. The linear mineral defects occur at sites of reversal lines; these can be found in normal bone, but are not so extensive.

Fig. A-9. Illustrating the microradiographic changes in abnormal bone: resorption, formation, and enlarged osteocyte lacunae. Iliac crest in hyperparathyroidism. Undecalcified, plastic embedded, ground section microradiographed at a thickness of 70 μm. ×154.

The scalloped surfaces indicate that resorptive activity has been taking place. Many of the low density surfaces are due to the fact that they are not at right angles to the film; this is true for the resorbed as well as the inert and forming surfaces and is an artifact much more frequent in cancellous than in cortical bone cut at right angles to its axis. Low mineral density occurs on the surface at the bottom of the photomicrograph, this is a forming and mineralizing site. There are two small knobs of bone on this surface that stained sections show are composed of woven collagen. As is common in immature bone, the osteocyte lacunae are particularly large. Elsewhere most of the osteocyte lacunae are irregular in size and some are relatively large—the smallest are of normal size and give a comparative value. Within the bone in the upper right-hand quadrant there is an intratrabecular resorption cavity. This may be interpreted as an agglomeration of enlarged osteocyte lacunae, or as a cavity originating from surface resorption above or below the plane of section.

Fig. A-10. Illustrating resorption and fibrous replacement of bone. Iliac crest biopsy in hyperparathyroidism. Decalcified, paraffin embedded section, stained with hematoxylin and eosin. ×154.

A trabeculum of bone has undergone central resorption, the space being filled by fibrous tissue. Polarized light would demonstrate short irregularly arranged collagen fibers, giving an appearance similar to that seen in the resorption cavity at the bottom of Fig. A-4. Osteoclasts are small polynuclear cells on one of the bone surfaces. The osteocyte lacunae are not enlarged. The marrow is distinctly shown and is free of fibrous tissue. The distinction between surface and intratrabecular resorption is without diagnostic significance and are the same process.

Fig. A-11. Illustrating resorption, fibrous replacement of bone and marrow, formation (both as surface apposition and membrane bone formation), and calcification front. Iliac crest in hyperparathyroidism. Undecalcified, plastic embedded, microtome section stained with solochrome cyanin. ×67.

Most of the bone trabecula (blue) have been resorbed. Fibrous tissue has replaced them and much of the adjacent marrow. The bone surfaces are either scalloped where resorption has occurred or are covered by osteoid where appositional formation is taking place. Osteoclasts are numerous but not clear in this photomicrograph; osteoblasts appear as a dark line overlying the osteoid; the dark band between osteoid and bone can be interpreted as calcification front. Within the fibrous tissue there are pale islands, sometimes outlined by a blue band of osteoblasts and sometimes containing a central bony (blue) focus. These are foci of membrane bone formation (once they are established their further increase in size is by appositional and not interstitial growth). A few osteocytes are evident in the trabecula as dark dots, but it is not possible to say more of their lacunae than that they are not obviously enlarged.

Fig. A-12. Illustrating reversal lines (mosaic pattern), resorption, formation, and lamellar and woven bone. Iliac crest in Paget's disease of bone. Undecalcified, plastic embedded, microtome section stained with hematoxylin and eosin. ×109.

The bone is blue in color. The reversal lines are dark and demarcate small areas, some of which are clearly lamellar, representing the original bone, whereas for the remainder the inference is that the collagen is woven in structure, which could be confirmed by examination in polarized light (see Fig. A-4). The relative proximity of reversal lines and their scalloped shape form the mosaic pattern. The bone surfaces show resorption and osteoid. Some mononuclear cells in resorption cavities must be regarded as osteoclasts, but osteoblasts are not seen.

Fig. A-13. Illustrating deficient collagen fibers in fibrogenesis imperfecta ossium, resorption and osteoid. Patella in fibrogenesis imperfecta ossium. Decalcified, paraffin embedded section, stained with hematoxylin eosin. ×155.

The normal bone is seen as a bright band of lamellar collagen fibers; it is interrupted by a resorption cavity whose surfaces are covered by osteoclasts. This bone is encased by other material with greatly reduced birefringence, which is both mineralized and unmineralized. The limits of the mineral can be seen in the lower edge at the tip of the bright line. It is not known whether the reduced birefringence is due to an absolute reduction in the number of collagen fibers or to an abnormal configuration of the collagen that is not anisotropic. This decalcified section was one in which the difference between bone and osteoid was preserved.

Fig. A-14. Illustrating tetracycline labeling of bone. Femoral cortex from rabbit following labeling with tetracycline on two occasions. Undecalcified, plastic embedded, ground section viewed in ultraviolet light. ×155.

Both cortical and trabecular bone are shown. Single and double labels are present, indicating the sites where mineralization was occurring when the tetracycline was administered. This can be used not only to confirm active mineralization but also to measure the quantity of bone produced in the time interval between labels. Owing to differences in the fluorescent color of various antibiotics, three or more labels can be used.

Fig. A-15. Illustrating the growth plate in mild rickets compared with normal. Iliac apophysis: undecalcified microtome sections. (a) Normal, age-matched control, solochrome cyanin. (b) Clinical rickets; solochrome cyanin. (c) Clinical rickets; unstained, ultraviolet light.

The most striking observation is the relative disorder of the cellular columns, whose cells are strung out and encompass a relatively wide zone. The diminution in blue staining of the cartilage suggests reduced mineralization. However, this is less evident in Fig. A-15 which shows the tetracycline label quite widely distributed here and in osteoid. Differences in the quantities of osteoid between Fig. A-15a and b cannot be established with confidence.

Fig. A-16. Illustrating the sclerotic bone of osteopetrosis. Iliac crest biopsy. Decalcified paraffin section, stained with hematoxylin and eosin viewed in partially polarized light. ×88.

The large amount of bone, due to broad trabecula, may be judged in comparison with other illustrations. This is not sufficient to encroach seriously on the narrow space. The bone structure is mainly lamellar, although some foci of woven collagen are present. The tissue encases cores of cartilage that have a diffuse low intensity birefringence without an obvious fiber structure. The surfaces have few cells and show little activity.

REFERENCES

Adams, P., Davies, G. T., and Sweetnam, P. (1970). *Q. J. Med.* **39**, 601.

Ali, S. Y. (1976). *Fed. Proc., Fed. Am. Soc. Exp. Biol.* **35**, 135.

Ali, S. Y., Sajdera, S. W., and Anderson, H. C. (1970). *Proc. Natl. Acad. Sci. U.S.A.* **67**, 1513.

Amprino, R., and Bairati, A. (1936). Z. Zellforsch. Mikrosk. Anat. 24, 439.

Amprino, R., and Engstrom, A. (1952). Acta Anat. 15, 1.

Amprino, R., and Sisto, L. (1947). Acta Anat. 2, 202.

Anderson, H. C. (1973). Hard Tissue Growth, Repair Remineralization, Ciba Found. Symp., 1972 p. 213.

Arnold, J. S., and Bartley, M. H. (1965). Fed. Proc., Fed. Am. Soc. Exp. Biol. 24, 554.

Arnold, J. S., Frost, H. M., and Buss, R. O. (1971). Clin. Orthop. Relat. Res. 78, 47.

Arnstein, A. R., Frame, B., and Frost, H. M. (1967). Ann. Intern. Med. 67, 1296.

Baker, S. L. (1956). J. Bone Joint Surg., Br. Vol. 38, 378.

Baker, S. L., Dent, C. E., Friedman, M., and Watson, L. (1966). J. Bone Joint Surg., Br. Vol. 48, 804.

Ball, J. (1960). In "Recent Advances in Pathology" (C. V. Harrison, ed.), 7th ed., Chapter 9. Churchill, London.

Ball, J., and Garner, A. (1966). J. Pathol. Bacteriol. 91, 563.

Barry, H. C. (1969). "Paget's Disease of Bone." Livingstone, Edinburgh.

Barzel, U. S., and Jowsey, J. (1969). Clin. Sci. 36, 517.

Baud, C. A. (1968). Clin. Orthop. Relat. Res. 56, 227.

Baud, C. A., and Anil, E. (1971). Acta Anat. 78, 321.

Bélanger, L. F. (1969). Calcif. Tissue Res. 4, 1.

Bélanger, L. F., Robichon, J., Migicovsky, B. B., Copp, D. H., and Vincent, J. (1963). In "Mechanism of Hard Tissue Destruction" (R. F. Sognnaes, ed.), p. 531. Publ. No. 75. Am. Ass. Advan. Sci., Washington, D.C.

Bingham, P., Brazell, I. A., and Owen, M. (1969). J. Endocrinol. 45, 387.

Bohr, H. H. (1967). In "L'ostéomalacie" (D. J. Hioco, ed.), p. 117. Masson, Paris.

Boothroyd, B. (1964). J. Cell Biol. 20, 165.

Bordier, P. J., and Tun Chot, S. (1972). "Clinics in Endocrinology and Metabolism" (I. MacIntrye, ed.), vol. 1 p. 197. Saunders, Philadelphia, Pennsylvania.

Bordier, P., Matrajt, H., Maravet, L., and Hioco, D. J. (1964). Pathol. Biol. 12, 1238.

Bourne, G. H. (1971). In "The Biochemistry and Physiology of Bone" 2nd ed., vol. 1 p. 211. Academic Press, New York.

Byers, P. D. (1962). J. Bone Joint Surg., Br. Vol. 44, 225.

Byers, P. D. (1963). J. Bone Joint Surg., Br. Vol. 45, 221.

Byers, P. D. (1975). In "Some Observations on the Training of a Surgeon" (L. Kessel and P. Byers, eds.), p. 10. Publ. No. 2. Institute of Orthopaedics, London.

Byers, P. D., and Jones, A. N. (1969). Br. J. Surg. 56, 262.

Byers, P. D., and Smith, R. (1967). Br. Med. J. 1, 682.

Byers, P. D., and Smith, R. (1971). Q. J. Med. 40, 471.

Cameron, G. R. (1930). J. Pathol. Bacteriol. 33, 929.

Cameron, J., and Sorensen, J. A. (1963). Science 142, 230.

Chalmers, J., and Weaver, J. K. (1966). J. Bone Joint Surg., Am. Vol. 48, 299.

Cochran, M., and Nordin, B. E. C. (1969). Br. Med. J. 2, 276.

Collins, D. H. (1966). "Pathology of Bone," p. 228. Butterworth, London.

Curtis, A. S. G. (1960). Med. Biol. Illus. 10, 261.

Dent, C. E., and Hodson, C. J. (1954). Br. J. Radiol. 27, 605.

Dent, C. E., and Watson, L. (1968). Lancet 2, 662.

Dent, C. E., Smellie, J. M., and Watson, L. (1965). Arch. Dis. Child. 40, 7.

Dequeker, J., Remans, J., Franssen, R., and Waes, J. (1971). Calcif. Tissue Res. 7, 23.

Dhem, A. (1966). Calcif. Tissues 1965, Proc. Eur. Symp., 3rd, 1965 p. 60.

Doyle, F. (1972). In "Clinics in Endocrinology and Metabolism" (I. MacIntyre, ed.), Vol. 1, p. 143. Saunders, Philadelphia, Pennsylvania.

Drury, R. A. B., and Wallington, E. A. (1967). Carleton's Histological Technique," 4th ed. Oxford Univ. Press, London and New York.

Dunnill, M. S., Anderson, J. A., and Whitehead, R. (1967). *J. Pathol. Bacteriol.* **94**, 275.

Editorial. (1971). *Lancet* **1**, 1168.

Engfeldt, B., Zetterstrom, R., and Winberg, J. (1956). *J. Bone Joint Surg., Am. Vol.* **38**, 1323.

Engstrom, A., Cosslett, V. E., and Pattee, H. H. (eds.) (1960). *Proc. Int. Symp. X-ray Microsc. Microanal., 2nd, 1960.*

Evans, D. J., and Azzopardi, J. G. (1972). *Lancet* **1**, 353.

Exton-Smith, A. M., Millard, P. H., Payne, P. R., and Wheeler, E. F. (1969). *Lancet* **2**, 1153.

Fairbank, H. A. T. (1951). "An Atlas of General Affections of the Skeleton." Livingstone, Edinburgh.

Feinstein, A. R. (1967). "Clinical Judgment." Williams & Wilkins, Baltimore, Maryland.

Flanagan, B., and Nichols, G. (1964). *Endocrinology* **74**, 180.

Fleisch, H., Bisaz, S., Care, A. D., Muhlbauer, R. C., and Russell, R. G. G. (1970). *Calcitonin Proc. Int. Symp., 2nd, 1969,* p. 409.

Frame, B., and Nixon, R. K. (1970). *In* "Osteoporosis" (U. S. Barzel, ed.), p. 238. Grune & Stratton, New York.

Frame, B., Frost, H. M., Pak, C. Y. C., Reynolds, W., and Argen, R. J. (1971). *N. Engl. J. Med.* **285**, 769.

Frost, H. M. (1959). *Stain Technol.* **34**, 135.

Frost, H. M. (1960a). *J. Bone Joint Surg., Am. Vol.* **42**, 447.

Frost, H. M. (1960b). *Henry Ford Hosp. Med. Bull.* **8**, 267.

Frost, H. M. (1960c). *Stain Technol.* **35**, 135.

Frost, H. M. (1962). *Henry Ford Hosp. Med. Bull.* **10**, 267.

Frost, H. M. (1963). "Bone Remodelling Dynamics." Thomas, Springfield, Illinois.

Frost, H. M. (1964). *Bone Biodyn., Proc. Symp., 1963* p. 315.

Frost, H. M. (1966). "The Bone Dynamics in Osteoporosis and Osteomalacia." Thomas, Springfield, Illinois.

Frost, H. M. (1969). *Calcif. Tissue Res.* **3**, 211.

Frost, H. M. (1973). *In Proc. Int. Symp. Clin. Aspects Metab. Bone Dis., 1972,* p. 124.

Gahm, J. (1968). *Zeiss Inf. Leafl.* No. 70, pp. 138–143.

Gaillard, P. J. (1965). *In* "The Parathyroid Glands" (P. J. Gaillard, R. V. Talmage, and A. M. Budy, eds.), p. 145. Univ. of Chicago Press, Chicago, Illinois.

Garner, A., and Ball, J. (1966). *J. Pathol. Bacteriol.* **91**, 545.

Haas, H. G., Muller, J., and Schenk, R. K. (1967). *Clin. Orthop. Relat. Res.* **53**, 213.

Hancox, N. M., and Boothroyd, B. (1963). *In* "Mechanisms of Hard Tissue Destruction" (R. F. Sognnaes, ed.), Publ. No. 75, p. 497. Am. Assoc. Adv. Sci., Washington, D.C.

Harris, E. E. (1970). "Hypothesis and Perception: The Roots of Scientific Method." Humanities Press, Inc., New York.

Harris, W. H. (1960). *Nature (London)* **188**, 1038.

Harris, W. H., Haywood, E. A., Lavorgna, J., and Hamblen, D. L. (1968). *J. Bone Joint Surg., Am. Vol.* **50**, 1118.

Hattner, R., Epker, B. N., and Frost, H. M. (1965). *Nature (London)* **206**, 489.

Heaney, R. P. (1962). *Am. J. Med.* **33**, 188.

Hennig, A. (1967). *Zeiss Werkzeitschr.* **30**, 78.

Herring, G. M. (1964). *Clin. Orthop. Relat. Res.* **36**, 169.

Heycock, C. T., and Neville, F. H. (1898). *Trans. Chem. Soc. London* **73**, 714.

Holley, K. J. (1969). M.D. Thesis, University of London, London.

Hong, Y. C., Yen, P. K.-J., and Shaw, J. H. (1968). *Calcif. Tissue Res.* **2**, 286.

Horsman, A. *et al.* (1970). *In* "Proceedings of Bone Measurement Conference" (J. R. Cameron, ed.), Conf. 700515. U.S. At. Energy Comm., Washington, D.C.

Hoyte, D. A. N. (1960). *J. Anat.* **94,** 432.

Jande, S. S., and Bélanger, L. F. (1971). *Calcif. Tissue Res.* **6,** 280.

Jee, W. S. S., Blackwood, E. L., Dockum, N. L., Haslam, R. K., and Kincl, F. A. (1966). *Clin. Orthop. Relat. Res.* **49,** 39.

Jenkins, D. H. R., Roberts, J. G., Webster, D., and Williams, E. D. (1973). *J. Bone Joint Surg., Br. Vol.* **55,** 575.

Johnson, L. C. (1964). *Bone Biodyn., Proc. Symp., 1963* p. 543.

Jowsey, J. (1960). *Clin. Orthop. Relat. Res.* **17,** 210.

Jowsey, J. (1963). *In* "Mechanisms of Hard Tissue Destruction" (R. F. Sognnaes, ed.), Publ. No. 75, p. 447. Am. Assoc. Adv. Sci., Washington, D.C.

Jowsey, J. (1964). *Bone Biodyn., Proc. Symp., 1963* p. 461.

Jowsey, J. (1966). *Am. J. Med.* **40,** 485.

Jowsey, J., and Riggs, B. L. (1970). *Acta Endocrinol. (Copenhagen)* **63,** 21.

Jowsey, J., Riggs, B. L., and Kelly, P. J. (1964). *Mayo Clin. Proc.* **39,** 480.

Jowsey, J., Kelly, P. J., Riggs, B. L., Bianco, A. J., Scholz, D. A., and Gershon-Cohen, J. (1965). *J. Bone Joint Surg., Am. Vol.* **47,** 785.

Jowsey, J., Massry, S. G., and Coburn, J. W. (1969). *Arch. Intern. Med.* **124,** 539.

Katz, A. L., Hampers, C. L., and Merrill, J. P. (1969). *Medicine (Baltimore)* **48,** 333.

Kaye, M., Chatterjee, G., Cohen, G. F., and Sagar, S. (1970). *Ann. Intern. Med.* **73,** 225.

Kerr, D. N. S., Walls, J. Ellis, H., Simpson, W., Uldall, P. R., and Ward, M. K. (1969). *J. Bone Joint Surg., Br. Vol.* **51,** 578.

Kim, D., Bell, N. H., Bundesen, W., Putong, P., Simon, N. M., Walle, C., and del Greco, F. (1968). *Trans. Am. Soc. Artif. Intern. Organs* **14,** 367.

Kirby-Smith, H. T. (1933). *Am. J. Anat.* **53,** 377.

Krane, S. M., Parsons, V., and Krunin, A. S. (1967). *In* "Studies on the Metabolism of Epiphyseal Cartilage in Cartilage Degeneration and Repair" (C. C. Andrew and L. Bassett, eds.), p. 43. Nat. Res. Counc., Natl. Acad. Sci., Washington, D.C.

Lamarque, P. (1938). *Br. J. Radiol.* **11,** 425.

Lee, W. R. (1963). M.D. Thesis, University of Manchester.

Lee, W. R. (1967). *J. Bone Joint Surg., Br. Vol.* **49,** 146.

Lloyd, E., and Hodges, D. (1971). *Clin. Orthop. Relat. Res.* **78,** 230.

Loe, H. (1959). *Acta Odontol. Scand.* **17,** Suppl. 27, 311.

Mankin, H. J., and Lipprello, L. (1969). *J. Bone Joint Surg., Am. Vol.* **51,** 862.

Matrajt, H., and Hioco, D. (1966). *Stain Technol.* **41,** 97.

Matrajt, H., Bordier, P., Martin, J., and Hioco, D. (1967). *J. Microsc. (Paris)* **6,** 499.

Mazess, R. B. (1971). *Invest. Radiol.* **6,** 52.

Meema, H. E. (1963). *Am. J. Roentgenol., Radium Ther. Nucl. Med.* [N.S.] **89,** 1287.

Melvin, K. E. W., Hepner, G. W., Bordier, P., Neale, G., and Joplin, G. F. (1970). *Q. J. Med.* **39,** 83.

Merz, W. A. (1967). *Mikroskopie* **22,** 132.

Merz, W. A., and Schenk, R. V. (1970). *Acta Anat.* **75,** 54.

Merz, W. A., and Schenk, R. K. (1970). *Acta Anat.* **76,** 1.

Meunier, P., Aaron, J., Edouard, C., and Vignon, G. (1971). *Clin. Orthop. Relat. Res.* **80,** 147.

Meunier, P., Bernard, J., and Vignon, G., (1971). *Israel J. Med. Sci.* **7,** 482.

Meunier, P., Vignon, G., Bernard, J., Edouard, C., and Coupron, P. (1973). *Proc. Int. Symp. Clin. Aspects Bone Dis., 1972,* p. 215.

Milch, R. A., Rall, D. P., and Tobie, J. E. (1958). *J. Bone Joint Surg., Am. Vol.* **40,** 897.

Miller, E. J., and Martin, G. R. (1968). *Clin. Orthop. Relat. Res.* **59,** 195.

Murray, R. O., and Jacobson, H. G. (1971). "The Radiology of Skeletal Disorders." Churchill, London.

Nichols, G., Jr., and Wasserman, R. H. (1971). "Cellular Mechanisms for Calcium Transfer and Homeostasis." Academic Press, New York.

Nordin, B. E. C. (1964). *Bone Biodyn., Broc. Symp., 1963*, p. 521.

Owen, M. (1970). *Int. Rev. Cytol.* **28**, 213.

Owen, M. (1972). *In* "The Biochemistry and Physiology of Bone" (G. H. Bourne, ed.), 2nd ed., Vol. 3, Chapter 8. Academic Press, New York.

Perry, W., Stamp, T. C. B., Allen, L. N., and Walker, P. G. (1976). In preparation.

Popowitz, M., and Johnston, A. D. (1971). *Clin. Orthop. Relat. Res.* **74**, 185.

Price, C. H. G. (1962). *J. Bone Joint Surg., Br. Vol.* **44**, 366.

Raina, V. (1972). *J. Clin. Pathol.* **25**, 229.

Ramser, J. R., Villanueva, A. R., and Frost, H. M. (1966). *Clin. Orthop. Relat. Res.* **49**, 89.

Rang, M., ed. (1969). "The Growth Plate and its Disorders." Livingstone, Edinburgh.

Rasmussen, H., and Bordier, P. (1974). "The Physiological and Cellular Basis of Metabolic Bone Disease." Williams & Wilkins, Baltimore, Maryland.

Reynolds, J. J. (1970). *Calcif. Tissue Res.* **4**, Suppl., 52.

Robichon, J., and Germain, J. P. (1968). *Can. Med. Assoc. J.* **99**, 975.

Robinson, R. A., and Cameron, T. A. (1956). *J. Biophys. Biochem. Cytol.* **2**, 253.

Rubin, P. (1964). "Dynamic Classification of Bone Dysplasias." Yearbook Publ., Chicago, Illinois.

Sandison, J. C. (1928). *Anat. Rec.* **40**, 41.

Saville, P. D. (1965). *J. Bone Joint Surg., Am. Vol.* **47**, 492.

Schenk, R. K., Merz, W. A., and Muller, J. (1969). *Acta Anat.* **74**, 44.

Schenk, R. K., Spiro, D., and Wiener, J. (1967). *J. Cell Biol.* **34**, 275.

Schenk, R. K., Olak, A. J., and Merz, W. *Proc. Int. Symp. Clin. Aspects Metab. Bone Dis., 1972*, p. 103.

Schmorl, G. (1932). *Virchows Arch. Pathol. Anat. Physiol.* **283**, 694.

Schorr, W. S. (1968). *Proc. Eur. Dial. Transplant Assoc.* **5**, 408.

Sedlin, E. D., Frost, H. M., and Villanueva, A. R. (1963). *Henry Ford Hosp. Med. Bull.* **11**, 217.

Sirois, J. (1963). *Can. Med. Assoc. J.* **89**, 1043.

Sissons, H. A. (1960). *In* "Bone as a Tissue" (K. Rodahl, J. T. Nicholson, and E. M. Brown, eds.), p. 3. McGraw-Hill, New York.

Sissons, H. A. (1966). *Clin. Orthop. Relat. Res.* **45**, 73.

Sissons, H. A., and Lee, W. R. (1964). *Bone Tooth, Proc. Eur. Symp., 1st, 1963*, p. 65.

Sissons, H. A., Holley, K. J., and Heighway, J. (1967). *In* "L'ostéomalacie" (D. J. Hioco, ed.), p. 19. Masson, Paris.

Sissons, H., Darby, A. J., Duggal, K., and Whyte, M. (1975). *In* "Modern Trends in Orthopaedic Surgery" (Z. Buzdeek, ed.), p. 27. Purkyně Univ. Med. Faculty, Brno.

Smeenk, D. (1961). *J. Clin. Invest.* **40**, 433.

Smith, R., Russell, R. G. G., and Bishop, M. (1971). *Lancet* **1**, 945.

Stanbury, S. W. (1968). *Am. J. Med.* **44**, 714.

Stanbury, S. W. (1972). *In* "Clinics in Endocrinology and Metabolism" (I. MacIntyre, ed.), Vol. 1, p. 239. Saunders, Philadelphia, Pennsylvania.

Swinson, D. R., Tam, C. S., Reed, R., Hoffman, D., Little, A. H., and Cruikshank, B. (1975). *J. Pathol.* **116**, 13.

Stanley, P., Baker, S. L., and Byers, P. D. (1971). *Br. J. Radiol.* **44**, 305.

Stewart, B. J. C., Sheppard, H. G., Preece, R. F., and Exton-Smith, A. N. (1972). *Age Ageing* **1**, 1.

Stewart, B. L. (1962). Ph.D. Thesis, University of London, London.

Takahashi, H., Hattner, R., Epker, B. N., and Frost, H. M. (1964). *Henry Ford Hosp. Med. Bull.* **12**, 359.

Talmage, R. V. (1969). *Clin. Orthop. Relat. Res.* **67**, 210.

Tam, C. S., Reed, R., Cruikshank, B. (1974). *J. Pathol.* **113**, 27.

Thomas, W. C., Jr., and Moore, T. H. (1968). *Trans. Am. Climatol. (Clin.) Assoc.* **80**, 54.

Tripp, E. J., and MacKay, E. H. (1972). *Stain Technol.* **47**, 129.

Trotter, M., and Peterson, R. R. (1967). *Clin. Orthop. Relat. Res.* **52**, 233.

Trotter, M., Broman, G. E., and Peterson, R. R. (1959). *Am. J. Physiol. Anthrop.* **17**, 19.

Underwood, E. E. (1970). "Quantitative Stereology." Addison-Wesley, Reading Massachusetts.

Vaes, G., and Nichols, G. (1962). *Endocrinology* **70**, 546.

van der Heul, R. O., van der Sluys Veer, J., and Smeenk, D. (1964). *In* "L'ostéomalacie" (D. J. Hioco, ed.), p. 25. Masson, Paris.

van der Sluys Veer, J., Smeenk, D., and van der Heul, R. O. (1964). *Bone Tooth, Proc. Eur. Symp., 1st, 1963,* p. 85.

Vaughan, J. M. (1970). "The Physiology of Bone." Oxford Univ. Press (Clarendon), London and New York.

Vilaghy, M. I. (1973). *Proc. Int. Symp. Clin. Aspects Metab. Bone Dis., 1972,* p. 152.

Villaneuva, A. R. (1967). *Am. J. Clin. Pathol.* **47**, 780.

Vitali, P. H. (1968). *Clin. Orthop. Relat. Res.* **56**, 213.

Wakamatsu, E., and Sissons, H. A. (1969). *Calcif. Tissue Res.* **4**, 147.

Weibel, E. R. (1963). *Lab. Invest.* **12**, 131.

Whitehouse, W. J. (1974a). *J. Microsc. (Paris)* **101**, 154.

Whitehouse, W. J. (1974b). *J. Microsc. (Oxford)* **101**, 169.

Williams, E. D. (1972). *Proc. R. Soc. Med.* **65**, 539.

Williams, J. A., and Nicholson, G. I. (1963). *Lancet* **1**, 1408.

Wilson, R. V., Ramser, J. R., and Frost, H. M. (1968). *Clin. Orthop. Relat. Res.* **49**, 119.

Woodhouse, N. J. Y. (1972). *In* "Clinics in Endocrinology and Metabolism" (I. MacIntyre, ed.), p. 125. Saunders, Philadelphia, Pennsylvania.

Woodhouse, N. J. Y., Reiner, M., Bordier, P., Kalu, D. N., Fisher, M., Foster, G. V., Joplin, G. F., and MacIntyre, I. (1971). *Lancet* **1**, 1139.

Woods, C. G., Morgan, D. B., Paterson, C. R., and Gossmann, H. H. (1968). *J. Pathol. Bacteriol.* **95**, 449.

Wills, M. R. (1971). "The Biochemical Consequences of Chronic Renal Failure." Harvey Miller & Medcalf, Aylesbury, England.

Wu, K., Schubeck, K. E., Frost, H. M., and Villaneuva, A. (1970). *Calcif. Tissue Res.* **6**, 204.

Zeiss, C. (1960). "Intergrating Eyepiece Leaflet," 40-195C. Oberkochen, West Germany.

5

Vitamin D, Rickets, and Osteomalacia

C. E. DENT AND T. C. B. STAMP

I. INTRODUCTION

Rickets and, to a lesser extent, its adult equivalent osteomalacia have been the scourge of mankind until recent times. A large proportion of the children in temperate climes would in the past have had rickets at some time, usually in early infancy and during the late winter. It was only about 50 years ago that the first reliable experimental production of rickets in dogs was achieved by Mellanby (1919). This quickly led the way to confirmation in man in postwar Vienna (Medical Research Council, 1923),

237

where it was unambiguously shown that the disease was mainly due to the dietary lack of an oil-soluble substance present in close association with vitamin A in cod liver oil. It was further shown that exposure of the skin to sunlight could also cure rickets. The most gracious acknowledgment by Professor Clemens Pirquet in the introduction to the report from Vienna summarizes most adequately the importance of the new discovery and the originality of these findings: "With regard to the etiology of rickets I held the view that it was an infectious disease, producing severe symptoms only in the case of those children who possessed special susceptibility as the result of an inherited tendency, of a faulty diet, or of defective general hygiene. I imagined rickets to be a disease comparable to some extent with tuberculosis. . . . The British workers succeeded with the accuracy of a laboratory experiment, in a city where rickets was extremely prevalent, in maintaining a large number of artificially fed babies free from the disease, and further, were invariably successful in healing children with rickets already developed." From then on rickets quickly became a rare disease in adequately developed countries, since the disease is ridiculously easy to treat once diagnosed. Public health measures of prophylaxis by repeated small doses of cod liver oil, or even by one large dose of high potency vitamin D given at the beginning of winter, effectively prevents its occurrence. This major landmark, however, had another effect that could not have been anticipated by the original workers. It became clear that in spite of the virtual disappearance of the common disease, there still remained a few rare cases, resembling rickets in most ways, in which the ordinary doses of cod liver oil were ineffective. In other words, the modern chapter was opened in which the many forms of rickets (and osteomalacia) due to metabolic causes could be identified. The nomenclature of these diseases has been confused, since terms such as "renal rickets" were later expanded into many others. Nomenclature has inevitably become more specific with time, and the meaning of terms such as "renal rickets" or "resistant rickets" cannot be interpreted without some knowledge of the dates when they were used. For these reasons the various forms of rickets (and osteomalacia) have been recently tabulated (Dent, 1970) into a form that recorded their decade of discovery since Mellanby's dog experiments in 1919. It is not possible here to deal in the same detail with rickets or osteomalacia from all these different causes. Full references to the original papers are given in a review by Dent (1970) and in a later supplement (Dent, 1971). In this chapter, however, we will be rather selective and emphasize the more common syndromes or those that, though rare, illustrate an important theoretical principle. The disease will be described according to an abbreviated nonhistorical classification. We wish first to emphasize the remarkable resemblance, as far as the bones are concerned, between all the various forms. X-Rays showing a ricketic metaphysis or a Looser zone of osteomalacia may be identical even when the cause varies as widely as in chronic renal disease, forms of malabsorption syndrome, excessive anticonvulsant therapy, or in a disease caused by a rare recessive gene (presumably caused by an enzymatic dysfunction). The same nonspecificity may also be noted in the bone histology and in the main relevant plasma biochemical determinations (calcium, phosphate, and alkaline phosphatase). Hence when an etiology is sought, a wide search must be made in other body systems for the finersubtleties of the clinical pattern of the bone disease itself. For example, age of onset, severity, body proportions and deformities, and presence or absence of myopathy or of associated bone disease (especially osteoporosis) and of primary or secondary hyperparathyroidism will all help to identify the precise etiology. The successful end of the search leads to correct treatment, since the bone disease can always be cured. There are only three necessary medications, almost always vitamin D in one of its forms, and occasionally sodium bicarbonate and disodium hydrogen phosphate, but the exact dose of any one required may be very critical. It may also have to be supplemented with treatment for a primary disease, for instance, a gluten-free diet in the relevant enteropathy, penicillamine in Wilson's disease, and surgery if, for example, obstructive uropathy appears remediable or if a parathyroid adenoma has to be removed. These aspects will later be described in more detail, taking advantage of the fact that the main signs and symptoms, at least of the bone disease, are identical in all cases and therefore need only one description. First, however, we must say something about the key compound in this group of diseases, namely, vitamin D.

II. VITAMIN D AND ITS METABOLISM

Our knowledge of the mode of action and metabolism of vitamin D has made rapid progress in the past few years (DeLuca, 1971, 1974, 1976). The discovery that ingested vitamin D undergoes transformation to a circulating metabolite, that this metabolite then undergoes further transformation into a more biologically active form, and that production of these metabolites may be subject to feedback control mechanisms has led to the recognition that vitamin D can be regarded as a hormone as well as a vitamin. This hormonal concept of the antirickets agent is far from new, since in 1919, the same year that Mellanby (1919) discovered that cod liver oil could cure rickets, Huldschinsky (1919) showed that ultraviolet irradiation of a single limb would cure rickets not only in the irradiated limb but in the other limbs as well; these findings already fulfilled the early criteria of a hormone as a substance that was synthesized at one site in the body and exerted a powerful metabolic effect at a distant site. The nature of this metabolic effect and its analogy with the steroid hormones in regulating DNA transcription and mediating *de novo* protein synthesis are now clearer. This section traces the developments and their bearing on problems in clinical medicine.

Vitamin D_3, the natural substance cholecalciferol, reaches the body in two dissimilar ways: first, by formation in the skin (possibly with other active compounds) from the action of ultraviolet light on the physiological precursor 7-dehydrocholesterol and, second, in diets containing oily fish, eggs, animal liver, and dairy products. When one considers the totally dissimilar nature of these two sources, it is easy to understand the great confusion that surrounded the causes and cures of rickets in the first two decades of this century. Since then further difficulties in interpreting human disease have continuously arisen with the discovery of bone diseases that closely resemble classic rickets and osteomalacia but which may be resistant to treatment with vitamin D in doses up to one thousand times the amount required to heal the simple nutritional disease. These diseases may be associated with disorders of intestines, liver, or kidney and also include a host of inborn and acquired errors of metabolism. More than thirty such diseases have been listed (Dent, 1970, 1971). While their discovery and description continue even now, their understanding has been greatly simplified by recent advances in the understanding of vitamin D metabolism, advances that have indicated the importance of different, seemingly unrelated organs in controlling the ultimate expression of vitamin D activity.

Much of our knowledge of the physiology of vitamin D is summarized in Fig. 1. Synthesis of the natural vitamin D precursor 7-dehydrocholesterol is active in skin, liver, and intestine (Gaylor and Sault, 1964), but the exact way in which its irradiation products are absorbed through the skin of man is uncertain. In early studies (Helmer and Jansen, 1937a,b) antiricketic material was recoverable from human skin washings, and it was shown that cholecalciferol could cure rickets when applied to unbroken animal skin. Although it is necessary for fur-bearing animals to secrete 7-dehydrocholesterol onto the skin surface, probably via the sebaceous glands (Gaylor and Sault, 1964) before effective irradiation can occur, there is evidence that this process may not occur in man. 7-Dehydrocholesterol appears maximally concentrated in the Malphigian layer of human skin (Wheatley and Reinertson, 1958) and it has been shown that a large proportion of ultraviolet light wavelength that includes the antiricketic range (290–320 nm) can readily penetrate the stratum corneum of Caucasian skin (Thomson,

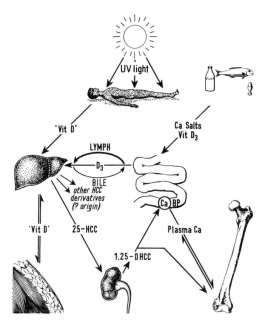

Fig. 1. Major pathways of vitamin D metabolism in man. Pathways are represented through skin, liver, small intestine, kidney, bone and storage reservoir of muscle and adipose tissue. Abbreviations: 25-HCC, 25-hydroxycholecalciferol; 1,25-DHCC, 1,25-dihydroxycholecalciferol; CaBP, calcium-binding protein.

1955; Loomis, 1967). While this penetration of ultraviolet light might conceivably be reduced in dark-skinned races owing to interference by melanin pigmentation, there is little direct evidence that vitamin D synthesis is reduced; artificial ultraviolet therapy rapidly cures nutritional rickets in dark-skinned Asian patients and rapidly raises circulating levels of the major vitamin D metabolite (Dent *et al.,* 1973a). Further work on skin synthesis and absorption of cholecalciferol, and possibly of other vitamin D metabolites, in man is thus required. Although some surface irradiation of 7-dehydrocholesterol may occur, frequent skin washing immediately before and after artificial ultraviolet irradiation has been shown not to delay healing of rickets nor notably to inhibit the rise in circulating vitamin D levels that occurs (Stamp, 1975).

Apart from certain oily fish such as tuna, mackerel, sardines, and salmon which contain large quantities of cholecalciferol (which they accumulate for reasons that are presently obscure), natural animal products are surprisingly deficient in vitamin D considering the natural connotations of the word ''vitamin'' (McCance and Widdowson, 1960). Thus, while all milk in the United States is fortified by the addition of 400 IU (0.01 mg) per quart, natural milk in Great Britain contains only approximately 5 units per pint. Long recommended intakes of 400 IU daily for children and 100 IU daily for adults are thus difficult to achieve without widespread fortification of foods with vitamin D. However, recent evidence, discussed further below, suggests that natural sunlight may be the more important source of vitamin D. Figure 1 shows vitamin D_3 (and calcium salts) from natural dietary sources entering the small intestine. Cholecalciferol is probably absorbed throughout the small intestine in humans, although the site of maximal absorption is still uncertain (Arnstein *et al.*, 1967). However, bile salts are necessary for its absorption in micelle form, although it is uncertain whether this requirement is absolute (Schacter *et al.*, 1964) or whether bile salts merely play a permissive role (Avioli, 1969; Thompson *et al.*, 1969; Stamp, 1974). At any rate, hepatic osteomalacia due to biliary obstruction can be cured by parenteral administration of physiological amounts (50 μg daily) of cholecalciferol (Dent and Stamp, 1970). Even so, osteomalacia is an uncommon complication of long-standing liver disease, and osteoporosis alone is much more commonly seen (Atkinson *et al.*, 1956). On the other hand, when rickets or osteomalacia is due to gluten-sensitive enteropathy (coeliac disease), the rickets may be resistant even to massive doses (1–2 mg) of vitamin D injected parenterally (Nassim *et al.*, 1959). Almost any form of steatorrhea may be complicated by rickets or osteomalacia, and the degree of resistance to treatment with vitamin D may vary considerably. The osteomalacia that sometimes follows partial gastrectomy is not infrequently due to self-restriction of vitamin D-containing fatty foods and may sometimes, therefore, respond to very small oral doses of vitamin D (Thompson *et al.*, 1966).

Major advances in our understanding of vitamin D metabolism have recently followed the use of isotopically labeled cholecalciferol of high specific activity. The first studies in this field were performed by Kodicek (1955), but it was not until 11 years later (Neville and DeLuca, 1966; Callow *et al.*, 1966) that it was possible to synthesize an isotope of high enough specific activity (20,000–26,000 dpm/IU) to clarify the pathways of vitamin D metabolism. After administration of the isotope to intact animals, chromatographic techniques were used to separate further discrete peaks of radioactivity corresponding to hydroxylated, and therefore more polar, metabolites of the parent vitamin. It was then shown that the major circulating form of the vitamin was a compound into which a second hydroxyl group had been introduced and this was identified as 25-hydroxycholecalciferol [25-OHD$_3$ (25-HCC, Fig. 2)]. Initial studies suggested that 25-OHD$_3$ itself was the biologically active form; it seemed to be synthesized only by the liver, and synthesis seemed closely regulated by a feedback control mechanism (DeLuca, 1971). Recent work has sug-

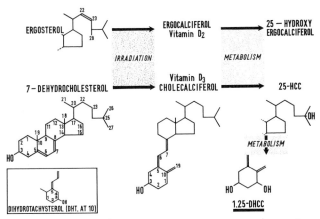

Fig. 2. Chemical transformations of vitamins D_2 and D_3 and their major metabolites. Ergosterol differs only in its side chain from 7-dehydrocholesterol, and only this side chain is shown. Similar changes are produced in both molecules by ultraviolet irradiation. Only the side chain of 25-hydroxycholecalciferol (25-HCC) and the A ring of 1,25-dihydroxycholecalciferol (1,25-DHCC) are shown.

gested, however, that some 25-hydroxylation of cholecalciferol may also occur in homogenates of chick kidney and intestine and that the process is not strongly inhibited in the presence of excess product (Tucker *et al.*, 1973). The possible physiological importance of other organs in the 25-hydroxylation of cholecalciferol and the enzymatic kinetics of the reaction may therefore require further study.

Vitamin D_2 (ergocalciferol), the well-known synthetic form of vitamin D, seems to be metabolized to 25-hydroxyergocalciferol (25-OHD$_2$) in identical fashion (see Fig. 2). Because both parent compounds have long been known to possess similar antiricketic activity in man, it may be assumed that in man both 25-hydroxylated derivatives also possess equal potency. The 25-hydroxy derivatives of both forms (together designated 25-OHD) can be measured by radio stereo assay (Haddad and Chyu, 1971). High concentrations of circulating 25-OHD are found in subjects with high occupational exposure to sunlight. Concentrations of 25-OHD increase rapidly during ultraviolet irradiation of the whole body, in spite of continuing vitamin D deficiency in the diet and in spite of the possession of a dark skin, which has popularly been supposed to lessen the transmission of ultraviolet light (Dent *et al.*, 1973a). 25-OHD$_2$ and 25-OHD$_3$ have been recently separated in human plasma; in the United States, where widespread fortification of foods with vitamin D_2 is practiced, plasma 25-OHD was still found to be composed largely of 25-OHD$_3$ (Haddad and Hahn, 1973). These findings indicate that the effect of sunlight on the skin, rather than the composition of the diet, provides the chief source of vitamin D in most human communities. Evidence is also forthcoming of marked seasonal variation in the plasma levels of 25-OHD in normal subjects in Britain, again indicating the major importance of summer (sunshine) in maintaining vitamin D nutrition (Stamp and Round, 1974). Mean 25-OHD levels in both normal adults and school children in London, England were about 13 ng/ml in early spring and 22 ng/ml in late summer. On an equivalence of 1 mg of 25-OHD$_3$ equals 50,000 IU vitamin D activity (DeLuca, 1971), these levels correspond to those levels of circulating antiricketic activity (measured in international units) in past bioassays of vitamin D in human plasma. The possibility that circulating antiricketic activity may thus be composed largely if not entirely of 25-OHD in normal human plasma is consistent with studies using isotopically labeled cholecalciferol which showed the virtual disappearance of isotopically labeled D$_3$ from the plasma within 2 to 5 days after injection, and showed the persistence of labeled 25-OHD$_3$ that resulted (Mawer et al., 1971). The actual rate of disappearance of isotopically labeled cholecalciferol and rate of appearance of 25-OHD and other more polar metabolites were shown to depend upon pool size in individual patients, that is on their state of vitamin D nutrition (Mawer et al., 1971).

The transporting proteins of cholecalciferol and 25-OHD$_3$ in the serum of various species have recently been studied (Edelstein et al., 1973). While chick serum contained two binding proteins, each relatively specific for one compound, the rat, pig, human, and monkey possessed a single binding protein responsible for the transport of both. In man, after intravenous injection of ^{3}H-D$_3$, significant binding of both ^{3}H-D$_3$ and ^{3}H-25-OHD$_3$ to lipoproteins was observed most noticeably at early time intervals after injection. At later stages virtually all binding was associated with an α-globulin. There is an enterohepatic recirculation of vitamin D and its metabolites, largely conjugated as glucuronides before secretion into the bile (Avioli et al., 1967), and bile fistula may thus also lead to vitamin D depletion. Earlier studies had shown that, following oral administration of cholecalciferol to ricketic rats, there was a 16–20 hour delay before increased calcium uptake by subsequently removed small intestine could be demonstrated in vitro (Zull et al., 1966). This time lag was reduced to about 6 hours when 25-OHD$_3$ instead of cholecalciferol was administered, but the continuing though smaller time lag suggested that further metabolism to a compound with immediate biological activity might be required. A further metabolite of vitamin D which had originally been first detected in intestinal cell nuclei (Lawson et al., 1969) was identified as 1,25-dihydroxycholecalciferol [1,25-(OH)$_2$D$_3$ (1,25-DHCC, Fig. 2] and was found to have immediate powerful action in promoting intestinal calcium absorption. This metabolite can be synthesized only by kidney (Fraser and Kodicek, 1970). Its structure and immediate powerful effect have been amply confirmed, and 1,25-$(OH)_2D_3$ is now regarded as the active hormonal form of the vitamin (Lawson *et al.*, 1971; Holick *et al.*, 1971; Myrtle and Norman, 1971). It is similar in structure to the steroid hormones, and it satisfies very well the criteria for classification as a hormone: it is rapidly active in minute concentrations, as low as $10^{-10} M$, in intestine and bone both *in vitro* and *in vivo* (Holick *et al.*, 1972a; Raisz *et al.*, 1972; Haussler *et al.*, 1971; Boyle *et al.*, 1972); recent evidence suggests that it binds initially to a specific cytosol receptor in the intestine (Brumbaugh and Haussler, 1973) and subsequently associates with a chromosomal receptor protein in the nuclear chromatin (Lawson *et al.*, 1969; Haussler and Norman, 1969). Early evidence concerning the subsequent course of events was a little conflicting, but there is now good evidence that 1,25-$(OH)_2D_3$, acting in a manner analogous to that of steroid hormones, regulates DNA transcription, inducing the synthesis of specific mRNA(s) that then mediate the *de novo* synthesis of calcium-binding protein (CBP) (Corradino and Wasserman, 1971; MacGregor *et al.*, 1971). This action of 1,25-$(OH)_2D_3$ is inhibited by actinomycin D (Corradino, 1973), as is its stimulation of bone calcium mobilization (Tsai *et al.*, 1973). Much more work is required to determine the possible physiological activity of the vitamin D metabolites in muscle, but the clinical evidence for such a specific action is strong.

What factors regulate the synthesis and function of this hormone? The mystery of the adaption to low calcium diets which occurs in growing animals began to unravel when it was shown that young rats respond to this situation by increasing the synthesis of 1,25-$(OH)_2D_3$ (Boyle *et al.*, 1971). It seemed likely at first that this response was mediated through falling concentrations of plasma calcium, and this association was then confirmed *in vitro* (Omdahl *et al.*, 1972). Furthermore, kidney tissue was found to secrete a second, apparently inactive, metabolite identified as 24,25-$(OH)_2D_3$ (Holick *et al.*, 1972b) in inverse proportion to the active compound. Because parathyroid hormone secretion is also controlled by variations in plasma calcium, the question then arose as to whether parathyroid hormone acts as a trophic hormone for 1,25-$(OH)_2D_3$ synthesis, and evidence has suggested such a role. In the experimental animal, parathyroidectomy may abolish 1,25-$(OH)_2D_3$ synthesis, and administration of parathyroid extract may restore it, opposite changes occurring as expected in the synthesis of 24,25-$(OH)_2D_3$ (Garabedian *et al.*, 1972). Corresponding changes in the responsible renal 1α-hydroxylase activity have also been shown, and these changes appeared in advance of the expected changes in plasma calcium which were also produced by parathyroidectomy or by the administration of parathyroid hormone (Fraser and Kodicek, 1973). 1,25-$(OH)_2D_3$ synthesis in isolated renal tubules was shown to be stimulated by cyclic AMP as well as by parathyroid hormone and to be inhibited by calcitonin (Rasmussen et al., 1972).

Precise theories were soon modified, however, when it became apparent that powerful control of 25-OHD_3 metabolism could also be exerted by inorganic phosphate. 1,25-$(OH)_2D_3$ synthesis, having been abolished by parathyroidectomy, was restored when increasing concentrations of plasma phosphate were reduced by dietary manipulation (Tanaka and DeLuca, 1973). Moreover, the ability of the kidney to secrete either 1,25-$(OH)_2D_3$ or 24,25-$(OH)_2D_3$ correlated with concentrations of both plasma phosphate and kidney cortex inorganic phosphate. At high concentrations of phosphate 24,25-$(OH)_2D_3$ was produced, and as phosphorus concentrations were reduced, synthesis switched to the active form. The low serum phosphate produced by low phosphorus-containing diets was found, as expected, to be associated with increased intestinal calcium transport (Tanaka et al., 1973). The independence of 1,25-$(OH)_2D_3$ production from that of parathyroid hormone has been confirmed (Larkins et al., 1973). Administration of cholecalciferol alone may reduce 1,25-$(OH)_2D_3$ synthesis (Galante et al., 1973), and it is open to speculation whether this too is mediated through changes in plasma phosphate. Regulation of 1,25-$(OH)_2D_3$ synthesis has in addition been attributed to intracellular calcium concentration in some component of the renal cell (Larkins et al., 1973; Galante et al., 1973), but, if so, calcium changes in this theoretical compartment are certainly not mirrored by similar changes in plasma calcium concentrations.

The physiological role of parathyroid hormone in control of vitamin D metabolism is, therefore, uncertain with regard to human biology and medicine. In the intact animal, it is still entirely possible that parathyroid hormone mediates control of vitamin D metabolism by the alteration of plasma and tissue inorganic phosphate which it produces. The species differences, with regard to calcium homoestasis, are fairly prominent, and variation with age within any given species may be equally prominent. For example, plasma calcium and phosphate concentrations are much more responsive to dietary manipulation in young animals; an additional mechanism, by which vitamin D metabolism is directly controlled by alteration in plasma phosphate concentrations, could thus be appropriate, at least in early life. Human hypoparathyroidism may be markedly resistant to treatment with vitamin D, a finding that is consistent with a requirement for parathyroid hormone in normal vitamin D metabolism. Although phosphate depletion alone is a very rare cause of osteomalacia in humans (Lotz *et al.,* 1964; Dent and Winter, 1974), the type of osteomalacia it produces is almost unique in its association with greatly enhanced calcium absorption and marked hypercalciuria (Lotz *et al.,* 1968). However, could this not also be due to the stimulated synthesis of 1,25-$(OH)_2D_3$?

Still more mysteries remain. Contrary to earlier beliefs, when 24,25-$(OH)_2D_3$ was administered experimentally, a slow but profound stimulation of intestinal calcium transport was observed, although bone calcium mobilization remained unaltered. This effect was the result of its conversion to a still more polar metabolite that localized in the intestinal mucosa and has been identified as 1,24,25-trihydroxycholecalciferol (Boyle *et al.,* 1973). If this metabolite has a physiological role, a therapeutic role may await the synthetic compound 1α-hydroxycholecalciferol (Haussler *et al.,* 1973). Its relatively easy synthesis has been described, and its effects, probably exerted subsequent to its *in vivo* 25-hydroxylation, seem as rapid and profound as administration of 1,25-$(OH)_2D_3$ itself. Synthesis of 1,25-$(OH)_2D_3$ by the kidney, its subsequent localization in the intestine, and the synthesis of calcium-binding protein, are represented in Fig. 1. Absorbed calcium is then transported to the osteoid seams and growing cartilage of bone where it is laid down with phosphate as hydroxyapatite in calcifying tissue.

A possible physiological requirement for vitamin D or its derivatives for normal calcification in bone is still uncertain. While the gross histological abnormality of osteomalacic bone, with its overall increase in osteoid tissue, continues to suggest that vitamin D may play a further part in normal calcification in addition to ensuring an adequate calcium $\times$ phosphorus solubility product in the blood, this has not yet been shown experimentally. *In vitro* studies have so far shown that certain vitamin D metabolites produce only increased bone resorption. Cholecalciferol was inactive in these systems; 25-OHD_3 and parathyroid hormone (also heparin and vitamin A) caused increased resorption (Reynolds, 1972), while 1,25-$(OH)_2D_3$ was 100 times more active in this respect (Raisz *et al.,* 1972). However, in the experimental animal, nephrectomy prevented the bone calcium mobilization response to 25-OHD_3 but not to 1,25-$(OH)_2D_3$ (Holick *et al.,* 1972a). These findings are thus consistent only with the clinical effects of vitamin D intoxication and to date do not implicate a direct role of vitamin D in normal calcification. The chemical formulae of cholecalciferol and the yeast vitamin ergocalciferol (vitamin D_2), together with their major metabolites, are shown in Fig. 2.

After formation in the human kidney, 1,25-$(OH)_2D_3$ appears in peripheral blood only in minute amounts that were at first only detectable by isotopic tracer methods (Mawer *et al.,* 1971a), but not in patients with chronic renal failure. Its synthesis has been localized to the renal tubule in rats (Shain, 1972). A radioreceptor assay for $1,25\text{-}(OH)_2D_3$ has now been developed (Brumbaugh *et al.*, 1974). Circulating levels in healthy subjects were approximately 60 pg/ml, but were low in patients with hypoparathyroidism and were undetectable in chronic renal failure. Failure of renal synthesis of $1,25\text{-}(OH)_2D_3$ thus provides an explanation of much of the mystery of renal rickets and the early occurrence of rickets in patients with severe renal tubular failure, but little glomerular failure as in the Lignac–Fanconi syndrome (cystinosis) with its early characteristic "swan-neck" deformity of the proximal renal tubule. Atrophy of the jejunal mucosa with consequent failure of the $1,25\text{-}(OH)_2D_3$ CBP system may provide part of the explanation for vitamin D resistance in gluten-sensitive enteropathy (coeliac disease).

The liver of man and animals has long been considered to be the major storage site of vitamin D, and indeed animal liver is the only meat product that contains significant amounts. Nevertheless, in patients who have received pharmacological amounts of vitamin D, necropsy and amputation studies (Lumb *et al.*, 1971) have revealed that skeletal muscle and adipose tissue may provide a large storage reservoir from which vitamin D may be slowly released as plasma levels fall. The form in which vitamin D is mainly stored in this reservoir, whether as the parent vitamin or as 25-OHD, is uncertain, since chemical analysis rather than bioassay must be applied.

Various therapeutic trials of $25\text{-}OHD_3$ in pharmacological dosage have been reported in the sex-linked form of vitamin D-resistant rickets, hypoparathyroidism, anticonvulsant osteomalacia, and chronic renal failure, and evidence suggests that in some situations it may be several times more potent on a weight basis than the standard preparations of vitamin D_2 or D_3 in current use (Balsan and Garabedian, 1972; Stamp *et al.*, 1972).

25-Hydroxylation of cholecalciferol and of ergocalciferol proceeds normally in patients with both the sex-linked variety of hypophosphatemic rickets and the recessively inherited vitamin D dependency rickets (Haddad *et al.*, 1973). The occurrence of rickets and osteomalacia due to long-term anticonvulsant therapy in epilepsy (Kruse, 1968; Dent *et al.*, 1970) was postulated to arise from hepatic enzyme induction leading to increased breakdown of vitamin D to inactive metabolites and thereby to increased vitamin D requirement in these patients. Confirmation of this theory has been assisted by the demonstration of abnormally low levels of 25-OHD in plasma from these patients (Stamp *et al.*, 1972; Hahn *et al.*, 1972a) and by the demonstration of phenobarbitone-induced alterations in vitamin D metabolism (Hahn *et al.*, 1972b, 1974). Other forms of hereditary or acquired vitamin D-resistant rickets (Dent, 1970, 1971) may well result from abnormalities of vitamin D metabolism, and clinical scientists are now poised to explore and clarify many of these poorly understood conditions. Meanwhile, many old established clinical pharmacological phenomena are already clearer. The delayed action of vitamin D_2, when given in large doses to heal metabolic rickets or to raise the plasma calcium in hypoparathyroidism, is clearly due to its required conversion to a more active form. This conversion may also be severely inhibited by the lack of parathyroid hormone. The more rapid action of dihydrotachysterol (DHT, AT 10) in raising plasma calcium may result from its steric configuration that in some ways more closely resembles $1,25\text{-}(OH)_2D_3$ (Fig. 2). This resemblance could permit its rapid action on bone resorption in hypoparathyroidism and, in high dosage, on the CBP system in various forms of resistant rickets. On the other hand, the inadequate conversion of DHT to a true hormonal form of the vitamin, such as $1,25\text{-}(OH)_2D_3$ or $1,25\text{-}(OH)_2D_2$, may explain its inadequacy in small dosage in the treatment of nutritional rickets. Synthetic analogues of vitamin D_3 and $25\text{-}(OH)_2D_3$, in which the A ring has been rotated through 180° so that it resembles the steric configuration of DHT in the position of the hydroxyl group (Fig. 2), have recently been found effective on bone and intestine in the absence of the kidneys, a situation where the natural compounds are without effect (Holick *et al.*, 1972a). The well-founded fear that most clinicians have of the occasional unpredictable effects of high-dosage vitamin D therapy, ranging from inactivity to sudden inexplicable intoxication, may be related to various steps in its metabolic feedback control. The pathways of vitamin D metabolism are thus affected by many at first seemingly unrelated extraneous factors that range from renal failure through intestinal mucous membrane atrophy to anticonvulsant therapy, and a host of inborn errors of metabolism. Our accumulating knowledge is helping to explain much of this, and, as the vitamin D metabolites themselves and their analogues become available for therapy, both powerful and safer new therapeutic weapons should lessen the worries of the practicing clinician. The therapeutic use of cholecalciferol and its analogues is further considered under headings of the individual syndromes.

III. ETIOLOGY, NOMENCLATURE, AND CLINICAL ASPECTS

There are now known to be over thirty causes of rickets and osteomalacia. An abbreviated classification of these causes suitable to the purposes of this chapter is shown in Table I. The original reviews should be sought for references and details of some of the very rare causes (Dent, 1970, 1971). Some of these particular diseases will be described in more detail later.

It is convenient to consider the clinical aspects of rickets under the two separate headings of rickets and osteomalacia, since although they are really the same disease, the manifestations differ considerably. The basis for adequate interpretation of the clinical changes of rickets in the growing child are the following:

1. The failure of adequate calcification mechanisms affects mostly those parts of the skeleton where bone growth is most rapid.

2. The most rapid bone growth is always in places where true bone formation is preceded by formation of calcified cartilage, that is mainly in the metaphyses of long bones. Only when rickets is very severe does defective subperiosteal calcification of bone formed in membrane occur, such as at the midshafts of long bones.

3. Note must be taken of which end of a long bone is its main growing end.

4. At different ages growth rates of particular bones vary, and age, therefore, affects the distribution of the severity of the rickets. At birth the skull grows faster than any other bone and craniotabes is, therefore, the main manifestation of congenital rickets. In the first year, the upper limb and ribs grow quickly leading to signs at the wrists and costochondral junctions (ricketty rosary). Later the legs grow faster, with most signs manifesting around the growing ends at the knees. There are many subtleties here to be noted; for instance, at the wrist the signs of rickets are usually worse at the ulnar rather than at the radial metaphysis. This is because, although both bones are growing side by side, the ulnar metaphysis actually has a faster growth rate since all growth in length occurs there (the other end is incorporated in the elbow joint and does not grow); the radius grows at both ends but grows more slowly at the wrist than the ulna.

5. Deformities in mild chronic rickets occur entirely due to damage from pressure on the widened cartilaginous growth plate. Only in very severe rickets, with subperiosteal undercalcification, do the shafts of the bones actually bend.

6. In many forms of rickets, signs of secondary hyperparathyroidism can occur. These are mainly radiological (see Section III) but, when the radiological signs are very severe, clinical signs occur at the metaphyses as a result of hyperparathyroid erosions. These are mainly collapsed deformities and acute angulations; they are often asymmetrical and related to stress. At the costochondral junctions, the appearance of a "ricketty rosary" may be mimicked.

TABLE I

Classification of Kinds of Rickets and Osteomalacia

1. Classic (dietary vitamin D lack and lack of solar irradiation)	Immigrant children and adults Fat-phobic adults Increased requirement in old age
2. Intestinal[a]	Coeliac disease (gluten-sensitive enteropathy) Small intestine diseases with malabsorption syndrome Partial or total gastrectomy Hepatic-biliary cirrhosis, other forms of cirrhosis, biliary fistula or atresia Pancreatic: chronic relapsing pancreatitis, chronic pancreatic insufficiency
3. Hereditary renal[a] (mainly renaltubular dysfunction with high PO_4 clearances)	Sex-linked hypophosphatemia-dominant inheritance Autosomal hypophosphatemia-dominant inheritance Pseudo-vitamin D-lack (''vitamin D dependent'') recessive inheritance Neurofibromatosis-child and adult presenting forms Fanconi syndromes: cystinosis, child and adult presenting forms without cystinosis, oculo-cerebrorenal (Lowe's) syndrome, tyrosinemia, Wilson's disease Distal renal tubular acidosis (nephrocalcinosis with renal rickets and dwarfism)

4. Acquired renal
  Mainly glomerular
  Mainly tubular
	Absolutely any cause of chronic renal failure
	Adult presenting hypophosphatemic osteomalacia
	Hypercalciuric rickets
	Fanconi syndromes: heavy metal poisonings, nephrotic syndrome, obstructive uropathy, gammopathies, myelomatosis
	Ureterocolostomy

5. Miscellaneous	Neonatal rickets Some cases of osteopetrosis Tumor rickets Anticonvulsant therapy Primary hyperparathyroidism Phosphate lack from aluminium hydroxide ingestion, or other nonabsorbable hydroxides

[a] Abbreviated and modified from Dent (1971).

7. Deformities before the age of 4 may largely correct themselves if the rickets remain healed; more severe deformities, especially at a later age, produce permanent deformities, mainly dwarfism and bow leg or knock knee, which can be recognized as such in later life.

8. "Late rickets" is usually a mild chronic form of rickets stimulated to clinical manifestations by the puberty growth spurt. It usually produces knock knee only.

9. The adult manifestations (Looser zones, codfish vertebrae) are only seen in young children when the rickets is very severe.

On the basis of these nine factors, the clinical signs of rickets can be sought, and their distribution and severity can be understood. The early signs are only those of the overproduction of cartilage at the metaphysis producing the well-known hard fusiform swellings; at first sight this might look like severe Still's disease, but on examination the swellings are not at the joints but at the bone ends. For instance, at the wrists they are proximal to the site of joint movement. Furthermore, movement at the joints can be elicited without pain. Pain is uncommon in the bones except around the knees on weight bearing or if very gross generalized rickets is present.

In severe classical rickets, and in some of the forms of metabolic rickets (see Section IV,B), a marked myopathy is present. The small child presents a weak floppy appearance that may be difficult to interpret, but in older children by testing of individual muscles it can be shown to be distributed as a proximal myopathy affecting mainly the muscles around the hips and shoulders, as is so typical in adults. The child has difficulty in rising from the knees-bent position, in going upstairs, and perhaps in raising the arms above the head. Appropriate treatment may cure the myopathy in 2–3 weeks, even while the bones are still largely unhealed. Of course when the child has been long immobilized, with consequent muscle atrophy, recovery takes longer.

All in all, rickets of any severity may be easy to diagnose owing to the deformities produced (Fig. 3). In the first months of life, the skull deformity is manifested as a frontal bossing with flattening at the back when it has been resting on the pillow. Later, a lateral collapse of both chest walls (Harrison's sulcus) and ricketty rosary are noted. Leg deformities are difficult to ascertain, since all young babies appear bow-legged, but after they have begun to stand the bowleg worsens instead of lessens, and children who sit cross-legged a great deal develop anterior bowing at the lower ends of their tibiae. The deformities of the upper limb are usually less than of the lower, owing to less stress of weight bearing. In a true late rickets (arising after 10 years of age) the limbs, which have until then

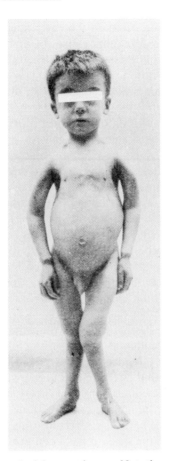

Fig. 3. Gross rickets, age and etiology not known. Note the prominent swollen epiphyses especially at the wrists, and other typical deformities (see text).

grown normally, are straight, and the angulation (now more often knock knee than bowleg) takes place entirely around the recently grown bone at the knees. At this age, it is important to look for other signs, such as dwarfism, anemia, and proteinuria, which might help to determine if the rickets is truly "late" and of recent onset or a manifestation of long-standing serious disease, such as renal failure. There is scarcely a more detailed and valuable description of the clinical and radiological signs of rickets than in the old report from Vienna (Medical Research Council, 1923).

In contrast to rickets, osteomalacia is very difficult to diagnose clinically, and this accounts for the fact that patients tend to be diagnosed only after having suffered years of considerable misery. The reason is simple, since no gross deformities occur in the early stages, and furthermore at this age there are innumerable other causes of similar aches and pains and muscular weakness. It can be assumed that the real duration of the disease is far longer than the duration of symptoms, since one must start with a normally formed skeleton, and the disease can only affect new bone laid down from then on. In adult life, all bone is formed in membrane and only develops from the ordinary continuous processes of bone formation and erosion. If about 5% of the skeleton is assumed to be newly laid down per year, it is clear that it must take many years for enough of the new undercalcified osteomalacic bone to cause real weakening of the skeleton. The eventual painful symptoms can be thought of as being due to bending on pressure, either from weight bearing or when considerable muscle pull is being exerted, since the periosteum is rather richly supplied with sensory nerve endings. When lying still the pain disappears, but may be elicited by direct pressure on the rib cage or by indirect pressure on turning in bed or coughing. Those bones whose strength mainly results from their internal trabecular structure rather than from their thick cortices are the first to become tender. This applies mostly to the vertebral bodies, especially the lumbar ones that carry more weight. Patients, therefore, get low backache on standing, and the ache is not localized to any particular level and is constant and reproducible under given circumstances. As the disease advances, the symptoms spread further up the back to include the ribs and later the feet and lower limbs. When a proximal myopathy is also associated with pain on weight bearing, very considerable crippling can result and can occur with no visible deformity whatsoever. Such patients may well be referred to psychiatrists for supposed imaginary symptoms. If the disease has been present for a long time, the vertebral bodies begin to collapse and a measurable loss of trunk height ensues; gross deformity such as kyphosis is usually a late sign. Osteomalacia, if developing for the first time in adult life, will occur in people of normal build and body shape. Most cases however are the result of longer lasting systemic disease, such as one of the forms of malabsorption syndrome, mild chronic renal damage, anticonvulsant therapy dating from childhood, or one of the forms of life-long hypophosphatemia. In such cases the patient is very likely to be dwarfed and may well show signs of mild childhood rickets, especially late rickets. Such rickets can heal spontaneously when growth ceases, only to recur much later as an otherwise typical osteomalacia, sometimes not until 70 or 80 years of age.

As in the case of rickets, associated nonskeletal signs will be present depending on the particular etiology in question, and will be obvious in most of the cases shown on Table I. Things to mention only briefly are other signs of malnutrition or of vitamin deficiencies, scars from abdominal operations, pigmented patches or neurofibromata, jaundice or other signs of chronic liver failure, a history of renal stones, and finally the presence in the urine of protein, glucose (with normal plasma glucose), cystine (as part of a generalized aminoaciduria), and a constant high pH and low osmolal concentration.

IV. RADIOLOGICAL AND LABORATORY DIAGNOSIS

The radiological signs in the bones are most important on account of their frequent specificity and because so many patients are first diagnosed from an X ray, frequently performed with other purposes in mind. Again it is convenient to deal with rickets and osteomalacia separately.

The cardinal signs of rickets, maximal at the fastest growing metaphyses (see Section III), are widening of the growth plate (owing to the fact as cartilage cells hypertrophy, they are not simultaneously being calcified and transformed into true bone) and the irregular appearance of the end of the metaphysis (which represents uneven invasion of the recently calcified cartilage by the adjacent bone tissue in the course of its transformation into bone). There is also apparently an excess production of cartilage (not visible on the X ray) in all directions, which accounts for the palpable bulging noted at the metaphyses. When affecting smaller diameter bones with rapid growth, such as the ulna, the more severe cases show widening of the metaphysis and a "cupping" concavity at its end (Figs. 4–6). These signs are quite specific for any of the causes of rickets, but do not distinguish between the many etiologies in question. Healing takes place, as would be expected, by calcification of the excess cartilage starting sometimes a little distance from the end of the metaphysis, and thus forming a line across the cartilage (Fig. 7) before fusing with the old bone and spreading toward the epiphyses eventually to produce a normal appearance with quite normal bone structure. The extent of such rickets is partly dependent on trauma, for example, from weight bearing, and after the age of 10 may be more marked, therefore, at the knees than at the wrists. It is difficult, however, to direct the X ray correctly at an exact right angle to the larger growth plate at the knees, so that its width and other appearances can be judged. Because more pressure is exerted at the knee medially when there is bowleg deformity, the rickets may appear more severe medially than laterally in the same growth plate (for instance, at the lower end of the femur). Conversely with knock knee deformity the rickets may appear worse laterally than medially in the growth plate. Rickets of fluctuating degree, as is almost always the rule when of dietary origin or when there is inconstant medical control in the metabolic cases, heals and recurs

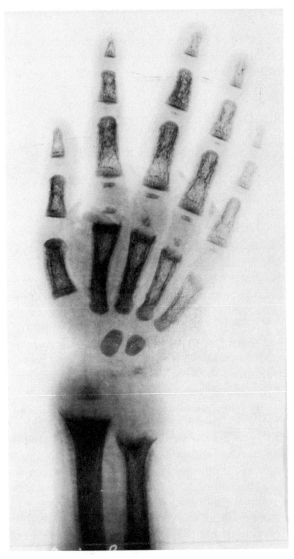

Fig. 4. Nutritional rickets. X Ray of wrists in a 14-month-old girl. See text for full description. Note identical changes in Figs. 5 and 6.

successively. This leaves behind in the shaft Harris lines of arrested growth and also transverse regions of irregular bone structure (Fig. 8). When very severe, subperiosteal bone tissue is also formed undercalcified, and gives the shafts of long bones a fuzzy outside margin surrounded by a fine line of the periosteum. Secondary hyperparathyroidism is commonly present in classic rickets, in renal rickets, and in some other forms, but in the isolated renal tubular hypophosphatemic cases it is hardly ever present. The hyperparathyroidism takes the form of irregular erosions of subperiosteal bone around certain metaphyses, especially the femoral neck, the medial sides of the proximal ends of the humeri, the medial sides of the femora and tibia at the knees, and the lateral aspects of the ulna and radius at the wrists. These are not the same regions of most rapid bone growth that dictate the main localization of rachitic lesions, but are presumably regions of maximal bone remodeling. The phalangeal signs of secondary hyperparathyroidism seen so well in adults are not so easily seen in younger children probably because the cortex of these bones is not yet well formed. Nor does one commonly see in children either the "cystic" form of the adult disease (in particular that form when only one or two such "cysts" are present in the absence of other signs) or the irregular rarefaction of the skull vault ("pepper-pot" skull).

As with the clinical signs, the radiological signs of osteomalacia are not

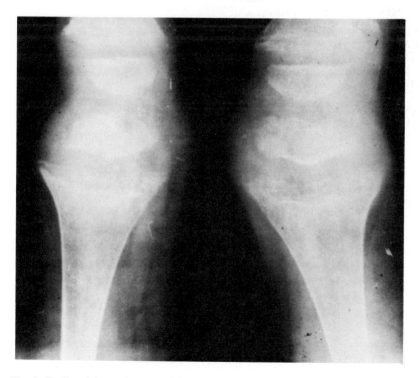

Fig. 5. Coeliac rickets (gluten-sensitive enteropathy). X Ray of knees in a 7-year-old boy.

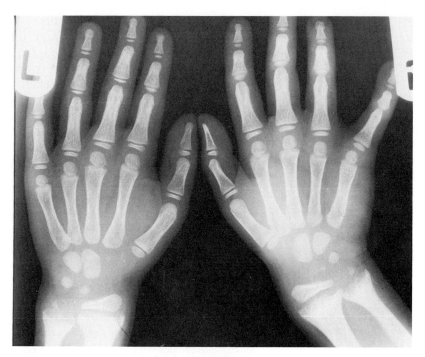

Fig. 6. Anticonvulsant rickets. X Ray of wrist in an 8-year-old boy. A little healing has taken place from previous vitamin D administration.

at all precise, probably for the same reasons as mentioned above, namely, the slow turnover rate of the adult skeleton. A patient can have severe symptoms of bone pain especially if the disease is severe and of relatively recent onset, with absolutely no clear X-ray changes in the bones (Medical Research Council, 1923). Often, however, one is greatly helped by the presence of Looser zones, also called pseudofractures or Milkman (1934) fractures.

These have been well described as "ribbonlike zones of rarefaction" and can occur in the shafts of most long bones and some flat ones, such as the lateral edge of the scapula (Figs. 9 and 10). It is essential to the description that the bones otherwise appear normal. Their origin is almost certainly a consequence of trauma, since the localization of these zones usually follows the well-known distribution of various forms of stress fractures occurring in normal skeletons. It must be supposed that small microfractures of cortical bone frequently follow successive strains in people with normal bones. They usually heal, especially if rested, and lead to no real disability. However, such a microfracture occurring in a patient with osteomalacia, however recent in origin, can only heal with the for-

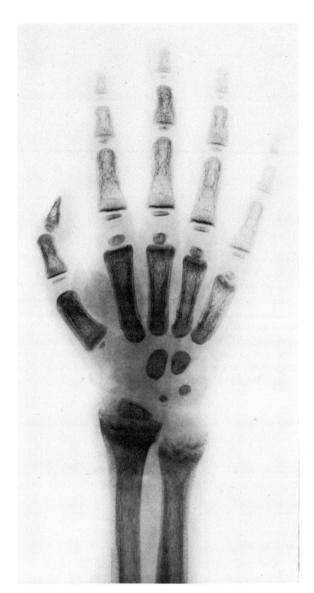

Fig. 7. Healing nutritional rickets in the same patient shown in Fig. 4. Note the line of calcification distal to the visible metaphysis (see text).

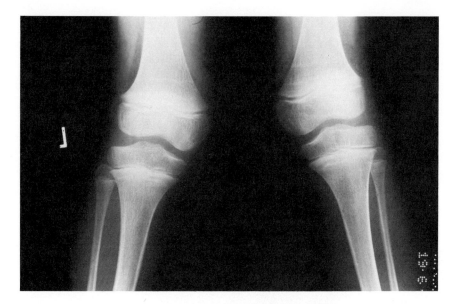

Fig. 8. Multiple Harris lines. X Ray of knees in a 6-year-old Indian girl (the sister of the boy whose data is shown in Fig. 15) with nutritional rickets taken on June 19, 1972. A previous X ray was available on March 1, 1972 which then showed active rickets in the region of the more distal Harris line of arrested growth. The subsequent growth of normal bone was spontaneous and presumably due to early summer sunshine. We presume the more proximal Harris line dates from a similar sequence of events the previous year (see text).

mation of uncalcified callus not visible of course on X ray. Such a site is a point of weakness that is liable to further fractures, which then eventually form the final Looser zone that may extend right across the shaft of the bone. This is the adult equivalent of rickets in childhood, which is more severe in the more rapidly growing bone (see Section III). In adults the only rapidly growing bone thus predisposed is the new bone formation following fracture.

It is useful to distinguish the relatively acute forms of osteomalacia ("acute" with bone disease means 1–5 year duration) with the fairly normal skeleton and perhaps some Looser zones (Fig. 11), from the more chronic forms ("chronic" here means more than 20 years or so duration) with very long-lasting osteomalacia that is perhaps milder, perhaps of fluctuating degree, and which may have begun in adolescence when the epiphyses have fused, though there is still more skeleton to be laid down. In the latter cases, clear evidence of deformities from bone softening may be found (indeed, this is what the word "osteomalacia" really means); thus the vertebrae are evenly squashed into a biconcave shape (Fig. 12), the pelvis is pushed in at the three pressure points, sacrum and both acetabulae, to produce the trefoil pelvis (Fig. 13), and even the shafts of long bones may bend. When they appear very soft such bones may not show Looser zones, since perhaps some brittleness is necessary to form the primary microfracture. Clearly, the described ''acute'' and ''chronic'' forms represent extremes, and in most cases a varying amount of one or the other is present. It is nevertheless useful to recognize these extremes,

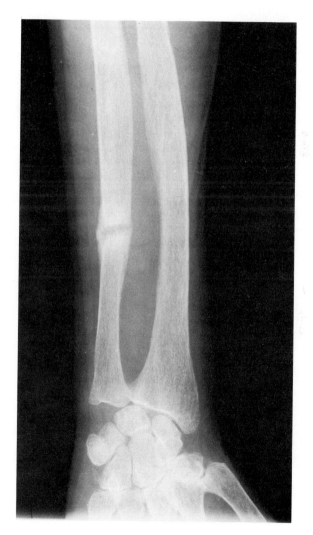

Fig. 9. Looser zone (Milkman's pseudofracture) in ulna of 72-year-old woman with coeliac osteomalacia (see text).

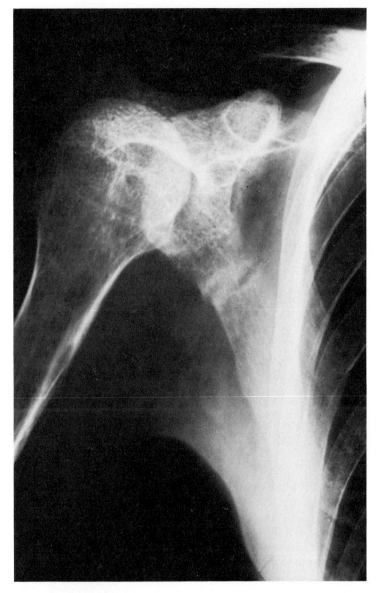

Fig. 10. Looser zone in lateral border of scapula of 31-year-old man presenting with adult hypophosphatemic osteomalacia (see text).

since it may help when trying to correlate this with the clinical history and probable etiology.

Secondary hyperparathyroidism is commonly seen in classical osteomalacia, and in renal disease (Volume II, Chapter 2). The most important sign is the presence of subperiosteal erosions that in mild cases are seen more on the thumb side of the middle phalanges of all the fingers. The normally fine periosteal margin is broken by gaps here and there, and the immediately underlying cortex is eroded to produce a wispy margin like small waves on the surface of water blown by the wind. The signs are obvious in advanced cases, and in early cases are best sought with a small hand lens. Another less useful sign is erosion of the outer line of the terminal phalanges. This is often difficult to see, since the terminal tuft normally has an irregular margin, but when normal, the line is not usually broken. Sometimes especially if the circulation to the fingers is impaired, this "tufting" may be much more grossly apparent than changes in the middle phalanges. Curiously, these bone changes in the hands are asymptomatic even in severe cases when the erosions affect the terminal phalangeal shafts and produce collapse of the bone and the appearance of "pseudoclubbing" (Fig. 14). The distribution of this collapse is asymmetrical and uneven. It affects the dominant hand more than the other and the

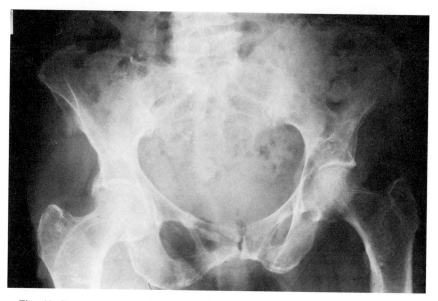

Fig. 11. Looser zone in pubic ramus of 88-year-old woman with senile osteomalacia (increased vitamin D requirement). The female pelvis is much more liable to this kind of fracture than the stronger male pelvis. Note absence of gross pelvic deformity.

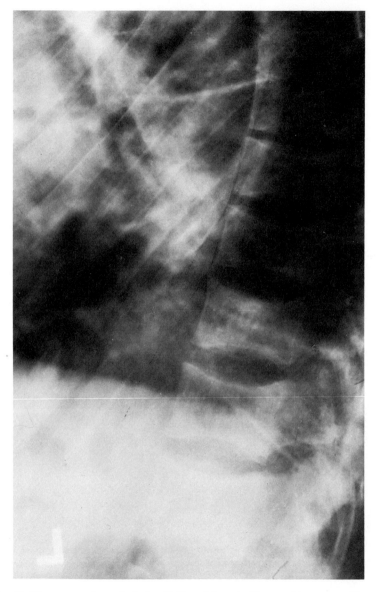

Fig. 12. Biconcave osteomalacic (codfish) vertebrae in 36-year-old woman with coeliac disease (see text).

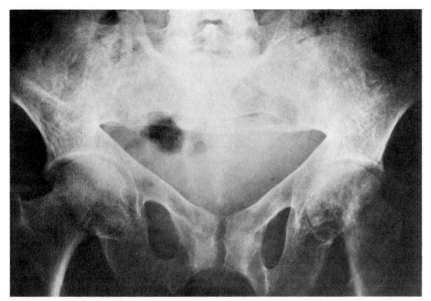

Fig. 13. Triangular ("trefoil") pelvis from coeliac osteomalacia. Same patient as in Fig. 12. Note the deformities of chronic osteomalacia (see text) in contrast to the pelvis of acute osteomalacia shown in Fig. 11.

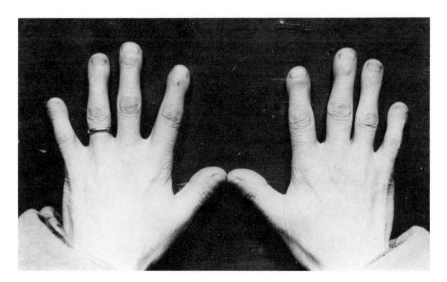

Fig. 14. Hands showing pseudoclubbing from hyperparathyroid erosions of terminal phalanges in a 50-year-old woman with secondary osteitis fibrosa from chronic renal failure (see text).

working fingers (index and thumb) the most, the ring fingers being less affected. In severe cases, long bone "cysts" (really osteoclastomas) also occur, especially in sites following trauma. Other radiological signs are the eroded appearance of the vault of the skull and a widening of the spaces at the symphysis pubis and sacroiliac joints.

These important radiological signs of disordered bone metabolism do not help one to determine the etiology and treatment. However, there are any other nonosseous signs that do help greatly in this respect. These are the size and shape of the kidney, especially the presence of nephrocalcinosis or renal stones, the detection of arterial or soft tissue calcification, distended gaseous intestines, and soft tissue shadows suggesting the presence of neurofibromata. X-Ray evidence is of special value since it means the whole skeleton can be surveyed and significance can be drawn sometimes only from findings of localized pathology, such as one bone "cyst" or one Looser zone. Since the expense and extra hazard of whole skeletal survey can hardly be justified, we recommend asking for X rays of an abbreviated "metabolic skeleton." These include most of the parts most likely to show important lesions and ensure that later X rays can be taken for comparison. Recommended views are the lateral aspect of the skull, posteroanterior chest, renal areas, both hands and wrists, pelvis and hips, lateral lumbar vertebrae, and both knees. Further views can be requested if clinically indicated.

A. Histology

The histological diagnosis of rickets or osteomalacia is described in detail in Chapter 4 so only a few clinically oriented points need be made here. The first is that although bone biopsy is of great value for its greater detail and specificity than, e.g., X-ray examination of the skeleton, biopsy is hardly to be undertaken as lightly as most of the other diagnostic techniques. It is, therefore, usually undertaken only in the more seriously ill patient in whom metabolic bone disease is already very strongly suspected. Bone biopsy has little application as a screening test. Also, repeated biopsies are difficult to justify so we do not usually have this means available in order to monitor response to treatment. The main diagnostic values of biopsy are in patients with "acute" osteomalacia when the biopsy may show gross pathognomonic changes when specific clinical and radiological signs are ambiguous or even absent. Rarely, patients with ambiguous biopsy evidence of osteomalacia have indeed recovered symptomatically when their physician has treated them rather empirically for this assumed diagnosis, and no other cause of various bone pains are likely to be discovered. The other negative or ambiguous biopsies in osteomalacia in our experience have been in patients with both marked osteoporosis and with osteomalacia first suspected early. They usually had a malabsorption syndrome or one of the hypophosphatemic syndromes. A possible explanation for this is that new bone formation was also slowed so that consequently fewer uncalcified osteoid seams appeared.

B. Biochemical Changes

Because of the easy availability of blood and urine, they can be used for routine screening as well as in specific cases. Table II summarizes the biochemical findings characteristically seen in patients with rickets or osteomalacia as well as in related diseases that have to be considered in the differential diagnosis.

Note that the same abnormalities in plasma calcium, phosphate, and alkaline phosphatase are common to all the forms of rickets and osteomalacia. However, certain further changes go part of the way in assigning the patient to one of the more specific syndromes. It is important to note that except in the hypophosphatemic syndromes, where the low plasma phosphate is permanent and not much affected by adequate treatment, the main findings (plasma calcium, phosphate, and alkaline phosphatase) all become normal on healing of the bone disease. Ambiguous chemistry may, therefore, be found in patients who have been partly treated. The rule in interpreting such cases is that plasma calcium and phosphate indicate the immediate status of the patient's bone metabolism. For instance, it will become normal in days in classical rickets after a single large dose of vitamin D and long before any X ray or symptomatic changes are noted. Conversely, on a vitamin D-free diet the plasma calcium and phosphate become abnormal long before radiological signs of rickets or osteomalacia appear. Such a patient may well appear with tetany as the only disease manifestation, his bones and phosphatase being normal, so it is possible for an unwary physician who has not taken a proper history to confuse it with some form of hypoparathyroidism. On the other hand, the plasma alkaline phosphatase rises and falls in direct relationship with the gross extent of the rickets, as seen radiologically. Lack of relationship between the plasma calcium and phosphate, on one hand, and plasma phosphatase and X-ray visible rickets, on the other, is most commonly seen in classic rickets, since the causal dietary lack of the vitamin D is so likely to vary greatly from time to time, as does also the amount of solar irradiation that can substitute for dietary vitamin D.

TABLE II

Main Biochemical Changes in Some Forms of Rickets and Osteomalacia and in Some Superficially Similar Bone Diseases

Diagnosis	Plasma Ca[a] (mg/100 ml)	Plasma P (mg/100 ml)	Plasma HCO$_3$ (mEq/liter)	Plasma urea (mg/100 ml)	Plasma alkaline phosphatase (KA units)	Urine Ca (mg/24 hours)
Normal adult	9.0–10.5 9.0–10.2 (fasting)	3.2–4.2	24–28	20–35	5–12 (♂) 3–10 (♀)	120–280 (♂) 120–220 (♀)
Normal children (1–16 years old)	9.0–10.5	4.0–6.0	20–26	15–30	15–25	10–100
Chondrodystrophies	Normal	Normal	Normal	Normal	Normal	Normal
Idiopathic osteoporosis	Normal	Normal	Normal	Normal	Normal	Normal
Hypophosphatemic rickets	Normal	1.0–2.5	Normal	Normal	Elevated	Low normal (high if in an active phase)
Classic and other forms of nonacidotic rickets	6.0–9.0	1.0–4.0	20–26	Normal	Elevated	10–100
Acidotic forms of rickets[b]	7.0–9.5	1.0–3.0	10–22	20–60	Elevated	150–350
Renal-glomerular osteodystrophy	5.0–9.0	4.0–10.0	10–20	100–500	Elevated	20–100
Primary hyperparathyroidism	10.2–16.0 (fasting)	1.0–3.0	20–26	Normal or elevated	Normal or elevated	150–600
Hypophosphatasia	9.0–14.0	3.0–5.0	20–28	20–100	1–2 (adult) 3–8 (infant)	Insufficient data, probably high normal
Hypohyperparathyroidism	5.0–7.0	4.0–7.0	22–26	Normal	Elevated	20–100

[a] All plasma Ca must be corrected for the protein content of the same specimen. For this we use the specific gravity determined by the CuSO$_4$ method. No correction is required if the specific gravity is 1027 which we take as normal. For every point above or below normal we subtract or add (respectively) 0.25 to the total Ca. This correction is valid only for small changes in specific gravity of up to 3→4, if the protein pattern is normal on electrophoresis, and if no other gross plasma change is present affecting the specific gravity (e.g., lipemia). It is not adequate to obtain the blood without venous compression and then assume the proteins will be normal and no correction will be necessary.

[b] Some of these cases are also associated with other signs of renal tubular dysfunction, such as renal-tubular proteinuria, renal glycosuria, and renal aminoaciduria.

V. DIFFERENTIAL DIAGNOSIS

The clinical signs of rickets are rather specific in the early age groups, especially when well marked. Any child who is dwarfed, with short, bowed long bones should have X rays taken. The child with achondroplasia will then at once be distinguished, since the growth plate has less rather than more cartilage, and there are other characteristic, gross morphological appearances that need not be summarized here. Hypophosphatasia sometimes causes diagnostic difficulty. Even the X-ray changes may appear as rickets, although the irregular, widened metaphyses are usually much more coarsely irregular than in rickets. In the milder cases of children presenting with bowleg or knock-knee after the age of 3, poor tooth structure is usually characteristic. Metaphyseal dysostosis, type Schmid, has often caused real difficulty (Dent and Normand, 1964); the clinical appearances are identical with those of a mild chronic rickets, except that the absence of myopathy narrows the list of possible causes. X Rays show widened growth plate and irregular metaphysis with splaying and cupping. The only difference at first presentation is that the irregular part of the metaphysis is denser than normal and appears more like healing than like active rickets, when density is often less than normal. Follow-up shows the maintenance of both a slow growth rate and of the "healing rickets." Furthermore, should osteotomy be necessary the bone shafts heal normally, since bone formation from membrane is quite normal, and only the formation from cartilage is deranged. Difficulty in differential diagnosis does not usually continue after biochemical investigations (see Table II).

In contrast with rickets, the differential diagnosis of osteomalacia in adults can be very large, especially in an early case of acute osteomalacia with severe bone pains, tenderness, and no other physical signs. Diffuse carcinomatosis of bone, as in multiple myeloma, can mimic osteomalacia closely and, of course, can be very extensive at a stage when there are no specific radiological signs. However, when spinal radiological signs do develop, they are those of osteoporosis rather than of osteomalacia (namely, irregular collapse of vertebral bodies and, sooner or later, a localized deposit in skull or long bone). The duration of the symptoms in cancer patients is usually relatively short (about 1 year), while in osteomalacia it is necessarily much longer than this owing to the slow rate of bone turnover as compared with the growth rate of most tumors. Needless to say, a search for primary growth needs to be carried out as well as determinations of plasma proteins, sedimentation rate, and other indirect tests for the presence of tumor. In practice, chronic backache from idiopathic or senile osteoporosis is more likely to cause some confusion, owing to its long duration and the good general health that goes with it. In osteoporosis the pain pattern is different. It comes acutely and leaves more slowly, in the early stages at least, with pain-free intervals. The pain is due to an acute impaction fracture of a vertebral body and is likely to be sharply localized to the region of the spine of the vertebra in question, often with radiation symmetrically round both sides of the trunk or down both legs if in the lower lumbar vertebrae. Healing takes about 3 weeks. The pain pattern is not associated with bone tenderness elsewhere. The more common causes of backache are, of course, prolapsed intervertebral discs and diseases of the joints and soft tissues. In joint and soft tissue disease, loss of stature is not noticeable, and the pains are related to movement, even if passive, rather than weight bearing.

Fortunately in any advanced case the spinal X rays should be diagnostic, and in milder early cases, we still have blood chemistry (Table II), which is abnormal only in osteomalacia. One must think of the diagnosis, however, before X rays and chemistry are ordered. There is no substitute here, especially if we wish to make the diagnosis as early as possible, for a good knowledge of the predisposing causes (Table I). Patients who have such a cause, for instance a partial gastrectomy, chronic pancreatitis, or malabsorption, should have their hospital notes so marked in a conspicuous fashion so that one can anticipate the possible development of osteomalacia. Patients diagnosed as having a hereditary form of osteomalacia must have their family fully screened to detect other asymptomatic cases if any; sibs only need be considered when the inheritance is by a recessive gene, other generations need to be considered if it is dominant.

VI. THERAPY

As all forms of rickets and osteomalacia however severe (except the form with congenital osteopetrosis) can be treated often with spectacular and always with gratifying results, the final response to the treatment serves as further confirmation of the diagnosis. Indeed, some lucky patients can be diagnosed so early in the development of the disease that many of the usual findings may be so slightly abnormal that they are not really diagnostic. Such patients, usually adults suffering from mild backache, can nevertheless be convincingly relieved of their symptoms, thus amply confirming the provisional diagnosis. We have seen this especially in early cases of renal osteodystrophy and in patients with the sex-linked form of chronic hypophosphatemia.

The nature of the treatment is simple and involves only a few drugs. It will be dealt with in more detail later under the particular syndromes, but it may be useful to summarize the main points in the form of a table (Table III). Clearly, other treatment, medical and surgical, may be required to

TABLE III

Main Lines of Medical Treatment of Rickets and Osteomalacia (Numbers as in Table I)

Kind of rickets or osteomalacia	Treatment of the bone disease[a]	Supplementary treatment of the cause
1. Dietary	Vitamin D (10–100 μg)	—
Senile	Vitamin D (50–500 μg)	—
2. Coeliac	Vitamin D (1–10 mg) till malabsorption controlled	Gluten-free diet Other vitamins as indicated
Idiopathic steatorrhea	Vitamin D (1–10 mg)	Other vitamins as indicated
Hepatic	Vitamin D (1–2 mg) orally or vitamin D (10–100 μg) parenterally	—
Pancreatic	Vitamin D (1–2 mg)	Pancreatic enzymes by mouth
3. Sex-linked hypophosphatemia	Vitamin D (1–2 mg) till growth ceases then again later in life when osteomalacia occurs	Inorganic phosphate
Pseudo-vitamin D lack	Vitamin D (1–2 mg) forever	1,25-$(OH)_2D$.
Cystinosis	Vitamin D (1–2 mg)	Sodium and potassium bicarbonates
Adult Fanconi syndrome	Vitamin D (1–2 mg) sodium bicarbonate (10–15 gm)	—
Wilson's disease	Vitamin D (1–2 mg) until osteomalacia healed	Penicillamine
Distal renal tubular acidosis	Vitamin D (1–2 mg) until healed, and continued sodium bicarbonate	—
4. Renal glomerular rickets	Vitamin D (1–2 mg)	Low protein diet, high Ca; 1,25-$(OH)_2D$; phosphate binding gels
Adult-presenting hypophosphatemia	Vitamin D (1–2 mg), disodium hydrogen phosphate (10–15 gm)	—
Ureterocolostomy	Vitamin D (1–2 mg) until healed, continued sodium bicarbonate (5–10 gm)	Urinary antibiotics
5. Tumor rickets	Vitamin D (1–2 mg) or removal of the tumor	—
Anticonvulsant	Vitamin D (0.1–1.0 mg)	—

[a] Measured in dosages per day by mouth. Note: Vitamin D = D_2 (perhaps D_3) not DHT.

deal with additional aspects related to other nonosseous tissues involved, and if bone deformities are present they may have to be corrected later by surgery when the bone disease is controlled.

The form of vitamin D used should usually be vitamin D_2 (ergocalciferol) and this is what is referred to in Table III. Vitamin D_3 (cholecalciferol) has very similar actions in similar doses, but we have inadequate experience of its use in many of the rare syndromes. Dihydrotachysterol (DHT, AT 10) is a little different, since it is much less effective in curing classic rickets and therefore should not be used for this. In most forms of metabolic rickets and osteomalacia (and in the treatment of tetany from hypoparathyroidism), DHT has been shown to be extremely effective, probably in about half the dose by weight as with vitamin D_2. However, we do not recommend it for general use yet in rickets and osteomalacia owing to insufficient published data.

Serious complications are still frequently seen from vitamin D intoxication. We stress that the only simple means of dosage is by constant daily oral dose. This does not appear to be equivalent to the same weight given daily by injection, and even less to a weekly injection of several times more. It is a great disadvantage that most preparations for oral route comprise tablets of 1.25 mg (50,000 IU) of vitamin D_2 or D_3. These are far too large for accurate dosage, and with the long delay in the maximum action, it is easy to become impatient at the apparent lack of response and double the dose that is an order of change not customary with other dangerous drugs when already being given in near-toxic doses. Furthermore, some tablets come on the market with "overage," that is additional vitamin (up to 20%) to cover possible slow deterioration on storage (Wiseman, 1972; Dent, 1972). We have been forced to make up in our own pharmacy preparations in low-peroxide arachis oil with 0.1% (w/w) hydroquinone as antioxidant. It is then encapsulated in sizes containing 0.25, 1.0, and 5.0 mg. With the stronger dihydrotachysterol a 0.1 mg size is also made.

Several mothers taking one of the three available forms of vitamin D (D_2, D_3, and DHT) for their metabolic bone disease, as well as for hypoparathyroidism, have become pregnant and delivered normal babies who have remained well on follow-up (C. E. Dent and T. C. B. Stamp, unpublished data). There have been 20 of these babies in our clinic and one other who had anencephaly that was probably unrelated to therapy. Our data on their neonatal plasma levels is incomplete. The mothers were all normocalcemic, and their pregnancy did not appear to affect their vitamin D requirement. It may be worse for the fetus if the mother were to become accidentally intoxicated, although we have no data on this.

VII. MAIN DISEASES AND SYNDROMES CAUSING RICKETS OR OSTEOMALACIA

A. Classic Rickets and Osteomalacia

While classic rickets can be found in a few children in well-developed communities if carefully looked for by the usual diagnostic means (biochemical, radiological, and pathological), such cases nearly always represent asymptomatic mild disease that is of consequence only to Public Health authorities who have to consider the effectiveness of their general prophylactic measures and educational programs. The condition is temporary and no harm is likely apart from the theoretical possibility of a slight growth check. There are, however, certain groups of high risk people that need special consideration. These comprise immigrants to Britain from sunnier countries who have not adapted to local dietary habits, local inhabitants on self-chosen restrictive diets, and old people. These will be considered in turn. We expect that similar situations will also occur in other developed countries.

The problem in immigrants has been serious in Britain over the last 10 years (Arneil and Crosby, 1963). Large numbers have arrived from India, Pakistan, and other Commonwealth countries who have been accustomed to live on largely vegetarian diets that are practically vitamin D-free. Presumably in their own countries this deficiency has been made up by skin exposure to sunlight. Certainly in Britain the ensuing wave of new cases of rickets has involved the 1- to 2-year-old age group, with the puberty growth spurt predisposing to the next most common age of incidence, and finally, more rarely still, there have been a few cases among adults of this immigrant group. Obtaining a clear dietary history has been a problem for many are able to obtain their accustomed foods, the analyses of which have not been included in the standard western textbooks on nutrition. Furthermore, different ways of cooking are employed: butter, for instance which may contain a little vitamin D, may be boiled before consumption thus probably destroying the vitamin. It is most important to distinguish classic rickets from one of the metabolic forms as the curative and safe dose of vitamin D may differ a hundredfold between them (Table III). In any case of doubt, a therapy trial with a small dose is essential, and for this we have used 50 μg (2000 IU) of cholecalciferol a day orally for about 3 weeks. In this time, a clear response, especially biochemical, will occur in classic rickets, but the dose is too small to have any effect on any of the metabolic forms of rickets. We have also used artificial ultraviolet rays for the same purpose. A mild erythema dose given daily to a large part of the skin surface will heal rickets just as quickly and will alter the calcium balance appropriately (Fig. 15). There is some controversy about the effectiveness of ultraviolet light in patients with pigmented skins. One theory is that melanin pigmentation largely prevents vitamin D synthesis on or in the skin. Indeed, it is claimed that the darker-skinned races who invariably populate equatorial regions avoid vitamin D intoxication by virtue of their dark skins, and that light skins have been developed by natural selection as man has moved to less sunny climes away from the equator (Loomis, 1970). The first half of this theory seems unusual to us, for we are unaware of any such instance of vitamin D intoxication occurring in a normal white-skinned person given excessive sun exposure. It is easier to believe that a dark skin is of value as a protection against sunburn and its long-term complications, such as rodent ulcer. The subject shown in Fig. 15 who responded quickly and well to his ultraviolet light was a very dark-skinned Indian boy. There is still a further problem in connection with immigrant rickets. Many workers having confidently made this diagnosis on the usual criteria, including diet history,

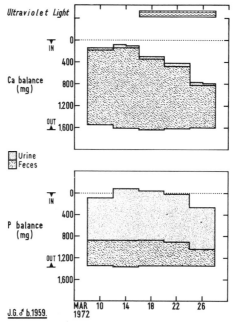

Fig. 15. Metabolic balance studies in a case of late childhood nutritional rickets. The patient was a dark-skinned Indian boy aged 13. Note the rapidly increasing positive calcium (and phosphorus) balances on treatment with whole-body ultraviolet irradiation. There was normalization of plasma calcium and phosphorus levels.

are reporting that the curative dose of vitamin D may at times be far larger than the dose of 50 μg daily recommended above for a therapy trial (Swan and Cooke, 1971). Obviously one has to look then for a double diagnosis, for many metabolic factors, mild renal failure, mild malabsorption, and perhaps hereditary predispositions can conceivably contribute to the vitamin deficiency. Further work is needed to clarify this problem.

The problem of rickets or osteomalacia occurring as the result of restrictive food habits in a person of western education is not a difficult one to determine so long as one knows of its existence (Dent and Smith, 1969). Such people are usually rather conspicuous food faddists, and in our experience have not always been strict vegetarians but rather what we describe as "fat-phobic." They dislike greasy fatty foods for various reasons, and their consequent diet, which can be otherwise very mixed, is necessarily vitamin D-free. This diet history is easy to elicit in practice. One of our patients, a lady of 59 years whose history was of avoiding fats since the age of 5, avoided previous overt bone disease and came to us with a first diagnosis of primary hyperparathyroidism. We think it likely that the parathyroid adenoma, then found and removed, might have arisen as a consequence of very long-term parathyroid hyperplasia from subclinical osteomalacia that was obvious on her bone biopsy. In other words, she had "tertiary" hyperparathyroidism. Epidemiological studies are needed to establish this possible long-term complication of chronic vitamin D deficiency.

Classic osteomalacia occurring in older people, say over 60 years of age, seems to occur more frequently than one would expect. Not all of these can be accounted for by dietary deficiency, and furthermore we have seen a small group whose signs and symptoms can only be cured by about 0.25 mg of cholecalciferol daily, a dose far higher than should be needed for dietary causes but still too low to affect most known metabolic forms of the disease. Mild malabsorption is common in old age and seems the most likely additional factor to predispose to the bone disease. These patients have been difficult to investigate, and further work is required. The important thing is to appreciate this possibility in old people even when on apparently adequate diets and to avoid treatment with vitamin D in the milligram dose range, since they easily become intoxicated. The term "senile osteomalacia" may be appropriate here.

B. Malabsorption Syndromes

1. Gluten-Sensitive Enteropathy

The odd thing here is that although gluten-sensitive enteropathy is very common, it is rarely complicated by rickets or osteomalacia. Even before gluten-sensitivity was recognized and therefore when coeliac disease was not adequately treated and ran a severe course for many years, the incidence of rickets was not high despite the occurrence of many other secondary deficiencies. In the first years of life, coeliac rickets is very rare indeed (Fig. 6) and most cases present later in the puberty age group. Such a child, usually knock-kneed, is nearly always dwarfed, a sign of a long-standing nutritional disturbance. Gastrointestinal manifestations in such cases are today usually inconspicuous, since otherwise diagnosis would certainly have been made sooner, treatment begun, and development of rickets prevented. An adolescent is likely to be sexually retarded and often gives a story of nocturia associated with lack of a normal diurnal rhythm of urine excretion and impaired excretion of water load. This superficially resembles renal rickets. The child often has severe iron deficiency-type anemia, other deficiencies being less common. This diagnosis must be carefully sought by the usual measures (fat output, intestinal biopsy, etc.) owing to the frequency of apparently normal gastrointestinal function as elicited by questioning. In the untreated state, the rickets is very resistant to both oral and parenteral vitamin D, sometimes even 10 mg a day having no effect. Once having responded to a gluten-free diet, normal vitamin D sensitivity returns. On beginning a gluten-free diet, a loading dose of vitamin D (about 5 mg daily) is therefore preferable, but dosage can be rapidly reduced within the next 1 or 2 months (to about 1 mg daily) and stopped entirely when the X-ray signs and the plasma alkaline phosphatase levels become normal. Long-term maintenance requires a gluten-free diet only. The response to this treatment can be most gratifying. As the patient usually has delayed puberty, rapid growth in stature as well as healing of the bones and normal body development can occur, even in the late teens (Fig. 16).

Adults can present with osteomalacic signs and symptoms at any stage, which is also odd for a disease we now believe to have been present from birth. Sometimes delayed onset can be related to the patient's choice of diet, since he may have noted that bread caused intestinal upset and thus largely have avoided it. One such person, the wife of a doctor, was not diagnosed until she was 72 years old, having had only 2 years of bone symptoms. This lady was dwarfed and did admit to occasional attacks of diarrhea all her life. Others may have shown instead short stature in childhood, late development of puberty, and continued slow growth until 21 or so years of age. The important point not always stressed is that a mild malabsorption, as measured biochemically, may lead to severe osteomalacia. In such cases the patient may be constipated with normal appearance of stools and have absolutely no other clinical signs of the disease. Tests for malabsorption, and perhaps a therapeutic trial on a

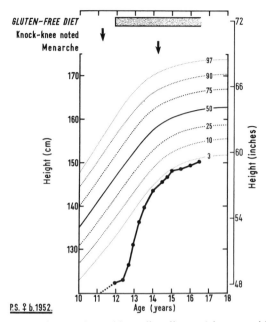

Fig. 16. Growth curve in a patient with coeliac disease (gluten-sensitive enteropathy). Note the early dwarfism and rapid "catch-up" growth after beginning a gluten-free diet (shaded bar). Menarche followed quickly after starting the diet. Numbers on curves are percentiles.

gluten-free diet, should be applied to any patient with no clear cause for their osteomalacia. Vitamin D treatment is given to the same schedule and in the same range of dosage as in children (see above). Most adults who do poorly are not keeping to the diet. A gluten-free diet is almost impossible to ensure when patients eat in public places. The British Coeliac Society is beginning to persuade food manufacturers to mark with an inconspicuous symbol tins of manufactured foods guaranteed to contain no wheat or rye protein. These are the two main offenders in the disease, although in certain patients the gluten-sensitivity also seems to involve other cereal sources.

2. Idiopathic Steatorrhea

However much we try to identify the etiology in a particular patient with a malabsorption syndrome, there still remain a few instances where no cause can be found even in the face of a severe malabsorption. We must treat such patients empirically, giving large amounts of whichever food factor they may be deficient in, almost any of the vitamins may be concerned as well as the minerals, in particular magnesium if the stool bulk is considerable (500–1000 gm/day). If the patient has osteomalacia, large doses of cholecalciferol of the order of 5–15 mg/day may be needed, intoxication being rare in these circumstances. Of course one should begin with smaller doses first and try to reduce from a higher dose when the stage of maintenance is reached.

3. Disorders following Gross Anatomical Changes and following Surgery

The etiology here usually presents no problem, especially when surgery has been undertaken. However, some physicians have considered that partial gastrectomy is not the cause of osteomalacia unless there are signs of gross malabsorption; this is not so. Many of our patients have been otherwise well enough nourished and have had fat outputs in the stool of only 4–7 gm/day, but nevertheless seem to have developed osteomalacia years later. Diet must be carefully checked, since it may have been inadvertently made vitamin D-deficient in the light of other requirements, such as a low fat diet. We have some patients with diarrhea and high fat excretions who have not developed osteomalacia after many years. We are not aware of this complication following simple excision of small intestine, although many of such patients develop other malabsorption complications.

Various spontaneous anatomical abnormalities, such as blind loops, small intestinal diverticulae, and acquired inflammatory disease, such as Crohn's disease or tuberculosis, can produce gross malabsorption syndromes with osteomalacia as one of the consequences. Obvious measures are surgical corrective procedures or medical care as in a case of idiopathic steatorrhea (above). Intestinal antibiotics may also have a place should gross secondary infection occur in parts of the intestine.

4. Hepatic Causes

Pathological fractures, for example, with severe lumbar back pain from vertebral collapse, may appear in any patient with long-standing liver disease. Metabolic bone disease from a malabsorption syndrome may thus complicate recurrent ascending cholangitis (for example following biliary surgery), primary biliary cirrhosis, and postnecrotic or alcoholic cirrhosis. Osteoporosis alone is appreciably more common (Atkinson et al., 1956) and results from severe calcium malabsorption in which fecal calcium excretion is higher than dietary calcium intake. However, bile salts may be an absolute requirement for optimal vitamin D and/or calcium absorption (Thompson et al., 1966), and bone disease may therefore result when there is an associated bile salt deficiency in the intestine. When osteoporosis is present it may be progressive and not respond to treatment.

However, if osteomalacia is a feature, these patients may be greatly improved by treatment with vitamin D, and it is therefore important to search for this complication by means of biochemical studies, X rays, and bone biopsy if necessary. Severe rickets and dwarfism may occur in the first year or two of life in infants with biliary atresia. There is also an enterohepatic recirculation of vitamin D and its metabolites, largely conjugated as glucuronides, and a biliary fistula (Fig. 17) may thus give rise to vitamin D depletion.

Osteomalacia may respond to physiological doses of vitamin D (50 μg daily) administered parenterally (Dent and Stamp, 1970), or they may require much larger doses (up to 5 mg daily as initial treatment) administered orally (Kehayoglou *et al.*, 1968). Maintenance oral dosage of vitamin

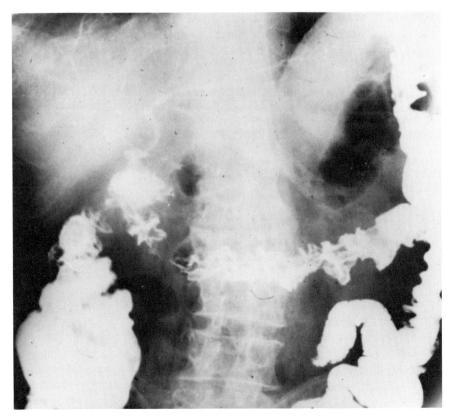

Fig. 17. Barium enema "cholangiogram" showing internal biliary fistula connected to hepatic flexure, from a presumed ruptured gallbladder (gallstones) in a 56-year-old man. The ensuing bile salt deficiency of the small intestinal contents caused osteomalacia and severe secondary osteitis fibrosa.

D may lie within the range 0.25–2.0 mg daily. It is theoretically possible that osteomalacia in severe hepatocellular disease may result from the failure of initial 25-hydroxylation of cholecalciferol, but this has not been established.

5. Pancreatic Insufficiency

The diagnosis of pancreatic insufficiency is difficult to establish as a cause of malabsorption syndrome, unless the pancreas is calcified or there is a history of clear-cut attacks of pancreatitis. The malabsorption may be very severe, with 50–80 gm of fat a day excreted in the stool. The patient usually loses a lot of weight, but hardly ever develops osteomalacia as do patients with milder malabsorption from other causes. Indeed rickets is also very rare in children surviving for years with fibrocystic disease of the pancreas. The two adults we have diagnosed and treated have responded to 1–2 mg a day of oral calciferol together with a suitable dose of pancreatic enzyme to take with their meals.

C. Hereditary Renal Causes

1. Sex-Linked Hypophosphatemic Rickets (SLHR)

In this condition (Dent et al., 1973) rickets develops in very early childhood between the ages of 1 to 3, usually soon after the infant begins to walk. The child is taking an adequate diet and remains healthy. Myopathy is never a feature of this disease. A positive family history, which must be consistent with sex-linked dominant transmission, is absent in about one-third of cases. These are presumed to be new mutations because they are inherited by half of the offspring in the sex-linked manner. The disease is of variable severity, and boys are more severely affected than girls; males are always dwarfed, but some female genotypes may escape all clinical manifestations and reveal only an isolated hypophosphatemia when they are tested (Burnett et al., 1964; Winters et al., 1958). The longer the condition remains undetectable and untreated, the greater the degree of dwarfism and permanent deformity (Fig. 18). Earliest possible diagnosis and treatment is therefore of the utmost importance, and, in the presence of a positive family history, existence of the abnormal gene can be predicted either with certainty or with fifty-fifty odds depending on the sex of the infant and of the affected parent because of the sex-linked inheritance. The disease usually heals after growth ceases, but may recur as osteomalacia later on in adult life.

X Rays show chronic rickets without secondary hyperparathyroidism; a special feature is that the bones are often excessively dense and the shafts

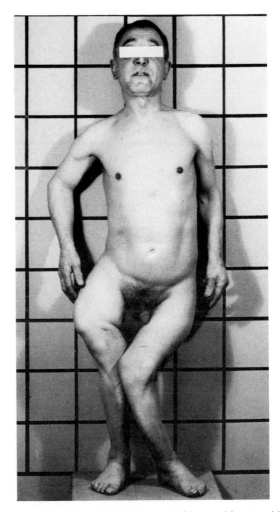

Fig. 18. Sex-linked hypophosphatemic rickets. A 54-year-old man with severe deformities. His illness in childhood antedated the known forms of medical treatment, but he did have osteotomies (see text).

of the long bones have thick cortices. More rarely, premature fusion of certain cranial sutures may give rise to skull deformities, with either an abnormally long head (which helps to produce the frontal bossing) or even less commonly, an abnormally short one. Under these conditions, and possibly through a rise in intracranial pressure, X rays of the skull may show a "copper beaten" appearance. Biochemically, the plasma calcium is always normal, the plasma phosphorus is always low, and the alkaline phosphatase (which correlates poorly with disease activity) may be variably raised. Urine calcium excretion is normal to low, and phosphorus excretion is normal. Net intestinal calcium absorption is poor. Except for the high renal phosphorus clearance and rarely diminished renal tubular glucose reabsorption, all other renal function is normal. Hypophosphatemia is constant, life-long, reproducible, and independent of clinical severity or treatment. Histology also reveals a characteristic perilacunar osteocyte resorption. (see Chapter 4).

Hypophosphatemia due to the isolated renal tubular phosphate leak is the fundamental abnormality, and rickets results partly from the low phosphorus. Hypophosphatemia has been shown not to be due to alterations in parathyroid function, which remains nearly normal (Arnaud *et al.*, 1971). Fundamental defects exist also in bone, however, as is shown by the characteristic histological abnormality that is never overcome, and in the intestine where calcium absorption is impaired.

Treatment with vitamin D_2 or D_3 should be started as early as possible (Dent *et al.*, 1973b). The presence of hypophosphatemia in affected infants can be confirmed as early as 3 to 6 months, and ideally vitamin D in the dosage of 0.25 mg should be started at that age, which is months before the appearance of rickets or of growth arrest. The requirement for vitamin D ranges between 0.5 to 2.0 mg daily, and a stable dosage schedule should be sought. The chosen dose of vitamin D should be such that rickets remains not quite completely healed on X ray. A permanent growth chart should be kept in order to assess long-term progress. Routine plasma calcium determinations at intervals not exceeding approximately 4 months are required because of the dangers of a vitamin D intoxication. This danger, although especially marked in the past because of the variable potency of "standard" vitamin D preparations and because the high dosage preparations were all restricted in dose range (only available as tablets or capsules containing 50,000 IU 1.25 mg), is still important today, and dangers arise from either overenthusiastic or underenthusiastic treatment. In addition, occasional sudden intoxication may occur in a patient whose dosage is apparently stable. Reasons for this are still unknown. If vitamin D intoxication is encountered, with plasma calcium levels rising above 10.5 mg%, vitamin D treatment should be stopped altogether until the plasma calcium returns to the normal range, which may take from 2 weeks to 2 months. Treatment may then be restarted at a dosage that has been reduced by 0.25–0.5 mg daily. Treatment can be stopped when growth has ceased, which occurs about the time that plasma alkaline phosphatase levels have reached the normal adult value (Figs. 19 and 20). This usually occurs between the ages of 16 and 17 in girls and between 18 and 20 in boys. A good result from adequate treatment and follow-up is illustrated

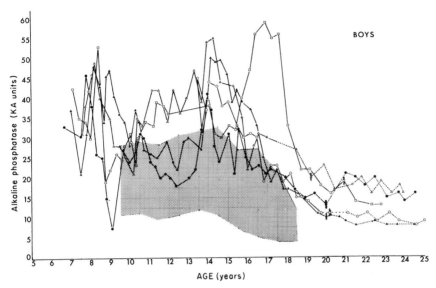

Fig. 19. Plasma alkaline phosphatase levels during long-term follow-up in 5 boys with sex-linked hypophosphatemic rickets, each represented by a different symbol. Broken lines indicate progress after stopping vitamin D treatment. Vertical bars on each line indicate cessation of growth in height. Normal range (shaded) defined by limits of $2 \times$ S.D. from the mean of 400 determinations in healthy school children after log transformation. (J. M. Round, unpublished observations.)

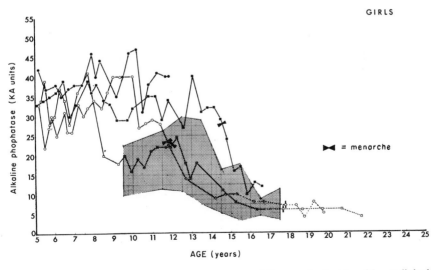

Fig. 20. Plasma alkaline levels during long-term follow-up in 4 girls with sex-linked hypophosphatemic rickets. Symbols as shown in Fig. 19.

in Fig. 21. Recrudescence of the disease as osteomalacia in adult life will necessitate restarting vitamin D or giving DHT in doses upward of 0.25 mg daily. Other forms of treatment that have not proved valuable in our hands include oral calcium alone, oral phosphate alone, human growth hormone, and corticosteroids.

Hypophosphatemic rickets inherited as both an autosomal dominant and an autosomal recessive characteristic has been described but must be

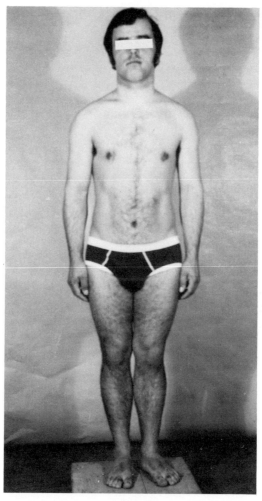

Fig. 21. Sex-linked hypophosphatemic rickets. Normally proportioned 23-year-old man after satisfactory medical treatment during childhood and adolescence. No surgery was required (see text).

excessively rare (Stamp and Baker, 1976). While the clinical pattern of this disease appears similar to the sex-linked form, too few patients have been available for comparative study, and since the abnormality is transmitted by a completely different gene, it is only sensible to classify the condition as a separate syndrome. Neurofibromatosis of nonosseous type is also transmitted as an autosomal dominant characteristic. Sporadic hypophosphatemic rickets or osteomalacia may sometimes develop in patients with neurofibromatosis with or without signs of neurofibromatosis bone disease (scoliosis, bone cysts, and bizarre growth pattern); the illness may present at any time of life—in infancy, later childhood, and in the adult. Effective treatment may require phosphate supplements in addition to high doses of vitamin D.

2. Pseudovitamin D Deficiency (Vitamin D-Dependent) Rickets

This disease (Dent *et al.*, 1968) is extremely rare but must be kept in mind, since if not properly treated the manifestations are very severe. However, treated adequately and early enough complete cure of the condition with the patient achieving normal stature and skeletal structure occurs. It is also theoretically important as an example of "true" vitamin D resistance: all signs (biochemical and clinical) mimic classic rickets in the untreated state and all become normal when the correct dose of vitamin D is given. As it is inherited as a mendelian recessive gene, it is very likely to be due to an enzymopathy. Another consequence of the homozygous state is that all cases closely resemble one another with regard to the various clinical features and their severity. This is quite different from sex-linked hypophosphatemic rickets with its dominant form of inheritance and great variability in severity even between affected members of the same family.

The disease presents at about 1 year of age as delayed standing and walking, with ricketlike deformities. Muscular weakness contributes to the delay in walking and may be quite severe. In one patient, respiration was difficult mainly because of the extreme softness of the ribs, and the child needed to be kept in an artificial lung until the vitamin D became effective about 6 weeks later. If not diagnosed and treated, gross dwarfism and bizarre bone changes develop, such as disappearance of ossification centers, flattening of vertebral bodies, and very severe osteoporosis and secondary hyperparathyroidism. This is certainly no more than the development of rickets that is so severe that most clinicians have little experience with it. Therefore, at this stage unwary physicians may ascribe the clinical and radiological findings to other causes and thus lead to disastrous delay in diagnosis. Most cases, however, are more fortunate since the patient tends to be diagnosed as "resistant rickets" and to be given appropriate treatment. The unusually good response may cause the doctor to flatter himself on the efficacy of the regime. The danger then arises after adolescence and cessation of growth, since the vitamin D may then be stopped as is correct in the sex-linked disease, and the patient, no longer in the hands of the pediatrician, slowly develops severe osteomalacia and proximal myopathy. In one of our patients, the disease was not recognized until the age of 27, by which time she had been chair- or bedridden for the last 10 years and had developed further deformities of severe chronic osteomalacia (Fig. 22). She is earning her living again as a secretary, but is only 112 cm tall and is very deformed and has required an osteotomy to straighten one femur.

When these patients are first seen at 1–2 years of age with their rickets, signs that may be noted which would indicate that this is not ordinary sex-linked hypophosphatemic rickets are (1) unusually low plasma calcium, (2) generalized aminoaciduria without the other signs of the Fanconi syndrome (see below), (3) myopathy, (4) and normal parents. In these circumstances a trial with 50 μg of cholecalciferol daily is indicated to exclude classic rickets. If no response occurs in plasma calcium and phosphorus levels in 3 weeks or so, the dose must be raised without delay to

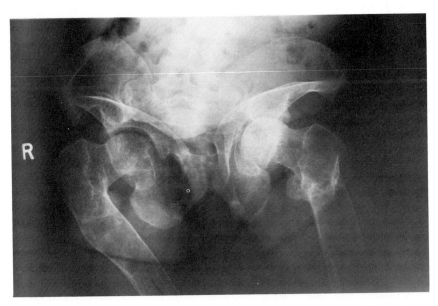

Fig. 22. Pseudovitamin D-deficiency rickets (vitamin D-dependent rickets). X Ray of pelvis in 30-year-old woman who had received no treatment for many years. She had been treated in childhood for "resistant rickets" (see text).

the milligram dosage range. A loading dose of up to 5 mg/day at first can be given if frequent plasma specimens are obtainable to ensure that the dosage is lowered at any sign of impending intoxication. The final maintenance dose 1 mg/day must be presumed to be a continual requirement. To monitor response to treatment, calcium balances are best but troublesome. Twice weekly plasma phosphorus before breakfast and 24-hour urine phosphorus on the same day can be used to plot renal clearance changes and are less difficult and almost as good as calcium balances. Finally, of course, the X rays must show healing, the raised phosphatase must fall to normal for the patient's age, and growth in stature should keep to the same percentile. In accordance with the theory that the disease is caused by an enzyme block in 1-hydroxylation of 25-OHD, an alternative treatment which looks promising is with 1–2 μg/day of 1,25-(OH)$_2$D or 1α-OHD (Fraser *et al.*, 1973).

3. Cystinosis

This is a disease with remarkably homogeneous manifestations which is inherited as a mendelian autosomal recessive gene (Seegmiller *et al.*, 1968). The baby appears quite normal at birth, and indeed a few studies have shown this to be true biochemically and with regard to the renal histology. After about 5 months of quite normal development a "failure to thrive" syndrome of increasing severity appears, and a watchful mother will note that considerable thirst is developing. Biochemically, in those few babies who have been watched during this period, all the signs of severe proximal renal tubular defect begin to develop after 4 to 5 months of age, namely, a renal–tubular proteinuria, a bicarbonate losing defect, renal glycosuria, renal aminoaciduria (involving all the common amino acids), and a high phosphate clearance. In addition, for reasons probably secondary to the above, the kidney tends to lose potassium, sodium, and its concentrating ability, so that the urine is usually watery pale and hypoosmolar. This is a nephrogenic diabetes insipidus and therefore uninfluenced by pitressin. The plasma, therefore, shows low potassium, bicarbonate, and phosphorus concentrations and an acid pH. After some months of practically no growth, the metaphyses begin to show the radiological changes of rickets and the plasma phosphatase rises. The rickets does not commonly develop quickly or with severe clinical signs. The child remains a proportional dwarf, mentally quite normal for its age, nearly always a beautiful child, and tends to be much fairer in skin and hair than would be expected in comparison with parents and sibs. If otherwise healthy and whether or not treatment (below) has been given, the child hardly grows any more and after about 5 years of useful activity, hampered mainly by the gross thirst and polyuria, renal glomerular failure appears and steadily worsens. The child then becomes hypertensive and dies of renal and left ventricular failure before 8 years of age. Before the immediate disease implications were understood, few such children reached this age. They died in infancy of dehydration and thirst-fever, of low potassium syndrome, or of inanition through failure to feed adequately in the face of difficulties from chronic mild electrolyte disorder. Some become hypothyroid and require thyroxine before death. The important pathology appearing after a few months of life consists of the development of a marked atrophy of the first part of the proximal tubule ("swan-neck deformity"); later more general atrophy and scarring occurs as in a chronic nephritis. The all important finding is the accumulation and crystallization of the rather insoluble amino acid cystine intracellularly (probably inside cell organelles) throughout the reticuloendothelial system. Analysis of spleen and lymph glands shows that about 3% (about 500 times normal) of the wet weight is cystine, 1% in the liver. The amount does not increase with the age of the child at death (C. E. Dent, unpublished data), and we have confirmed that it is L- and not D-cystine. Curiously enough the cells that contain most of the material do not appear to be damaged by it, and the tissues, especially kidney, that are most damaged by the disease do not contain very much cystine. No treatment can yet reduce the amount of cystine thus stored in the tissues. The cornea also has cystine crystals deposited in it, presumably also intracellularly; this is best seen using the slit lamp. This does increase with age and appears as a visible ocular cloudiness in older survivors. A milder form of the disease presenting with dwarfism usually around 7 to 11 years of age has been recently described and is presumably caused by an allelic gene. The biochemical findings are identical and progressive, although slower. Glomerular failure also occurs.

Treatment of the electrolyte complications is most satisfactory. Five grams per day of sodium bicarbonate and 5 g of potassium bicarbonate can usually be given in drinks and, with a suitable large fluid intake, will usually prevent the need for intravenous resuscitation. The rickets respond well to vitamin D in doses of 1–2 mg/day; perhaps even better to much smaller doses of 25-hydroxycholecalciferol. The only known likely cure at the moment is renal allograft. Donated kidneys so far have not developed progressive renal failure and are functioning as well as grafts into more normal children (Mahoney et al., 1972). However the problems of organ grafting in very young children remain, and not the least is the problem of when to do it. Should transplant be performed early in an active but dwarfed child, who has no serious complications yet, or should one reserve it as a dramatic rescue operation when the child is sick from uremia, has hypertension, and has other pathology? Only one thing is easy in the disease, that is to prognosticate once an unequivocal diagnosis has been made. All patients die young, often with distressing cardiac asthma.

4. Adult Presenting Fanconi Syndrome

The name "Fanconi syndrome" is usually used to describe a severe form of proximal renal tubular failure similar to that discovered first in cystinosis and manifested by renal glucosuria, phosphaturia, amino-aciduria, and associated rickets or osteomalacia resistant to treatment with vitamin D in the microgram dosage range. After an adult patient had been noted with a similar tubular dysfunction, and with osteomalacia as would be expected, he was diagnosed by Dent and Stowers (1947) as having "adult Fanconi syndrome." However, we have confidently re-diagnosed him now as having had Wilson's disease with a secondary Fanconi syndrome (Dent and Stowers, 1965). We now suggest that the name above be reserved for a form of the disease, inherited as an autosomal recessive gene, which presents around the age of 40 with signs and symptoms of either hypopotassemia or of osteomalacia, or both, and in which no other systemic disease can be discovered. They do not have cystine crystallization in their tissues.

Our first case of primary Fanconi syndrome was diagnosed in 1949, after 10 years of increasing bone pains and muscular weakness thought mainly to be of psychiatric origin (Dent and Harris, 1951). A routine chest X ray had shown the presence of many Looser zones, and further skeletal X rays showed over 40 of these in the usual places. The urine contained glucose and a heavy concentration of all the common amino acids as the main findings, and further tests showed that there was a fully developed Fanconi syndrome. She was treated with vitamin D and sodium bicarbonate, which was followed by the slow disappearance of pain and muscular weakness, healing of her Looser zones, and a rise in plasma potassium. The whole family was then surveyed, and over 40 specimens of urine obtained from the near relatives. Three of her four sibs, at that time symptom-free, were found to have gross aminoaciduria and on further testing all the other signs in blood and urine of a Fanconi syndrome. All the others including the parents and some half-sibs, had normal urine and were not further investigated. The three symptom-free affected sibs were followed as out-patients, and one after the other developed characteristic bone pain, one or more Looser zones, and a rise in alkaline phosphatase and were then treated and cured. We used this sibship to try the different forms of vitamin D (D_2, D_3, and DHT), and with experience of a few other cases (the disease is very rare), we can come to some conclusions about treatment. First, this disease requires treatment with both alkalis and vitamin D in the milligram dosage range. The alkali can usually be given as sodium bicarbonate in a dosage throughout of 10–15 gm/day. If the potassium does not become normal, some of this can be substituted by the less palatable potassium bicarbonate. The osteomalacia does not heal properly without simultaneous alkali, which is also required on subsequent maintenance to correct the acidosis and potassium loss. One of our patients who lived alone in a remote country district ran out of her alkali and became paralyzed again as she had been on first presentation. She spent 3 days struggling on her own until she remembered she had some baking powder ($NaHCO_3$) and cured her paralysis by consuming large quantities. Vitamin D can be given in a loading dose (5 mg/day) at first for quicker healing, but the maintenance dose is of the order of 0.5–1.0 mg/day of vitamin D_2 and D_3 and about 0.25–0.5 mg/day of DHT. All three forms work about the same in appropriate dosage, and with all three we have had clear recurrences of osteomalacia when lowering the dose to determine the minimum requirement.

The patients under appropriate maintenance do extremely well and manage to continue in full-time employment, one being a manual laborer. Very slow deterioration in glomerular function does seem to be occurring in the two survivors of our original sibship and perhaps in some later cases that have not of course been followed for such a long time. The original sibship of four cases shows a tendency to develop carcinoma, which, however, we have not yet noted in other cases. A sister aged 46, died in 1952 of a carcinoma of the cervix. Her postmortem examination gave us the opportunity to confirm that, as in cystinosis, her kidney tubules showed the swan-neck deformity. The proband, although still alive and well at the age of 63 years, has had a carcinoma of the vulva removed, it is feared, incompletely. A brother, now aged 65 years, who is still alive and the most uremic, has had two rodent ulcers removed from his face (he is always suntanned) and recently had an adenocarcinoma removed from his small intestine. The other brother died of a cardiac infarct at age 52 years and was apparently free of cancer. Our oldest patient is 73-years-old having been under treatment for 21 years. She is extremely well and active. None of our patients have developed nephrocalcinosis.

The hereditary Fanconi syndromes also include the oculocerebrorenal (Lowe's) syndrome with additional manifestations of congenital glaucoma, cataracts, and mental deficiency; tyrosinemia in which cirrhosis and hepatosplenomegaly are associated with increased urinary excretion of tyrosine and tyrosyl derivatives; glycogen storage disease; and Wilson's disease (hepatolenticular degeneration). Fuller descriptions should be sought among works devoted to the individual syndromes (see references cited in Dent, 1971).

5. *Distal Renal–Tubular Acidosis*

This is our preferred name for the disease described by Albright in his classic paper as "renal-tubular-insufficiency-without-glomerular-insufficiency" (Albright and Reifenstein, 1948). This long word is useful to pinpoint the main type of renal dysfunction and thus to distinguish it from the commoner forms of renal disease that have marked glomerular damage and a totally different etiology, treatment, and prognosis. However, Albright can hardly be blamed for not realizing at that time that his long word would quickly lose its diagnostic value as many more forms of renal tubular dysfunction came to be discovered. The other name he used, "hyperchloremic nephrocalcinosis with renal rickets and dwarfism," was far more precise. However, most people today refer to it as renal tubular acidosis (RTA). We like to suggest that the word "distal" be added to this term, owing to the recent discovery of a quite distinct "proximal" RTA that can rarely exist as a disease in its own right, but more commonly occurs as part of the other tubular defects in the Fanconi syndrome.

There are many puzzling features about distal RTA. It seems to be inherited sometimes as a dominant gene with very variable penetrance. In some families asymptomatic members may be detected by X-ray surveys that show them to have early nephrocalcinosis. Even when occurring in two brothers of similar age, very gross difference in disease manifestation may be noted (Fig. 23). This means that when occurring seemingly sporadically, we cannot be sure whether this is a true mutation or whether it was inherited from a symptomless parent. Furthermore, we are not too aware of the natural evolution of the untreated disease, since few patients are picked up early in the disease and those detected later with symptoms are usually easily diagnosed and treated. Treatment in this condition is fully effective and not only interrupts the course of the disease but may improve renal function and even lessen nephrocalcinosis. Most patients present with one of three main complications of the disease, hypopotassemic paralysis, renal stones, or rickets (or osteomalacia). By this time the patient usually has clear nephrocalcinosis detectable on X ray, low blood pH, low potassium, low bicarbonate, and high chloride. The urine does not usually contain microorganisms, contains a trace of protein (which is albumin), is always above pH 6.0 even after ammonium chloride administration (Wrong and Davies, 1959), and contains normal ammonium. There is usually a marked inability to concentrate the urine, which is unaffected by pitressin. Glomerular filtration is not greatly reduced. The disease is easy to treat, and 5–10 gm/day of sodium bicarbonate is all that is usually required. When gross osteomalacia is present, it is healed much more rapidly if high dosage vitamin D is added (15 mg/day), although vitamin D

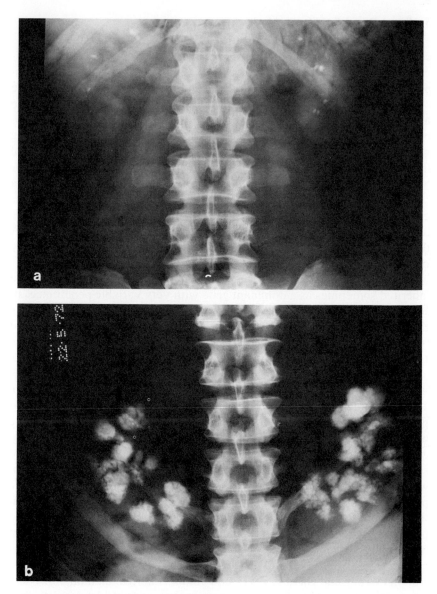

Fig. 23. Distal renal tubular acidosis. X Rays of renal areas in two brothers aged 41 (a) and 38 (b) showing marked difference in the degree of nephrocalcinosis (see text).

is not required for maintenance therapy when the osteomalacia has healed. The literature is very confusing regarding the role of vitamin D in distal RTA. Figure 24 illustrates the healing of a Looser zone with sodium bicar-bonate alone in a few months in one of our patients who also had gross nephrocalcinosis. Her bone pains were mild and quickly lessened so we were under no pressure to add vitamin D. Many workers on noting the spectacular healing of bone lesions with vitamin D added to the alkali are thus reluctant to stop the vitamin D therapy later and also continue to use it routinely with new cases. We advise that eventual stopping of the vitamin should always be done, owing to the hazard of vitamin D intoxication and since we believe it is no longer required. Our first patient diagnosed in 1947 when he had symptoms of osteomalacia, having previously had low potassium paralysis and renal colic, is living today, aged 62 years, and is quite symptom-free on a current dose of 10 gm daily of sodium bicarbonate. Vitamin D was stopped over 20 years ago without harm. Perhaps the confusion about vitamin D arises since we tend to think always of the more common renal-glomerular osteodystrophies. In these diseases vitamin D alone is effective and is essential to cure the bone lesions. Alkalis are usually not necessary even when the patient is very acidotic. It may be that a patient with distal RTA who has been diagnosed late, after much glomerular damage has occurred, may also need vitamin D as well as alkalis for maintenance, and this could lead to some confusion. There is confusion too in interpreting the early features of the renal dysfunction. It should be borne in mind that one would not expect a hereditary renal tubular dysfunction that only caused chronic acidosis to produce rickets, since rickets does not occur in many other forms of even more severe chronic acidosis, for instance, in glycogenosis. It seems reasonable, therefore, that the rickets only occurs as a consequence of further secondary renal tubular damage. This damage usually coincides with the appearance of nephrocalcinosis. We then have to presume that alkalis alone cure the rickets not because they heal the acidosis but because their administration reverses some progressive tubular damage, probably connected with the metabolism of vitamin D to 1,25-dihydroxycholecalciferol. However, as the tubular damage increases, the additional need for vitamin D becomes apparent. This need is at first temporary, but in the end becomes permanent in order to maintain a normal skeleton. We have tried to express these confusing thoughts in Table IV, where we imagined the evolution of the disease on the basis of fragments of our short-term clinical observations in many patients.

One thing is fairly clear. The variable onset of the disease from early childhood to late middle age could be easily explained on the basis of the alkalinity or acidity of the patients self-chosen diet. One patient with the

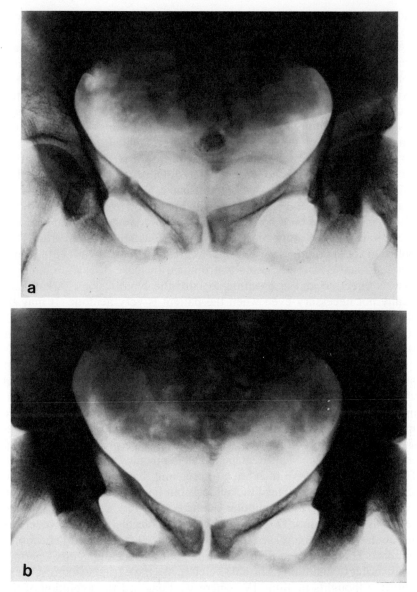

Fig. 24. Distal renal tubular acidosis with osteomalacia. X Ray of pelvis in a 28-year-old woman showing healing of a Looser zone after 6 months treatment with sodium bicarbonate 5 gm daily as sole treatment. (a) Before treatment, (b) after treatment (see text).

TABLE IV

Hypothesis with Regard to the Natural History of Distal Renal Tubular Acidosis

	Stage 1	Stage 2	Stage 3	Stage 4	Stage 5
	Primary defect of distal tubular H⁺ excretion, congenital and lifelong. Normal NH₄ excretion		No change in H⁺ excretion →		
			Slowly worsening NH₄ excretion →		
State of kidney function and appearance	Otherwise normal	Early defect in urine concentration, microscopic nephrocalcinosis	Definite urine concentration defect, X-ray nephrocalcinosis	Previous things worse; GFR begins to fall	GFR now low
Plasma findings	Mild acidosis, diet dependent	More definite acidosis, low K developing	Clear acidosis, low K, phosphate rising	Previously worse	Previously worse
Bone status	Normal	Normal	Early rickets or osteomalacia	Overt rickets or osteomalacia	Rickets or osteomalacia, secondary hyperparathyroidism
Clinical state	Normal	Normal	Slow development of various disease manifestations if left untreated →		
Treatment and response	Sodium bicarbonate corrects acidosis and prevents progression to later stages	As for stage 1	Sodium bicarbonate alone cures all disease manifestations and causes some reversal to stage 2	Sodium bicarbonate alone cures bone disease slowly, faster with vitamin D; maintains subsequent normality when given alone	Both sodium bicarbonate and vitamin D now needed for healing of bones and for long term maintenance

fully developed syndrome was diagnosed some years ago. She refused to come to the hospital; while waiting she had been persuaded to become a vegetarian and was so well in consequence that she saw no reason for more investigation. Clearly, such an alkaline ash diet would be as good as taking sodium bicarbonate. Conversely, heavy meat eaters could be expected to become more acidotic and to develop the complications sooner.

D. Acquired Renal Disease

1. Chronic Renal Failure

Metabolic bone disease is probably inevitable in any patient with progressive generalized renal damage provided they survive long enough (see Volume II, Chapter 2 for specific details). Etiology of the renal disease may be irrelevant and includes chronic glomerulonephritis or pyelonephritis, polycystic kidneys, obstructive uropathy, ureterocolostomy, renal dysgenesis, or any known toxic or inflammatory process. Renal osteodystrophy is a complex mixture of varying proportions of rickets (osteomalacia), osteitis fibrosa generalista, and osteosclerosis. We do not understand what determines the relative proportions of these components, but our knowledge of the renal tubular production of 1,25-dihydroxycholecalciferol (see Section II) has at least clarified the etiology of renal rickets; a simple concept of the development of renal bone disease can thus be formulated (Fig. 25). Since the clinical pattern of renal disease also depends on whether the lesion is concentrated in the glomerulus or in the tubule, it has therefore been convenient for present purposes to subdivide

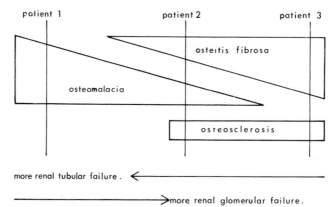

Fig. 25. Schematic illustration of range of bone manifestations in renal osteodystrophy. Vertical lines indicate the composition of bone disease in 3 hypothetical patients. Osteoporosis is not a significant feature of the disease.

the classification on the basis of whether the disease is mainly glomerular or mainly tubular in its effects (Table I). In this way it has also been possible to include under the latter heading some diseases in which an acquired etiology is presumed and in which there is little or no evidence of histological damage.

2. Adult Presenting Hypophosphatemic Osteomalacia (Dent and Stamp, 1971)

Rare cases of hypophosphatemic osteomalacia present after childhood in the absence of any family history and in the absence of any stigmata of childhood rickets which would otherwise suggest a recrudescence of sex-linked hypophosphatemic rickets (SLHR) (see Section VII,C,1). Males and females are equally affected, and the disease may occur at any time from adolescence to middle age. In contrast to SLHR, but in company with all other forms of metabolic rickets, myopathy is probably always present. Presenting symptoms are bone pain or muscle weakness, or both with occasional recurrent long-bone fractures. Loss of height due to trunk shortening from vertebral collapse may be severe and reach 10–20 cm. Early diagnosis and adequate treatment are, therefore, extremely important, but both have too often been delayed for years probably owing to the rarity of the condition. We stress that misdiagnosis in patients with little more than severe myopathy has too often led to disaster. For example, large doses of steroids have been given for "polymyositis," which has then superimposed severe acute osteoporosis. Plasma calcium levels are always normal, sometimes near the upper limit, and alkaline phosphatase levels are usually raised, but this is not always so marked as would be expected from this severity of the bone disease. Hypophosphatemia is the cardinal biochemical abnormality and is due to a renal tubular phosphate leak. The hypophosphatemia is constant, reproducible, and changes negligibly with treatment. There is usually no evidence of the mild proximal renal tubular acidosis due to secondary hyperparathyroidism that is often found in other forms of osteomalacia. Diminished tubular glucose reabsorption is infrequently seen, but an isolated increase in urinary glycine excretion is revealed on urine amino acid chromatography in about two-thirds of cases and should be regarded as a further characteristic of the syndrome. Pathogenesis is uncertain, and it is not known whether life-long hypophosphatemia may antedate the presentation of osteomalacia in adult life (analogous to the situation in sex-linked rickets where osteomalacia may recrudesce after a long period of clinical inactivity). Although genetic factors are not yet implicated, too few children of affected parents have been available for study, and it is still possible that the disease may be due to a rare mutant gene with dominant inheritance.

Satisfactory treatment of the condition requires not only vitamin D in high dosage but also phosphate supplements in order to heal the osteomalacia fully. Treatment should be started with 5 mg daily of calciferol, 10 gm daily of dibasic sodium phosphate ($Na_2HPO_4 \cdot 10 H_2O$) (or equivalent, e.g., phosphate Sandoz), and a calcium supplement providing approximately 1000 mg daily. The maintenance dose of vitamin D is under 2 mg/day and calcium supplements may be withdrawn after a year or so. Oral phosphate supplements are probably required for life in addition to vitamin D.

3. Fanconi Syndromes

At first sight the patient with an acquired Fanconi syndrome may closely resemble those described above with the hereditary form. Age may give the clue. For instance a boy of 15 years who presented with rickets and Fanconi syndrome was too young for the usual hereditary adult form. He later developed neurological signs and Kayser–Fleischer rings and could then be easily diagnosed as an unusual manifestation of Wilson's disease. Our original "adult Fanconi syndrome" patient whose osteomalacia appeared at the age of 34 years had no specific neurological signs; however, he had cirrhosis of the liver and died with liver failure and primary hepatoma. He had osteotomy scars from childhood late rickets. He is now also thought to have had Wilson's disease. A new adult case had ambiguous neurology that was thought at first to be disseminated sclerosis. The treatment for all these patients is with vitamin D in the milligram dosage range together with treatment, if any, for the primary disease. When the latter is reversible, the vitamin D can be stopped and the Fanconi tubular dysfunction may largely disappear. This has happened with our latest adult case of osteomalacia and Wilson's disease who is maintained only on penicillamine.

If a Fanconi syndrome manifests itself in an atypical manner, its cause is more likely to be acquired than hereditary. For instance, a current patient with gammopathy, secondary Fanconi tubule, and osteomalacia has early nephrocalcinosis, a finding not yet reported in the primary disease. Multiple myeloma has been clearly associated with a Fanconi syndrome (Horn et al., 1969). Many heavy metals, such as cadmium (Adams et al., 1969), lead, and uranium, damage the renal tubular cells nonspecifically to produce a Fanconi tubule. Also other toxins and chemicals are proved or suspect, and nephrotic syndromes have also been associated with these characteristic biochemical patterns. The tubule may bear the main brunt in conditions such as obstructive uropathy and after ureterocolostomy, and these patients may thus present with rickets or osteomalacia and little clinical evidence of glomerular failure. A wide search must, therefore, always be made, since although the bone disease can always be cured, failure to deal with the cause of the tubular dysfunction leads to progressive glomerular as well as fully irreversible tubular damage.

One form of Fanconi syndrome presents in early childhood as "resistant rickets" without cystine crystallization in the tissues. Treatment with alkali and vitamin D gives excellent results, and progressive glomerular damage does not appear to occur in up to 10 years of follow-up. We do not know yet whether it is inherited or acquired. It is important not to confuse this with cystinosis and thus give a poor prognosis.

A separate condition, namely, hypercalciuric rickets, lies outside this category but is conveniently considered here. Patients manifest renal tubular proteinuria, renal aminoaciduria, hypercalciuria, and phosphaturia (Dent and Friedman, 1964). Treatment requires vitamin D in a dosage of about 0.25 mg daily.

E. Miscellaneous Causes

1. Tumor Rickets

Various forms of cancer are now known to produce polypeptide hormones closely akin to the natural ones, with consequent development of the clinical endocrine syndromes (e.g., Cushing's syndrome from many cancers, especially oat-cell bronchial carcinoma). Only relatively recently have certain tumors (so far benign ones) been observed to cause hypophosphatemic rickets and osteomalacia. The first report was by Prader et al. (1959) when rickets was noted in a child with a reparative granuloma of a rib. On removal of the granuloma, the rickets healed without further treatment. There have been a few further descriptions more recently, and these tumors have usually been described as angiomas with sclerosis or calcification. We have recently been referred a patient whose osteomalacia came and went as a breast carcinoma developed and was removed. The findings in adults exactly mimic those in adult presenting hypophosphatemic osteomalacia, so it seems likely that some of these latter patients may eventually be shown to have tumor rickets. Tumors should, therefore, be carefully sought in all such patients, but especially in children because the spontaneous hypophosphatemic rickets akin to that in adults is not yet described. The bone disease in tumor rickets responds to high dosage vitamin D and oral phosphate, so this can be given if surgery is delayed. The pathogenesis of this metabolic complication is still obscure, but could well be of great theoretical interest. The disease may be much more common than present data suggest. The dying cancer patient is not always fully investigated, and odd aches and pains can be dismissed with other explanations: indeed we have known well-marked Looser zones to be interpreted as being due to metastatic deposits.

2. Anticonvulsant Rickets and Osteomalacia

In recent years the occurrence of rickets and osteomalacia has been recognized among epileptic patients taking long-term, high-dosage anticonvulsant therapy (Dent *et al.*, 1970). Rickets may present as early as 20 months of age after 18½ months of anticonvulsant therapy or in later childhood with knock-knee; osteomalacia may present at any stage of adult life. Muscle weakness from the associated myopathy, bone pains, or pathological fractures that do not heal may be prominent features. In these patients who may often be physically and mentally slow and who, in any case, are expected to suffer sometimes from fractures during seizures, the possibility of osteomalacia may be overlooked. Its detection is particularly important, however, because the associated hypocalcemia may worsen the frequency of seizures and lead to a higher and higher requirement for anticonvulsant drugs, thereby creating a vicious circle (Stamp, 1974). Conversely, correction of hypocalcemia with vitamin D has been shown to lessen the frequency of seizures and to diminish the requirement for anticonvulsant drugs. Patients who develop this condition are usually on at least two of the major antiepileptic drugs, both in fairly high dosage.

Low plasma calcium levels (less than 9.0 mg per 100 ml) have been reported in 20–25% of institutional epileptic patients, and hypocalcemia is therefore the main biochemical abnormality. It may be an apparently isolated finding in patients with no histological evidence of osteomalacia. Plasma phosphorus levels are normal or low, and the alkaline phosphate is usually slightly raised (in the region of 15–20 KA units). Bone biopsy often gives evidence of secondary hyperparathyroidism. Radiological appearances may be somewhat misleading; in adults there may be no visible Looser zones (pseudofractures), and appearance may resemble osteoporosis alone with Schmorl's nodes and irregular vertebral collapse (Dent *et al.*, 1970). More regular biconcavity of the lumbar vertebrae may, on the other hand, suggest the correct diagnosis, and early subperiosteal and phalangeal tuft erosions may indicate secondary hyperparathyroidism. Florid rickets may appear in children (Fig. 6), but the disease may also more closely resemble idiopathic juvenile osteoporosis with severe metaphyseal rarefaction. Unequivocal idiopathic osteoporosis alone has been recognized in some epileptic patients for some time. This may be also related to their anticonvulsant therapy.

The disease is believed to result from hepatic enzyme induction under the influence of anticonvulsant drugs. The enzymes produced are mostly hydroxylases and conjugases and constitute the major hepatic detoxication mechanisms (Kuntzmann, 1969). Hydroxylation of cholecalciferol to inactive metabolites occurs (Hahn *et al.*, 1972b), plasma levels of 25-hydroxycholecalciferol fall (Stamp *et al.*, 1972; Hahn *et al.*, 1972a), and the daily requirement for dietary vitamin D may therefore be considerably increased. With this moderate resistance to vitamin D, oral doses of at least 0.25 mg daily are required for a prompt response. On the other hand, physiological amounts of 25-hydroxycholecalciferol (less than 50 μg daily) are rapidly curative, as is exposure to ultraviolet irradiation to the limits of tolerance (Stamp *et al.*, 1972; Stamp, 1974). As has been stated above, restoration of normal plasma calcium values may lead to a diminished requirement for anticonvulsant drugs.

3. Primary Hyperparathyroidism

Most cases of this disease present with renal stones and appear to have normal bones on X ray. About 20–30% present with bone pains, usually without stones, and X-ray examination of the skeleton reveals osteitis fibrosa generalisata with its usually pathognomonic signs. Much more rarely, the symptomatology rather exactly resembles osteomalacia with a proximal myopathy as well as the appropriate aches and pains. On X ray and bone biopsy, changes of osteomalacia are superimposed. Rarely, osteomalacia alone may be present with multiple Looser zones, wide osteoid seams, and all the biochemical changes except that the plasma calcium is high instead of normal or low. We have shown that some of these patients actually have tertiary hyperparathyroidism, having first had chronic osteomalacia and later developing a parathyroid adenoma from one of the previously hyperplastic glands (Dent *et al.*, 1975). Gluten-sensitive enteropathy has usually been the cause in these latter patients. In other cases, no cause for chronic osteomalacia has been found, and we are left wondering why a parathyroid adenoma has formed and why it appears to have caused the bones to develop osteomalacia instead of one of the more usual syndromes. In either case, the correct treatment is not difficult. The parathyroid adenoma must be removed, and the osteomalacia then treated appropriately. When healed and if medical treatment can be discontinued, it will be important to observe if either condition recurs. Primary hyperparathyroidism is very rare in children, and we are aware of only one case of rickets due to this cause (Wood *et al.*, 1958)—in a boy of 11 whom we are still observing now at the age of 27. His hyperparathyroidism has recurred several times since his first operation, suggesting that the original adenoma was really a carcinoma of low grade malignancy. Most cases of hyperparathyroid osteomalacia have been in much older people.

4. Other

Phosphate depletion following prolonged ingestion of nonabsorbable antacids, which bind phosphate in the intestines, has been associated with osteomalacia, particularly in patients with chronic renal failure (Dent *et al.*, 1961), but also in patients with normal renal function taking large doses by self-medication for dyspepsia (Lotz-*et al.*, 1964; Dent and Winter, 1974). This may be a particular danger in patients on long-term hemodialysis who may have a tendency to hyperphosphatemia and therefore given aluminum hydroxide gels (Baker *et al.*, 1974). In very premature babies, X-ray appearances of rickets may possibly be due to calcium deficiency alone, as can also be produced in young experimental animals, but it is important to remember that calcium deficiency is otherwise never a cause of rickets or osteomalacia. Temporary rickets may be found in other neonates and is perhaps of renal origin owing to relative immaturity of tubular function. Finally, rare cases of otherwise typical infantile osteopetrosis may exhibit all the biochemical findings of rickets and also show a zone of ragged and defective calcification at the ends of their "marble bones."

VIII. CONCLUSION

Osteomalacia and rickets are a large group of diseases that are not difficult to diagnose, but it is often difficult to relegate the cause accurately and to prescribe optimal treatment. This review has not attempted to include all the known forms of the disease, and more forms are being discovered all the time. This chapter is no substitute for comprehensive indexes (McKusick, 1968) and original papers (Frame *et al.*, 1973). We do, however, stress the importance of giving full descriptions of all their various aspects when describing new phenomena. Too many current cases, e.g., of alleged adult-presenting hypophosphatemic osteomalacia, are being described with no record of patients height, body proportions, or presence or absence of old deformities. A brief description under each successive heading as in this chapter (clinical, radiology, etc.), must be the minimum for an important case history.

REFERENCES

Adams, R. G., Harrison, J. F., and Scott, P. (1969). *Q. J. Med.* **38,** 425.
Albright, F., and Reifenstein, E. C. (1948). "The Parathyroid Glands and Metabolic Bone Disease." Williams & Wilkins, Baltimore, Maryland.
Arnaud, C., Glorieux, F., and Scriver, C. (1971). *Science* **173,** 845.

Arneil, G. C., and Crosby, J. C. (1963). *Lancet* **2**, 423.

Arnstein, A. R., Frame, B., and Frost, H. M. (1967). *Ann. Intern. Med.* **67**, 1296.

Atkinson, M., Nordin, B. E. C., and Sherlock, S. (1956). *Q. J. Med.* **25**, 299.

Avioli, L. V. (1969). *Am. J. Clin. Nutr.* **22**, 437.

Avioli, L. V., Lee, S. W., McDonald, J. E., Lund, J., and DeLuca, H. F. (1967). *J. Clin. Invest.* **46**, 983.

Baker, L., Ackrill, P., Cattell, W. R., Stamp, T. C. B., and Watson, L. (1974). *Brit. Med. J.* **3**, 150.

Balsan, S., and Garabedian, M. (1972). *J. Clin. Invest.* **51**, 749.

Boyle, I. T., Gray, R. W., and DeLuca, H. F. (1971). *Proc. Natl. Acad. Sci. U.S.A.* **68**, 2131.

Boyle, I. T., Miravet, L., Gray, R. W., Holick, M. F., and DeLuca, H. F. (1972). *Endocrinology* **90**, 605.

Boyle, I. T., Omdahl, J. L., Gray, R. W., and DeLuca, H. F. (1973). *J. Biol. Chem.* **248**, 4174.

Brumbaugh, P. F., and Haussler, M. R. (1973). *Biochem. Biophys. Res. Commun.* **51**, 74.

Brumbaugh, P. F., Haussler, D. H., Bressler, R., and Haussler, M. R. (1974). *Science* **183**, 1089.

Burnett, C. H., Dent, C. E., Harper, C., and Warland, B. J. (1964). *Am. J. Med.* **36**, 222.

Callow, R. K., Kodicek, E., and Thompson, G. A. (1966). *Proc. R. Soc., Ser. B* **164**, 1.

Corradino, R. A. (1973). *Nature (London)* **243**, 41.

Corradino, R. A., and Wasserman, R. H. (1971). *Science* **179**, 402.

DeLuca, H. F. (1971). *Recent Prog. Horm. Res* **27**, 479.

DeLuca, H. F. (1974). *Am. J. Med.* **57**, 1.

DeLuca, H. F. (1976). *J. Lab. Clin. Med.* **87**, 7.

Dent, C. E. (1970). *Proc. Roy. Soc. Med.* **63**, 401.

Dent, C. E. (1971). *Birth Defects, Orig. Artic. Ser.* **7**, No. 6, 79.

Dent, C. E. (1972). *Pharm. J.* (Sept. 23), p. 280.

Dent, C. E., and Friedman, M. (1964). *Arch. Dis. Child.* **39**, 240.

Dent, C. E., and Harris, H. (1951). *Ann. Eugen.* **16**, 60.

Dent, C. E., and Normand, I. C. S. (1964). *Arch. Dis. Child.* **39**, 444.

Dent, C. E., and Smith, R. (1969). *Q. J. Med.* **38**, 195.

Dent, C. E., and Stamp, T. C. B. (1970). *Lancet* **1**, 857.

Dent, C. E., and Stamp, T. C. B. (1971). *Q. J. Med.* **40**, 180.

Dent, C. E., and Stowers, J. M. (1947). *Q. J. Med.* **26**, 275.

Dent, C. E., and Stowers, J. M. (1965). *Br. Med. J.* **1**, 520.

Dent, C. E., and Winter, C. (1974). *Br. Med. J.* **II**, 520.

Dent, C. E., Harper, C. M., and Philpot, G. R. (1961). *Q. J. Med.* **30**, 1.

Dent, C. E., Friedman, M., and Watson, L. (1968). *J. Bone Joint Surg., Br. Vol.* **50**, 708.

Dent, C. E., Richens, A., Rowe, D. J. F., and Stamp, T. C. B. (1970). *Br. Med. J.* **4**, 69.

Dent, C. E., Round, J. M., Rowe, D. H., and Stamp, T. C. B. (1973a). *Lancet* **1**, 1282.

Dent, C. E., Round, J. M., and Stamp, T. C. B. (1973b). *In* "Clinical Aspects of Metabolic Bone Disease" (B. Frame, A. M. Parfitt, and H. Duncan, eds.), Int. Congr. Ser. No. 270, p. 427. Excerpta Med. Found., Amsterdam.

Dent, C. E., Jones, P. E., and Mullen, D. P. (1975). *Lancet* **i**, 1161.

Edelstein, S., Lawson, D. E. H., and Kodicek, E. (1973). *Biochem. J.* **135**, 417.

Frame, B., Parfitt, A. M., and Duncan, H., eds. (1973). "Clinical Aspects of Metabolic Bone Disease," Int. Congr. Ser. No. 270. Excerpta Med. Found., Amsterdam.

Fraser, D. R., and Kodicek, E. (1970). *Nature (London)* **228**, 764.

Fraser, D. R., and Kodicek, E. (1973). *Nature (London)* **241**, 163.

Fraser, D. R., Kook, S. W., Kind, H. P., et al. (1973). *N. Eng. J. Med.* **289**, 817.

Galante, L. S., Colston, K. W., Evans, I. M., Byfield, R. G. H., Matthews, E., and MacIntyre, I. (1973). *Nature (London)* **244**, 438.

Garabedian, M., Holick, M. F., DeLuca, H. F., and Boyle, I. T. (1972). *Proc. Natl. Acad. Sci. U.S.A.* **69**, 1673.

Gaylor, J. L., and Sault, F. M. (1964). *J. Lipid Res.* **5**, 422.

Haddad, J. G., and Hahn, T. J. (1973). *Nature (London)* **244**, 515.

Haddad, J. G., and Chyu, K. J. (1971). *J. Clin. Endocrinol. Metab.* **33**, 992.

Haddad, J. G., Chyu, K. J., Hahn, T. J., and Stamp, T. C. B. (1973). *J. Lab. Clin. Med.* **81**, 22.

Hahn, T. J., Hendin, B. A., Scharp, C. R., and Haddad, J. G. (1972a). *N. Engl. J. Med.* **287**, 900.

Hahn, T. J., Birge, S. J., Scharp, C. R., and Avioli, L. V. (1972b). *J. Clin. Invest.* **51**, 741.

Hahn, T. J., Scharp, C. R., and Avioli, L. V. (1974). *Endocrinology* **94**, 1489.

Haussler, M. R., and Norman, A. W. (1969). *Proc. Natl. Acad. Sci. U.S.A.* **62**, 155.

Haussler, M. R., Boyce, D. W., Littledike, E. T., and Rasmussen, H. (1971). *Proc. Natl. Acad. Sci. U.S.A.* **68**, 177.

Haussler, M. R., Zerewekh, J. E., Hesse, R. H., Rizzardo, E., and Pechet, M. M. (1973). *Proc. Natl. Acad. Sci. U.S.A.* **70**, 2248.

Helmer, A. C., and Jansen, C. H. (1937a). *Stud. Inst. Divi Thomae* **1**, 83.

Helmer, A. C., and Jansen, C. H. (1937b). *Stud. Inst. Divi Thomae* **1**, 207.

Holick, M. F., Schnoes, H. K., and DeLuca, H. F. (1971). *Proc. Natl. Acad. Sci. U.S.A.* **68**, 803.

Holick, M. F., Garabedian, M., and DeLuca, H. F. (1972a). *Biochemistry* **11**, 2715.

Holick, M. F., Schnoes, H. K., DeLuca, H. F., Gray, R. W., Boyle, I. T., and Suda, T. (1972b). *Biochemistry* **11**, 4251.

Horn, M. E., Knapp, M. S., Page, F. T., and Walker, W. H. C. (1969). *J. Clin. Pathol.* **22**, 414.

Huldschinsky, K. (1919). *Dtsch. Med. Wochenschr.* **45**, 712.

Kehayoglou, A. J., Agnew, J. E., Holdsworth, C. D., Whelton, H. J., and Sherlock, S. (1968). *Lancet* **1**, 715.

Kodicek, E. (1955). *Biochem. J.* **60**, 25.

Kruse, R. (1968). *Monatsschr. Kinderheilkd.* **116**, 378.

Kuntzmann, R. (1969). *Annu. Rev. Pharmacol.* **9**, 21.

Larkins, R. G., MacAuley, S. J., Colston, K., Evans, I., Galante, L., and MacIntyre, I. (1973). *Lancet* **2**, 289.

Lawson, D. E. M., Wilson, P. W., and Kodicek, E. (1969). *Biochem. J.* **115**, 269.

Lawson, D. E. M., Fraser, D. R., Kodicek, E., Morris, H. R., and Williams, D. H. (1971). *Nature (London)* **230**, 228.

Loomis, W. F. (1967). *Science* **157**, 501.

Loomis, W. F. (1970). *Sci. Am.* **223**, 76.

Lotz, M., Ney, R., and Bartter, F. C. (1964). *Trans. Assoc. Am. Physicians* **77**, 281.

Lotz, M., Zisman, E., and Bartter, F. C. (1968). *N. Engl. J. Med.* **278**, 409.

Lumb, G. A., Mawer, E. B., and Stanbury, S. W. (1971). *Am. J. Med.* **50**, 421.

McCance, R. A., and Widdowson, E. M. (1960). *Med. Res. Counc. (G.B.), Spec. Rep. Ser.* **SRS-297.**

MacGregor, R. R., Hamilton, J. W., and Cohn, D. B. (1971). *Clin. Orthoped. Rel. Res.* **78**, 83.

McKusick, V. A. (1968). "Medelian Inheritance in Man, Catalogues of Autosomal Dominant, Autosomal Recessive and X-linked Phenotypes," 2nd ed. Johns Hopkins Press, Baltimore, Maryland.

Mahoney, C. P., Stricker, G. E., Fetterman, G. H., and Marchiovo, T. L. (1972). *In* "Enzyme Replacement in Genetic Diseases." Williams & Wilkins, Baltimore, Maryland.

Mawer, E. B., Schaefer, K., Lumb, G. A., and Stanbury, S. W. (1971b). *Clin. Sci.* **40**, 39.

Medical Research Council. (1923). "Studies of Rickets in Vienna 1919–1922." MRC Spec. Rep. Ser. No.77. HM Stationery Office, London.

Mellanby, E. (1919). *Lancet* **i**, 407.

Milkman, L. A. (1934). *Am. J. Roentgenol. Radium Ther.* [N.S.] **32**, 622.

Myrtle, J. F., and Norman, A. W. (1971). *Science* **171**, 79.

Nassim, J. R., Saville, P. D., Cook, P. B., and Mulligan, L. (1959). *Q. J. Med.* **28**, 141.

Neville, P. F., and DeLuca, H. F. (1966). *Biochemistry* **5**, 2201.

Omdahl, J. L., Gray, R. W., Boyle, I. T., Knutson, J., and DeLuca, H. F. (1972). *Nature (London)* **237**, 62.

Prader, A., Illig, R., Uehlinger, E., and Stahler, G. (1959). *Helv. Paediatr. Acta* **14**, 554.

Raisz, L. G., Trummel, C. L., Holick, M. F., and DeLuca, H. F. (1972). *Science* **175**, 768.

Rasmussen, H., Wong, M., Bikle, D., and Goodman, D. P. B. (1972). *J. Clin. Invest.* **51**, 2502.

Reynolds, J. J. (1972). *In* "Calcium, Parathyroid Hormone and the Calcitonins" (R. V. Talmage and P. L. Munson, eds.), Int. Congr. Ser. No. 243, p. 454. Excerpta Med. Found., Amsterdam.

Schachter, D., Finkelstein, J. D., and Kowarski, S. (1964). *J. Clin. Invest.* **43**, 787.

Seegmiller, J. E., Friedmann, T., Harrison, H. E., Wong, V., and Schneider, J. A. (1968). *Ann. Intern. Med.* **68**, 883.

Shain, S. (1972). *J. Biol. Chem.* **247**, 4393.

Stamp, T. C. B. (1974). *Proc. Roy. Soc. Med.* **67**, 64.

Stamp, T. C. B. (1974). *Lancet* **ii**, 121.

Stamp, T. C. B. (1974). *Proc. Nutr. Soc.* **34**, 119.

Stamp, T. C. B., and Baker, L. R. I. (1976). *Arch. Dis. Child.* **51**, 360.

Stamp, T. C. B., and Round, J. M. (1974). *Nature (London)* **247**, 563.

Stamp, T. C. B., Round, J. M., Rowe, D. J. F., and Haddad, J. G. (1972). *Br. Med. J.* **4**, 9.

Swan, C. H. J., and Cooke, W. T. (1971). *Lancet* **1**, 456.

Tanaka, Y., and DeLuca, H. F. (1973). *Arch. Biochem. Biophys.* **154**, 566.

Tanaka, Y., Frank, H., and DeLuca, H. F. (1973). *Science* **181**, 564.

Thompson, G. R., Lewis, B., and Booth, C. C. (1966). *Lancet* **1**, 457.

Thompson, G. R., Ockner, R. K., and Isselbacher, K. J. (1969). *J. Clin. Invest.* **48**, 87.

Thomson, M. L. (1955). *J. Physiol. (London)* **127**, 236.

Tsai, H. C., Midgett, R. J., and Norman, A. W. (1973). *Arch. Biochem. Biophys.* **157**, 339.

Tucker, G., Gagnon, R. E., and Haussler, M. R. (1973). *Arch. Biochem. Biophys.* **155**, 47.

Wheatley, V. R., and Reinerston, R. P. (1958). *J. Invest. Dermatol.* **31**, 51.

Winters, R. W., Graham, J. B., Williams, T. F., McFells, V. W., and Burnett, C. H. (1958). *Medicine (Baltimore)* **37**, 97.

Wood, B. S. B., George, W. H., and Robinson, A. W. (1958). *Arch. Dis. Child.* **33**, 46.

Wrong, O., and Davies, H. E. F. (1959). *Q. J. Med.* **28**, 259.

Zull, J. E., Czarnowska-Misztal, E., and DeLuca, H. F. (1966). *Proc. Natl. Acad. Sci. U.S.A.* **55**, 177.

6

Osteoporosis: Pathogenesis and Therapy

LOUIS V. AVIOLI

I. DEFINITION

Although first described by Pommer (1885, 1925), osteoporosis is not unique to modern man, having been documented in prehistoric man living within the third millenium BC (Perzigian, 1973; Moseley, 1965; Berg, 1972; Dewey *et al.,* 1969). Osteoporosis is a generic term used currently to define a specific form of generalized "osteopenia," a term initially introduced by Bauer (1960) as equal to "too little calcified bone." However, it is herein redefined as signifying a reduction in bone mass below that which normally characterizes the skeleton for the age, sex, and race of an individual.

307

As such it is a description of a state not a disease. According to classic histological criteria, osteoporosis is characterized by a reduction in trabecular bone mass in relation to the total area of the histological section and a ratio of mineral to organic matrix which approximates that of normal bone. Osteoporosis must be differentiated from osteomalacia (see Chapter 5) in which the ratio of mineral to organic matrix is by definition low, although total bone mass (i.e., osteoid plus mineral) may be normal, decreased, or even increased (Fig. 1). In most instances (i.e., in the absence of pseudofractures) the distinction between osteoporosis and osteomalacia is only established with certainty by bone biopsy (usually of the rib or iliac crest) and inspection of appropriately stained, undemineralized, histological sections (LeMay and Blunt, 1949; Steinbach *et al.*, 1959). The distinguishing histological features of osteomalacia observed on trabecular surfaces or newly forming haversian systems are wide osteoid seams and an increased number of surface seams per unit area of bone. In addition to these changes one classically finds a decreased rate of osteoid mineralization or so-called "appositional rate" at the calcification front, as shown by either special staining (see Chapter 4) or tetracycline labeling techniques. These combined histological criteria are essential to the diagnosis of osteomalacia per se, since other pathological osteopenic disorders characterized by elevated appositional rates (i.e., hyperthyroidism, Paget's disease, or primary hyperparathyroidism) may also lead to an increase in the surface area occupied by osteoid seams (see Chapter 4) despite ample evidence of osteoid mineralization. Histological confirmation of osteoporosis as the primary underlying form of osteopenia is considered most essential for the institution of appropriate therapy. Without appropriate bone biopsy documentation, therefore, a variety of proposed therapeutic "cures" for osteoporosis may, in fact, simply represent a remineralization of an associated osteomalacic process. Not infrequently osteoporosis and some degrees of osteomalacia occur together without the so-called classic laboratory "hallmarks" of osteomalacia (see Chapter 5) (Johnson *et al.*, 1971; Haas *et al.*, 1963). Moreover, osteomalacia makes an important contribution to the increased incidence of femoral neck fractures in elderly individuals (Aaron *et al.*, 1974a). Serum "antirachitic activity" (Smith *et al.*, 1964) and 25-hydroxycholecalciferol (Corless *et al.*, 1975) may be significantly lower in elderly females with symptomatic skeletal osteopenia. Variations in sunlight exposure (Aaron *et al.*, 1974b), nutritional inadequacy (Exton-Smith *et al.*, 1966), and acquired defects in the metabolism of 25-hydroxycholecalciferol have been invoked as potential etiological factors (Lund *et al.*, 1975a).

To the radiologist, osteoporosis represents increased radiolucency of bones (particularly of the vertebrae), usually associated with biconcavity

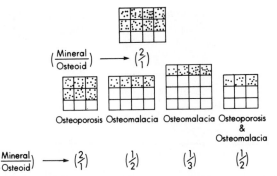

Fig. 1. Schematic representation of bone mass and mineral–osteoid relationships in osteoporosis and osteomalacia. Each large block represents a hypothetical bone segment. The stippled areas denote mineralized osteoid and the clear areas, poorly mineralized or nonmineralized osteoid. The total number of small blocks in each hypothetical bone segment represents individual bone units. Note that bone mass is always decreased in osteoporosis, although the mineral–osteoid ratio is normal. Although bone mass may be normal, increased, or (when associated with osteoporosis) decreased in osteomalacia, the mineral–osteoid ratio is always decreased.

of vertebral bodies or ballooning of the intervertebral discs; with advanced rarefaction some degree of vertebral collapse may occur (Fig. 2). When judged by relatively insensitive roentgenographic criteria alone, the incidence of osteoporosis of the spine of women between the ages of 45 and 79 has been estimated as 29% (Smith *et al.*, 1960), whereas only 18% of ambulatory elderly males are similarly affected (Urist, 1960). Despite attempts to refine radiographic techniques (McFarland, 1954), this definition is somewhat crude and misleading since a loss of over 30% of bone mineral is apparently necessary before the trained radiologist is certain of abnormal demineralization (Lachman, 1955; Wray *et al.*, 1963), and radiological criteria, such as ballooning of the vertebral discs, have been shown to be of little value in assessing the amount of bone loss (Doyle *et al.*, 1967). Moreover, the amount of demineralization necessary for the radiological diagnosis of osteopenia varies widely in different bones and in different parts of the same bone depending on the structural composition of the area in question (Lachman and Whilan, 1936). Decreased bone mass is more readily visible in bone characterized by an increased trabecular content and relatively thin cortices. There are also individuals with excessive loss of vertebral trabecular bone without associated vertebral collapse as well as those with traumatic wedge fractures with a normal complement of trabecular bone. There is also a lack of correlation between central (i.e., vertebral column and iliac crest) and peripheral (i.e., proximal ends of ulnar and femur and small tubular bones of hands and feet) bone loss

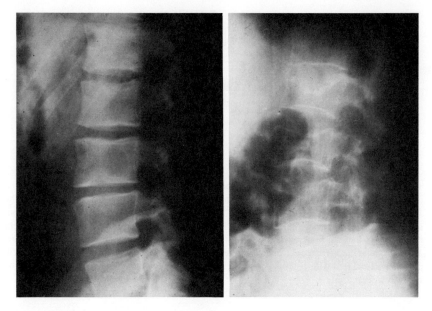

Fig. 2. Lumbar vertebrae of a 29-year-old asymptomatic female on the left and that of 55-year-old female with progressive osteopenia on the right.

(Garn *et al.,* 1969). Obviously the propensity toward vertebral collapse and fracture depends not only on the mineral integrity of the skeletal site in question but also on the intensity of the mechanical forces applied to the area.

Terms such as "postmenopausal" and "senile" osteoporosis, although well entrenched in the medical literature for decades, have also led to false assumptions regarding etiologic determinants for the disease. In 1941, the term "postmenopausal osteoporosis" was proposed to describe cases that presented between menopause and age 65. Those cases that occurred after age 65 were arbitrarily assigned to a "senile osteoporosis," category although fundamentally the underlying pathological processes were considered similar (Albright *et al.,* 1941). Clinical descriptions of osteoporosis in terms of pathological criteria such as "back pain" or "crush fracture syndrome" may also prove inadequate for the aging individual with non-symptomatic progressive osteopenia and intact vertebrae. It seems appropriate, therefore, to reserve the term "osteoporosis" for disorders with a radiologically documented reduction in bone volume, where the reduction in skeletal mass is histologically characterized by a normal degree of osteoid mineralization and a loss of bone greater than that anticipated for the age, race, and sex of the individual.

II. PHYSIOLOGICAL OSTEOPENIA

Bone affords an enormous depot of calcium that, when appropriately stimulated by a variety of hormones and metabolic agents, serves as the guardian of the circulating calcium pool. Unlike the mineral of tooth enamel that is relatively inert, bone undergoes constant remodeling and turnover. The dynamic process of bone turnover normally results in the resorption and deposition of approximately 400–600 mg of calcium per day. Calcium is gradually deposited in the fetus during the early gestational period. During the final trimester, fetal accumulation of calcium is accelerated, and approximately two-thirds of the calcium in the neonatal skeleton is deposited during this period. The total calcium content of a full-term child weighing 3500 gm approaches 30 gm or about 1% of the body weight. X-Ray diffraction analysis of bones obtained from newborn infants reveal that both the apatite crystals and collagen are poorly oriented. This random pattern is converted to a highly oriented apatite–collagen relationship as the limbs are used and the skeleton is alternately stressed and relaxed (Chatterji et al., 1972).

The turnover of skeletal calcium varies with age. It has been estimated to be 100% per year in infants up to 1 year, decreasing with age to a turnover rate of 10% in older children (see Volume II, Chapter 7). The skeleton weighs approximately 100 gm at birth and actually doubles in weight during the first year of life. Skeletal growth during childhood involves calcium retention of not more than 150 mg/day until after the first decade. During the peak adolescent growth "spurt," bone development is at its maximum. At this time calcium accumulation or "accretion" in bone may amount to between 275–500 mg/day, and bone mineral content increases by about 8.5% annually (Mazess and Cameron, 1971). Thus, there are two periods of most rapid bone gain, that of infancy (through the second year) and that of adolescence (from 10 through 16, depending upon sex and maturity rate). The adolescent spurt in subperiosteal new bone formation is earlier in girls (from 10 through 16 years of age) than in boys (from 12 through 16 years of age). The ratio of bone cortical area (i.e., second metacarpal) to total surface area is very similar to that of the 50th percentile curves of weight-for-age for all children aged 2–18 years (Gryfe et al., 1971). By the age of 18, however, the ratio of cortical area to body weight is approximately 20% lower in girls than boys. This relatively lower bone mass in girls in early adult life may be one of the factors leading to a higher incidence of osteoporosis in postmenopausal women. Blacks have more bone and a heavier skeleton at nearly all ages (Trotter et al., 1960). This bone difference is significant and reflects a greater net formation relative to net resorption and a larger skeleton mass. These observations are also consistent with observations documenting advanced skeletal development in black children (Garn *et al.*, 1972a) and others citing the important influence of genetic factors in control of bone development (Smith *et al.*, 1973). Children and young adults from impoverished areas or those suffering malnutrition characteristically exhibit a significant decrease in the amount of new bone formation during these periods (Garn, 1972). Although ossification status (i.e., development of ossification centers) is not retarded by acute protein–calorie malnutrition, at comparable "bone age" this acute insult leads to a dramatic decrease in compact cortical bone (Garn *et al.*, 1964b). Subperiosteal growth in simple malnutrition is comparable to normal bone growth, but slower and with less bone formed. Bone growth in severe protein-calorie malnutrition malabsorption states and in some disorders of oxygen transport is slower, but in addition endosteal bone resorption is accelerated. Bone "recovery" may also occur in adolescence in a variety of disorders, including osteogenesis imperfecta, vitamin D-resistant rickets, hypophosphatasia, and Down's syndrome (Garn and Poxnanski, 1970; Garn *et al.*, 1972b).

The rate of bone turnover is highest in cancellous or trabecular bones (i.e., vertebrae and ribs) than in compact bone, such as the skull and mandible. The age-related remodeling processes of the skull probably differs from those of other skeletal parts, since skull bones are composed of two cortical layers, the outer and inner tables, separated by cancellous or diploe bone. As such, the bones in cross section from outside to within are characterized by two periosteal-lined surfaces, two compact layers of bone, and both endosteii interspersed between diploic bone. This dual periosteal nature of the cranium leads to an increase in bone thickness. In contrast, the decreased thickness of round bones (i.e., rib, femur, and metacarpal) results from endosteal resorption exceeding periosteal apposition. It is still unclear whether or not either of the skull tables become thinner with age, a phenomenon that typifies the fate of comparable structural units (i.e., rib, femur, and metacarpal cortex) (Steinbach and Obata, 1957). In adults, after epiphyseal closure and longitudinal growth have ceased, skeletal turnover does not entirely cease, since there is both continuing subperiosteal bone formation and a continuation of the later adolescent shift to endosteal bone formation or apposition. At this time, the skeletal maintenance requires the deposition of approximately 180 gm of calcium per year, or 15% of the total skeletal content. The skeleton is in a relatively steady state, since bone formation equals bone resorption with no net change in skeletal mass. Epidemiological surveys in varied populations with wide ranges in calcium intake demonstrate a shift in this equilibrium between the third and fourth decades, with bone resorption dominating; this results in a loss of skeletal mass, especially in the vertebrae and long bones (Arnold, 1964; Garn *et al.*, 1969; Khanna and Bhargava, 1971; Smith *et al.*, 1972) (Figs. 3 and 4). The age-related bone loss most probably effects the entire skeleton, although it is far from uniform, proceeding at different rates in different parts (Morgan and Newton-John, 1964; Adams *et al.*, 1970). Thus, the amount of cancellous trabecular bone of the vertebral bodies begins to decrease by the age of 25–30 years, whereas the loss of cortical bone occurs much later in time. Furthermore, the rates of bone resorption in various cancellous bones are also different, since vertebral bodies atrophy sooner than the calcaneum (Weaver and Chalmers, 1966). Age-related decreases in mandibular alveolar bone also lead to diminution of tooth support, fenestration of the roots, and ultimate loss of teeth (Israel, 1967).

There are certain other characteristics of this universal loss of skeletal mass with age: (1) The rate of bone loss does not increase with age in that there appears in persons aged 30–40 years to be a linear fall in the average amount of bones of 8% per decade in women and 3% per decade in men. (2) In well-nourished individuals with calcium intakes greater than 700–800 mg/day, the decrease in bone mass is unrelated to calcium intake. (3) Among young adults, the skeletal mass is greater in males than females and greater in blacks than whites. (4) The loss begins earlier in females than in males. (5) Taller subjects of both sexes lose bone less rapidly (Garn and Hull, 1966). (6) Although the onset of loss in the females antedates the menopause, the rate of skeletal loss in some females is distinctly accelerated after menopause. Thus, since the maximum skeletal maturity is less for the white female than for the white male or the black male or female and because the loss begins earlier in the female and proceeds at a more rapid rate after menopause, net skeletal mass is lowest in the postmenopausal white female. Genetic and epidemiological factors all appear to play important roles in determining the total bone mass of adult populations. Striking low levels of compact bone and vertebral density have been observed in prepubertal children with the XO variety of gonadal dysgenesis (Levin and Kupperman, 1961; Keats and Bruns, 1964; Finby and Archibald, 1963; Beals, 1973) in American-born and Asiatic-born Chinese and Japanese (Garn *et al.*, 1964a), women of Anglo-Saxon origins (Smith and Rizek, 1966), and American Eskimos (Mazess, 1970). In this last group the demineralization has been associated with a ''benign'' systemic ketoacidosis that results from the Eskimo's high protein acid-ash diet (Cahill, 1974). Childhood osteopenia is seen in inherited disorders associated with abnormal hemoglobins, in patients with pseudo-pseudohypoparathyroidism (see Volume II, Chapter 3), inherited forms of pseudogliomatous blindness (Neuhaüser *et al.*, 1976) and in subjects with chromosomal reduplications such as Klinfelters syndrome (XXY) (Garn

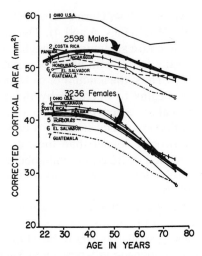

Fig. 3. Age-associated decrease in the metacarpal cortical area of males and females from 7 countries (a total of 5834 subjects). The overall trend of bone loss for all subjects is depicted by the heavy black lines that represent pooled weighted mean values. (Reprinted from Garn *et al.*, 1969; with permission of authors and publisher.)

and Poznanski, 1970). Osteopenia also exists in young XXXY and XXXXY individuals and in Down's syndrome. In the last instance, the osteopenia may be evident as early as the first year of life, but, unlike patients with XO Turner's syndrome, is reversible with dramatic improvement during pubescence (Garn and Poznanski, 1970). Studies of omnivores ingesting predominantly acid-ash diets with low calcium–phosphate ratios and of individuals with habitual excessive alcoholic intakes also demonstrate significant losses in bone mass when compared to age- and sex-matched vegetarians (Ellis *et al.*, 1972) or nonalcoholics (Nilsson and Westlin, 1973), respectively. Moreover, since external mechanical forces and skeletal muscle mass condition the structural integrity of bone (Shamos and Lavine, 1964; Doyle *et al.*, 1970; Friedenberg *et al.*, 1973; Siemon and Moodie, 1973; Bassett *et al.*, 1964; Nilsson and Westlin, 1971; Steinberg *et al.*, 1968; Meema *et al.*, 1973), the age-related loss of muscle mass (Allen *et al.*, 1960; Forbes and Reina, 1970; Myhre and Kessler, 1966) depicted in Fig. 5 combined with the gradual assumption of relatively sedentary lifestyles probably also contribute to the progressive decrease in skeletal mass that attends the aging process. One must also consider age-related changes in the intestinal absorption of calcium as another potential causative factor. Although there is reportedly no correlation between calcium intake and either the thickness of the second metacarpal (Garn, 1970; Garn *et al.*, 1967) or "spinal osteoporosis"

(Smith and Frame, 1965), as estimated from routine radiographic analyses, more specific quantitative radiographic densitometric measurements demonstrate a significant negative correlation between calcium intake and vertebral mineralization (Hurxthal and Vose, 1969) in individuals 40 to 70+ years of age. Moreover, a negative linear correlation also exists between calcium absorption and age in both men and women (Alevizaki *et al.*, 1973; Avioli *et al.*, 1965; Bullamore *et al.*, 1970; Ireland and Fordtran, 1973), and the adaptive efficiency of the intestine to a decreased calcium intake is impaired by the aging process (Ireland and Fordtran, 1973) (Fig. 6). These factors together with the subtle alterations in renal function that

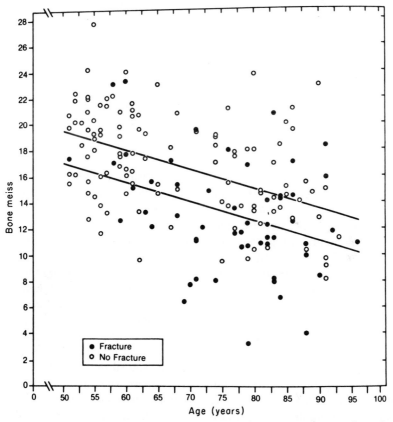

Fig. 4. Forearm trabecular bone mass (ordinate) in white women >50 years of age plotted versus age (abscissa). Upper regression line is that for nonfracture patients; lower line is for fracture patients. The photon absorption technique by Cameron and Sorenson (1963) was used to quantitate bone mass. (Reprinted from Smith *et al.*, 1972; with permission of authors and publisher.)

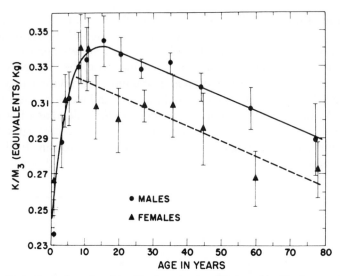

Fig. 5. Variation in the ratio of total body potassium (K) to residual body mass (M₃) as a function of age and sex. Whole body K was determined by whole body counting of ⁴⁰K. Residual body mass (M₃) is defined as the residual mass of the body after removal of bone mineral, fat, and water from the gross body mass. (Reprinted from Allen *et al.*, 1960; with permission of authors and publisher.)

characterize the aging process may lead to a chronic stimulated release of parathyroid hormone and perpetuate the accelerated rate of bone loss of aging individuals (Joffe *et al.*, 1975; Berlyne *et al.*, 1974).

Other factors that may be implicated in the age-related bone loss phenomenon include progressive decrease in osteoblastic activity (Courpron *et al.*, 1973) and alterations in the quantity of the bone matrix (Little *et al.*, 1962). The changes in vertebral density in aged individuals appear to correlate sufficiently well with alterations in the texture and collagen structure of skin (McConkey *et al.*, 1963; Hamlin *et al.*, 1975) and connective tissue. A number of studies on experimental animals and human subjects have shown that the amounts of soluble (or immature) collagen in tissues and the rates of collagen synthesis and degradation decrease with age (Kivirikko, 1970). More detailed analyses reveal that both lysyl- and prolylhydroxylysine activities in human skin decrease with advancing age (Anttinen *et al.*, 1973). Although the qualitative estimate of bone collagen is unaltered during the aging process, a significant qualitative change does occur in that the insoluble, highly cross-linked fraction (see Chapter 1) increases proportionally with age and with decreasing bone mass (Dequeker and Merlevede, 1971). The relationship between these age-dependent qualitative changes in bone collagen and skeletal mass, and other changes, demonstrating age-related alterations in the excretion of other bone matrix components such as the glycosaminoglycans (Murata, 1973; Pedrini-Mille *et al.*, 1974), are consistent with the hypothesis that the progressive loss of bone mass that attends the aging process represents an acquired alteration in the orderly sequence of skeletal (both mineral and matrix) metabolism, which initially characterized the first two to three decades of life. It has been well documented that in all populations bone density increases from childhood throughout adolescence to maturity, remains approximately constant through the second and third decades, and universally falls thereafter at varying rates. Factors that appear to play influential roles in this regard include race, diet, sex, ethnic origin, socioeconomic status, physical activity, and geographic area. The critical level of skeletal mass at which osteoporosis becomes radiological or symptomatically manifest will be reached much earlier in the individual who failed to acquire the full complement of bone in adolescence. The individual with relatively lower skeletal mass at the time of maturity will not only be more susceptible to the complications of physiological osteopenia at an earlier age but also to the skeletal manifestations of any acquired metabolic bone diseases that may result in a net loss of bone in excess of that attributable to the aging process.

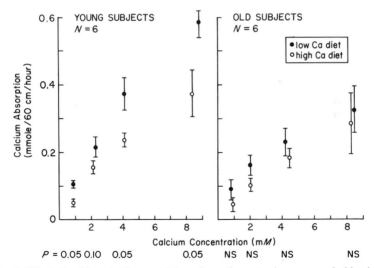

Fig. 6. Effect of calcium intake on calcium absorption rates in young and old subjects. Each subject was studied twice, once on a low and once on a high calcium diet. The rate of calcium absorption in the old subjects was significantly less than that observed in younger individuals and the intestinal response of old individuals to calcium deprivation blunted. NS, no significant difference. In this study the urinary calcium was higher in the older subjects despite the fact that they absorbed less calcium. (Reprinted from Ireland and Fordtran, 1973; with permission of the authors and publisher.)

III. DIAGNOSTIC AIDS

A. Radiology

Since bone mass is normally gradually decreasing with age in all adults, before osteoporosis is attributed to some other cause, the degree of osteopenia must be shown to be inappropriate for the age and sex of the individual. This distinction is often quite difficult, since estimates of the amount of mineral that must be lost to be evident to the trained radiological eye have ranged from 20–60%; various radioisotopic absorptiometric methods utilizing monoenergetic radiation sources and more sensitive columnated detection devices have led to more precise determinations and the detection of mineral losses of substantially less than 8% (Cameron *et al.*, 1968; Zimmerman *et al.*, 1973; Hahn *et al.*, 1974; Smith *et al.*, 1972). Regional bone mass measurements (radius and humerus) utilizing photon absorption densinometric techniques have also been shown to correlate quite well with total bone mineral mass and presently show promise for accurately predicting total body mineral content (Manzke *et al.*, 1975; Smith *et al.*, 1972). This method, however, cannot be relied on for accurate diagnosis of osteoporosis in individual cases (Shapiro *et al.*, 1975). Furthermore, even when lack of mineral can be clearly determined, it may be impossible to differentiate senile or postmenopausal osteoporosis from osteomalacia (Rose, 1964), malignant disorders with skeletal involvement, such as multiple myeloma (Fig. 7), or primary hyperparathyroidism (Dauphine *et al.*, 1975).

Fortunately, one need not depend on uncertain estimates of diminished density, for there are a number of "geographic" changes in bone roentgenograms that, although detectable only when a significant amount of bone has been lost, are indicative of osteoporosis (Rose, 1964; Dent and Hodson, 1954; Garn *et al.*, 1971). In the vertebrae, generally corresponding to the severity of the disorder, one may see accentuation of end plate shadows and preservation and perhaps intensification of vertical trabeculae and biconcave compressions, localized to one or two vertebrae, usually with expansion of the intervertebral discs (Figs. 8 and 9). In most forms of osteoporosis the vertebral cortex is thin and uninterrupted and gives the false impression of increased density because of the loss of trabeculae in the main body. Erosion of the cortex is rare in osteoporosis and should lead one to suspect malignant disease. The superior and inferior vertebral cortices are usually thickened or eburnated in excess corticoid-induced osteoporosis (Murray, 1960; Wang and Robbins, 1956) (Fig. 10). As the disease progresses, the trabecular pattern is accentuated because of the loss of horizontal trabecular structure and maintenance of

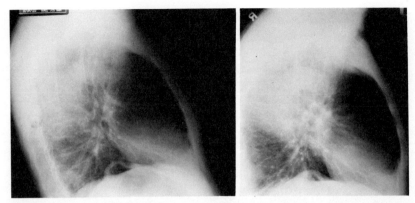

Fig. 7. Progressive vertebral osteopenia in a 56-year-old male with multiple myeloma over a 14-month period. Initially (left) the "osteoporosis" was reflected radiologically by vertebral compression fractures and diffuse vertebral demineralization. Progressive disease (right) resulted in further loss of vertebral mass and rounded kyphosis in the thoracic portion of the vertebral column. At no time were the classic "punched out" lytic lesions of myeloma detected radiologically.

vertebral trabeculae according to the structural lines of stress (Vernon-Roberts and Pirie, 1973; Atkinson, 1967). Further progression of the osteoporotic process may result in biconcave compression of the end plates by the pressure of the intervertebral discs on the hypomineralized vertebrae resulting in "codfish" vertebrae and "ballooned" intervertebral discs (Figs. 2, 10, and 11). Localized herniations of the nucleus pulposus into the vertebral body, producing a concave mushroom-shaped defect in the upper or lower surface of the involved vertebrae or "Schmorl's nodes" (Fig. 11) may also be observed, although there is no association between Schmorl's nodes and the incidence of osteoporosis (Boukhris and Becker, 1974). Progressive vertebral demineralization leads subsequently to wedge or compression fracture. In osteoporosis, the apex of a wedge fracture affecting mainly thoracic vertebrae is typically anterior. Posterior wedging strongly suggests a different underlying disease process, such as Paget's disease, trauma, or metastatic malignancy.

The osteoporotic spine with irregularly spaced biconcave vertebral bodies containing Schmorl's nodes can often be distinguished from osteomalacia, the latter characteristically leading to biconcavity of the majority of vertebrae with expansion of the intravertebral spaces without Schmorl's nodes (Fig. 12). These differences may be useful features for distinguishing the changes of osteoporosis and osteomalacia in the vertebral column with the following exceptions: (1) The vertebrae of osteoporotic children reveal the regular shape changes described as characteristic

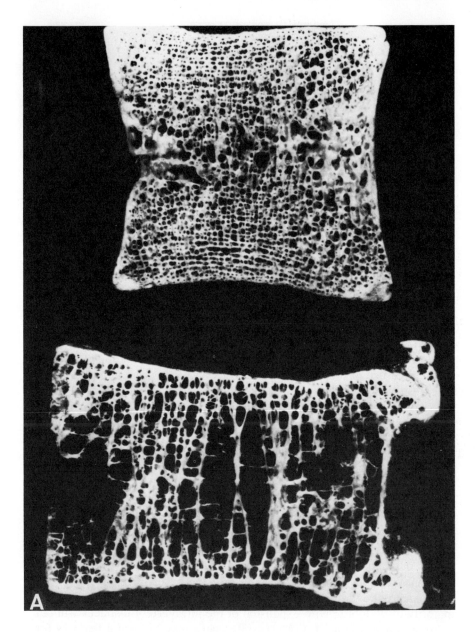

Fig. 8(A). Midsagettal view of a lumbar vertebrae of a young (upper) and elderly (lower) female.

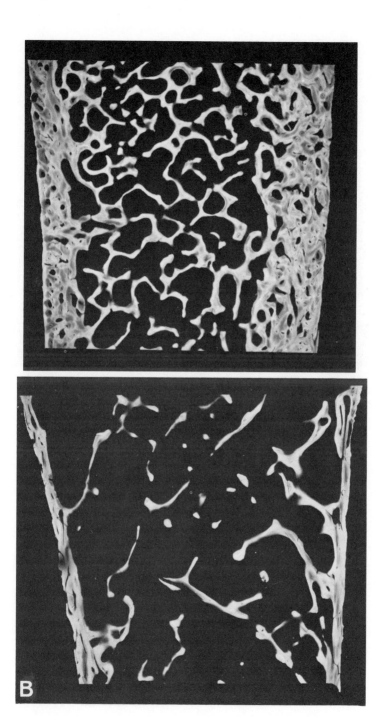

Fig. 8(B). Microradiograph of an iliac crest biopsy of a young (upper) and elderly (lower) female.

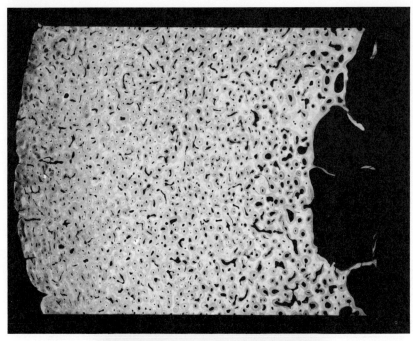

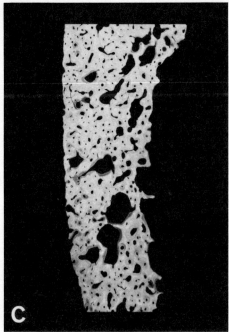

Fig. 8(C). Microradiograph of the femoral cortex obtained postmortem in a young (upper) and elderly (lower) female. Courtesy of Jennifer Jowsey.

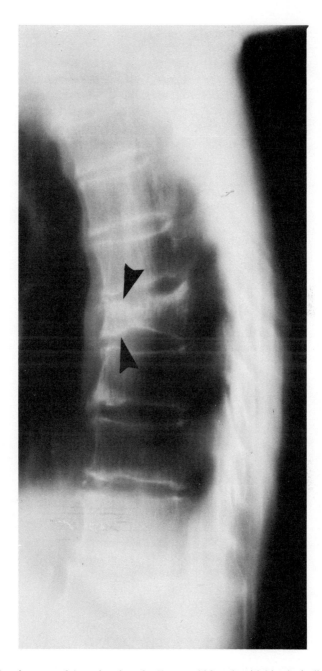

Fig. 9. Laminogram of thoracic spine of a 60-year-old female with histologically confirmed osteoporosis. Note the accentuation of the vertical trabeculae and the areas of radiographic opacification (arrowheads) resulting from compression by the intervertebral discs and subcortical microfractures.

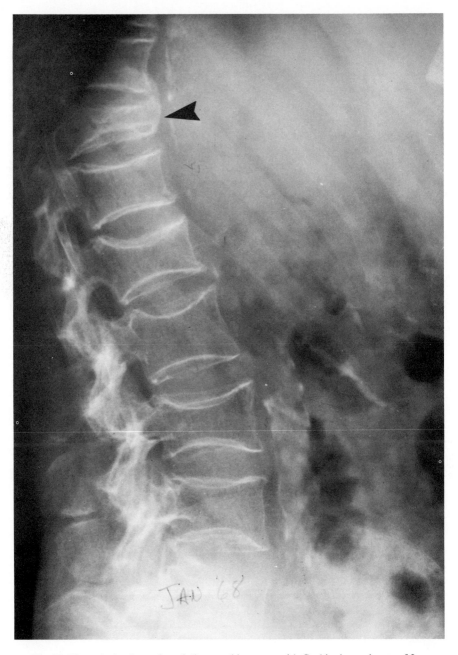

Fig. 10. Thoracic–lumbar spine of 40-year-old woman with Cushing's syndrome of 2-year duration. Note the generalized vertebral osteopenia with accentuation of the cortical margins and the compression fracture of T_{11} (arrowhead).

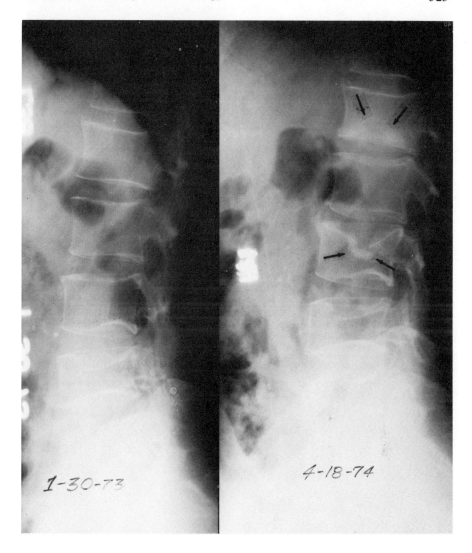

Fig. 11. Progressive osteoporosis (histologically confirmed) in a 55-year-old man. Note the "ballooning" intervertebral discs leading to localized herniations (arrows) into the vertebral bodies (i.e., Schmorl's nodes).

for osteomalacia (Rose, 1964), and (2) when osteoporosis and osteomalacia coexist in the same individual, the appearance of the spine may be classically that of osteoporosis. The presence of vertebral fractures in osteoporosis are highly correlated with the coexistence of other radiographic indications of osteoporosis, the association being particularly

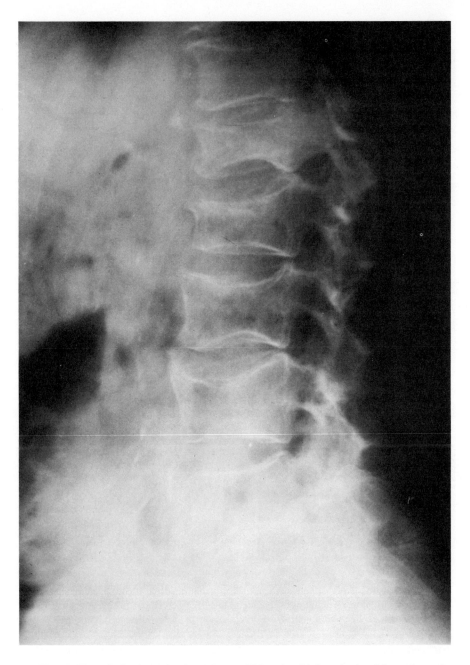

Fig. 12. Thoracic–lumbar spine in a 46-year-old female with intestinal malabsorption and histologically confirmed osteomalacia. Note the diffuse osteopenia and generalized "ballooning" of the intervertebral discs and the absence of Schmorl's nodes or compression fractures.

strong for the white female (Boukhris and Becker, 1973). The female with a vertebral fracture (most commonly the twelfth thoracic and first three lumbar vertebrae) has a 98% likelihood of having coexistent generalized osteoporosis as opposed to the male, in whom the coexistence is approximately 70%. Fractures above the sixth thoracic vertebrae without concomitant disease below this level are rarely due to the loss of bone mass which attends senescence. Spontaneous fractures above the fourth thoracic vertebrae should suggest metastatic cancer or septic spondylitis. Black individuals with vertebral fractures of the lower spine should always be considered to have generalized skeletal osteopenia until otherwise determined (Boukhris and Becker, 1973).

Radiographic changes, when apparent in peripheral skeletal sites, include cortical thinning of the long bones (Fig. 8) with irregularities of endosteal surfaces and diffuse demineralization. Thinning of the tables of the calvarium is rare but when present is usually diffuse. Occasionally, the demineralization in the skull is spotty, resembling multiple myeloma or metastatic carcinoma. These changes, seen usually only in advanced cases of osteoporosis, may be associated with decreased density of the floor and dorsum of the sella turcica. Pelvic and femoral involvement are characterized by a thin rim of well-mineralized cortex and a decreased amount of trabecular or cancellous bone (Fig. 8). The remaining trabecular pattern in the pelvis and femoral necks reflect the lines of stress applied to the skeleton and may actually appear more dense (Fig. 13). In this regard, some have advocated simple radiographic quantitation of trabecular content in the femoral heads as a reliable method of categorizing various degrees of osteoporosis (Singh et al., 1970). An estimate of the severity of the osteoporotic process can also be obtained by measurements of cortical thickness of the femur, metatarsal, metacarpal, and phalangeal bones in relation to the total width of the shaft (Exton-Smith et al., 1969; Gryfe et al., 1971). Combined thickness of the two cortices of less than 45% of the shaft width is considered to represent objective evidence of a significant decrease in bone mass (Barnett and Nordin, 1960, 1961). When the development of the osteoporotic process has been relatively rapid, as in severe forms of extreme immobilization, the earliest sign of demineralization may be a submetaphyseal band of rarefaction in the distal ends of the femora or tibiae. Only. 1.5–2.5% of total body calcium loss (i.e., 20–30 gm), when localized to the long bones, is readily detected radiographically in cases of paralytic poliomyelitis (Whedon and Shorr, 1957). This localized osteoporosis was detected as early as 2–3 months after the initiation of immobilization. Related roentenographic features of limited diagnostic value are the absence of less than usual amount of osteophytosis or spur formation along the vertebrae, a process which normally accompanies the

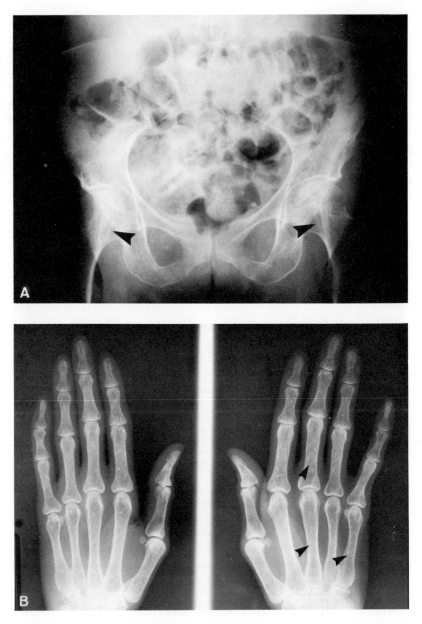

Fig. 13. Radiographs of the pelvis (A), both hands (B), and right upper extremity (C) in a 65-year-old female with histologically documented osteoporosis. Cancellous bone of the right distal humerus, both femoral heads, and tubular bones of the hands have lost most of the trabeculae components (arrowheads). Remaining trabeculae, representing those in the lines of stress, are increased in density and width.

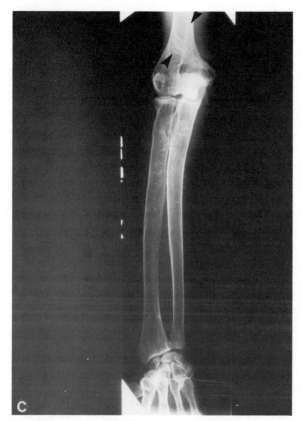

Fig. 13(C)

aging process (Smith and Rizek, 1966), and a relative increase in calcification of the aorta compared with that expected for the age of the patient (Boukhris and Becker, 1972, 1973).

B. Clinical Characteristics

Most patients with osteoporosis are asymptomatic despite the presence of one or more vertebral fractures. When present, back pain is usually localized and of two types. Coincident with a vertebral fracture, the patient may experience sudden onset of sharp severe pain, aggravated by motion and located directly over a vertebral process. The pain may be spasmodic and characteristically radiates anteriorly around the flank into various portions of the abdomen, legs, or pelvis. In contrast to osteomalacia, generalized skeletal pain is uncommon and, between episodic bouts of vertebral fracture, the patient is usually completely free of pain. Nerve root and spinal cord compressions are also exceedingly rare complications of spinal osteoporosis, despite the presence of severe spinal deformities. With rest and with slight hyperextension of the back if necessary, the pain gradually subsides within 2 or 4 weeks regardless of any other treatment. The other, more commonly observed pain is dull and aching, of long duration, and located several centimeters to one or both sides of the midline in the lower thoracic or lumbar region. These symptoms are often attributed to "rheumatism" or "lumbago." Careful palpation usually detects associated spasm of the paravertebral muscles. The pain is apt to be exacerbated by sitting or standing for some time or by the Valsalva maneuver, and is usually relieved by lying down.

The history may also reveal a gradual loss of height over a period of years or sometimes only months. The loss of height in osteoporosis is due to vertebral compression, most marked in the lumbar vertebrae although it is also seen in the thoracic vertebrae. Clinically, the loss of height can be shown to be above the pubis by demonstrating that the distance from pubis to heel minus the distance from crown to pubis is greater than 2 inches, while the pubis-to-heel dimension is still one-half the span from fingertip to fingertip. Stepwise decline in height and an associated lower dorsal kyphosis (commonly referred to as the "Dowager's" or "Widow's hump") are reliable clinical signs of progression of the osteoporotic process (Figs. 7 and 14). Progressive spinal deformity usually leads to downward angulation of the ribs and a narrowing of the normal gap between the lower ribs and the iliac crest, which may become so severe that patients complain of rubbing together of the iliac crest and lower ribs. At this point, measurable reduction in height usually ceases, since it would be difficult for any further reduction in vertebral compression to occur. For this reason, changes in linear height as a reflection of therapeutic responsiveness should be interpreted with caution (Henneman and Wallach, 1957; Hernberg, 1960). Intestinal distention and prominent horizontal skin creases are also seen across the abdomen resulting from an accordian-like folding of the torso (Fig. 14). In severe forms of the disease, the loss of the anterior lumbar curve may produce a forward pelvic tilt, hamstring contractures, permanent hip joint flexion, stiff ankles, and pronated feet so that the patient walks with a shuffling, unsteady gait, and a broad stance. Common sites of fracture other than vertebrae are the distal end of the radii, i.e., Colles' fracture, and the femoral neck. At these sites, the fracture incidence is closely related to age and diminished bone density as seen radiologically (Alhava and Puittinen, 1973; Newton-John and Morgan, 1970; Foss and Byers, 1972; Iskrant, 1968).

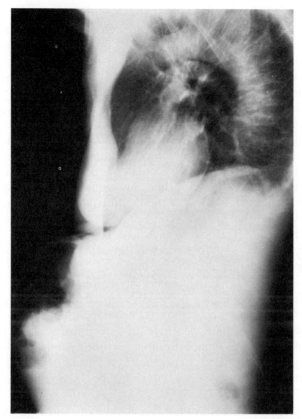

Fig. 14. Severe thoracic kyposis in a 70-year-old osteoporotic woman resulting in abdominal distention.

C. Laboratory Testing

Calcium and inorganic phosphate in the plasma are characteristically normal for the age of the patient; elevated phosphate values are usually seen in the prepubertal age in both sexes and may be noted in the postmenopausal female (Greenberg *et al.,* 1960; Kelly *et al.,* 1967, 1969). Occasionally, severe osteoporosis associated with hyperthyroidism or acute immobilization may be present with a mild hypercalcemia and hyperphosphatemia (Cook *et al.,* 1959; Harden *et al.,* 1964), the former due to rapid resorption of skeletal mineral reservoirs and the latter possibly to parathyroid suppression induced by the hypercalcemia. Diagnostic significance has been attributed to the serum phosphate level in postmenopausal forms of osteoporosis, and a direct correlation has been observed between circulating phosphate values and bone-resorbing surfaces quantitated microradiographically (Kelly *et al.*, 1967). Occasionally, states of adrenal corticoid excess may result in hypocalcemia (Hockaday and Keynes, 1966) and hypophosphatemia, the latter resulting from the phosphaturic effect (either direct or indirectly because of associated elevations in circulating parathyroid hormone) of glucocorticoids on the kidney (Schartum and Nichols, 1961). Mild hypocalcemia and hypocalciuria with all other signs indicative of osteoporosis suggest coexistent osteomalacia. Serum alkaline phosphatase is usually normal in osteoporosis and if elevated suggests associated osteomalacia, healing fractures (Nilsson and Westlin, 1972a), or hypercortisolism. Occasionally, patients with osteogenesis imperfecta tarda demonstrate elevations in serum alkaline phosphatase and acid phosphatase (McKusick, 1972a), although these changes are not characteristic for the disease (Ginsberg, 1962). Immunoreactive parathyroid hormone (iPTH) levels have also been reported as low or high in certain individuals with hypercortisolism or the postmenopausal variant of osteoporosis (Riggs *et al.*, 1973a; Fujita *et al.*, 1972; Berlyne *et al.*, 1974, 1975; Joffe *et al.*, 1975; Teitelbaum *et al.*, 1976).

Although urinary calcium is usually normal in elderly patients with osteoporosis and there is no demonstrable endocrinopathy, hypercalciuria has been observed in situations where the osteoporosis results from a clear etiologic factor, such as immobilization, cortisone administration, multiple myeloma, castration, and hyperparathyroidism. Hypercalciuria may occur in patients with so-called "juvenile" or "idiopathic" osteoporosis (Rose, 1967; Fanconi *et al.*, 1966).

In selected instances, the author has noted hypercalciuria with histological documentation of osteoporosis in the middle-aged female with functional defects in the aging kidney (Friedman *et al.*, 1972) and what appears to be an occult form of acquired distal renal tubular acidosis (Adler *et al.*, 1968). This diagnosis can only be established with certainty by recording urinary pH for 2–3 consecutive days, and determining the response to NH_4Cl (0.1 gm/kg body weight). Normally, the urine pH should fall below 5.6 during this maneuver. Urinary hydroxyproline, an indirect measurement of bone collagen turnover, is also generally normal in osteoporotic subjects (Guggenheim *et al.*, 1971; Moskowitz *et al.*, 1965). It must be emphasized that the adult urinary hydroxyproline normally decreases with increasing age (Dequeker *et al.*, 1972) and that a "normal urinary hydroxyproline" may, in fact, reflèct accelerated bone resorption in individuals with reduced skeletal mass (Smith and Nordin, 1964; Nordin *et al.*, 1976). Increased hydroxyproline excretion usually attends the "osteoporotic-like" skeletal changes seen in patients with hyperthyroidism, hyperparathyroidism, osteogenesis imperfecta tarda, acromegaly, Cushing's syndrome, and immobilization (Lee and Lloyd, 1964; Prockop and Kivirikko, 1967).

IV. CLASSIFICATION

The classification of the osteoporotic states listed in Table I represents a heterogenous group of disorders that may become clinically manifest as osteopenia radiologically and, in some instances, histologically confirmed as osteoporosis. Although longitudinal growth ultimately terminates, cancellous and cortical bone are constantly remodeled during life. A reduction in bone mass may, however, develop at any rate of skeletal remodeling. Despite the well-documented "coupled response" between bone formation and bone resorption (Harris and Heaney, 1969), osteoporosis ultimately develops when resorption is more active than formation regardless of their individual rates (Fig. 15).

A. Senile and Postmenopausal

Although a variety of diseases characterized by metabolic or hormonal imbalances result in osteoporosis, the majority of patients thus afflicted

TABLE I

Differential Diagnosis of Radiologically Detectable "Osteoporosis"

Senile and postmenopausal osteoporosis[a]	Sudeck's atrophy[a]
Thyrotoxicosis	Transient osteoporosis[a]
Acromegaly[b]	Hepatic insufficiency
Hypercortisolism[a]	Cystic fibrosis[a]
Ovarian agenesis (Turner's syndrome)[a]	Down's syndrome
Male hypogonadism (Klinefelter's syndrome)[a]	Heparin therapy[a]
	Systemic mastocytosis[a]
Osteogenesis imperfecta	Chronic pulmonary disease[a]
Adult hypophosphatasia	Immunosuppressive therapy[a]
Homocystinuria	Rheumatoid arthritis[a]
Marfan's syndrome	Waldenstrom's macroglobulemia
Ehlers–Danlos syndrome	Lymphoma and leukemia
Menkes syndrome	Multiple myeloma
Riley–Day syndrome	Hyperparathyroidism
Vitamin D-resistant rickets	Osteomalacia (in the absence of
Juvenile (idiopathic) osteoporosis[a]	pseudofractures)
Immobilization[a]	

[a] Histologically (iliac crest or rib biopsy) the lesion is reflected primarily by a decrease in skeletal mass with a normal osteoid:mineral ratio.

[b] Osteoporosis, when detected radiographically, associated with either pluriglandular syndrome and/or hyperparathyroidism or consistent with the age of the patient.

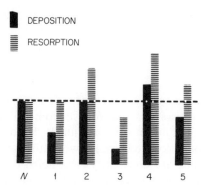

Fig. 15. Representation of five (1–5) different combinations of bone deposition and resorption rates that result in osteopenia. Despite varied rates of bone turnover or varying changes in either bone resorption or deposition (or both), the relative increase in bone resorption results in osteopenia in each instance. "N" refers to the normal state of bone turnover when bone deposition and resorption are equal producing a hypothetical state of homeostatic skeletal balance (as reflected by the horizontal dashed line). (Reprinted from Eisenberg, 1969; with permission of the author and publisher.)

are postmenopausal women. It has been estimated that of the approximately one million fractures experienced each year by women aged 45 years or older in the United States, about 700,000 are incurred by women with osteoporosis (Iskrant and Smith, 1969). In 1968, falls were the leading cause of nontransport accidental deaths in all persons and the leading cause of all accidental deaths in elderly white females in the United States. Approximately three-quarters of all deaths from falls occur in patients aged 65 and over with a female: male fracture incidence ratio of 8 : 1 (Iskrant, 1968). The rate (per 1000 population per year) of hip fractures in white women due to minimal trauma increases from 2.0 at ages 50 to 64, to 5.0 at ages 65 to 74, to 10 at ages greater than 75 years (Bollet *et al.*, 1965).

Since the gradual decrease in bone mass that accompanies aging in both sexes necessarily distorts the structural integrity of strategical, weight-bearing skeletal foci, such as the neck of the femur or vertebral bodies, the increased fracture rate that attends senescence should be anticipated. Why then is the postmenopausal female particularly at risk in this regard? Although there are reports that negate a direct causative relationship between accelerated bone loss and the menopause (Donaldson and Nassim, 1954; Saville, 1967; Ruikka *et al.*, 1968; Newton-John and Morgan, 1970; Krokowski, 1973), there is evidence that cessation of ovarian function results in an acceleration of the age-related bone loss phenomenon in some individuals (Albright *et al.*, 1941; Smith *et al.*, 1960; Nordin, 1971; Aitken *et al.*, 1973a; Davis *et al.*, 1966; Meema and Reid, 1969; Mazess and Cameron, 1973; Dalen *et al.*, 1974; Meema, 1966).

It should be emphasized that the majority of data collected to date defining age-related changes in bone mass and the effect of either natural or artificially induced cessation of normal ovarian function thereon are cross sectional and obtained by quantitating cortical bone content of peripheral tubular bones from radiographs or trabecular content of distal sites of the forearm (i.e., radius) densitometrically. Changes in appendicular skeletal mass may not always reflect the mineral content of the axial skeleton (Cameron *et al.*, 1968; Goldsmith *et al.*, 1971; Dalen and Lamke, 1974; Manzke *et al.*, 1975; Morgan and Newton-John, 1969). Definitive conclusions regarding the effect of age and the menopause on vertebral mineral content currently await the development of more sensitive and reproducible techniques applicable to the vertebral column and prospective longitudinal analyses. In one study utilizing photon absorptiometric measurements of bone mineral content in the proximal end of the shaft of the radium, two distinct phases of bone loss were noted in females: a rapid process accounting for a 10–15% loss per decade between 45 and 70 years, and a slower process accounting for a 4% loss per decade after age 50. In contrast, the rate of bone loss in males aged 50 to 80 years was constant at 5% per decade (Mazess and Cameron, 1973). The bone density of men with symptomatic osteoporosis is abnormally low when compared to either unaffected age-related men or older men (Meema and Meema, 1969). One must also account for the fact that the rate of cortical and trabecular bone loss in a population of symptomatic postmenopausal osteoporotic females with vertebral fractures appears to be equal to that of age-matched asymptomatic females without vertebral fractures (Fig. 4), although at any age the trabecular bone content is less in the females with symptomatic fractures (Smith *et al.*, 1972; Meema and Meema, 1969). Postmenopausal females who develop symptomatic "osteopenia" may simply represent those selected individuals who approach the menopause with the smaller skeletal mass in the normally distributed population at ages 45–50 years. In fact, both "postmenopausal" and "senile" osteoporosis are probably no more than the clinical and radiological expression of the lower limits of presenile and senile osteopenia (Courpron *et al.*, 1973; D. M. Smith *et al.*, 1975). Of note in this regard is the observation that the density of the ulnar of clinically normal women over 45 years of age follows a bimodal distribution pattern with 37% demonstrating bone densities in the preosteoporotic range (Selle and Jurist, 1966a,b; Jurist, 1970). As a consequence of the accelerated bone mineral loss that attends the postmenopausal years in all females (Mazess and Cameron, 1973), those females with lower bone densities should become susceptible to fractures earlier.

Documented seasonal variations in bone mineral content after the menopause with increments from winter to summer and decrements from summer to winter should also be considered (Aitken *et al.*, 1973b). Not only does the surface area of osteoid in bones increase with age in women after the fourth decade (Frost, 1962), but serum vitamin D activity in some postmenopausal women is higher in the summer than the winter (Smith *et al.*, 1964). The possibility that subclinical vitamin D deficiency and resultant osteomalacia might be another contributing factor to the increased fracture ratio incidence in some women with postmenopausal osteoporosis should also be entertained (Epstein *et al.*, 1973), since the combination of both histological defects in over 30% of postmenopausal osteopenia females has been documented (Johnson *et al.*, 1971; Lund *et al.*, 1975b; Aaron *et al.*, 1974a; Melsen *et al.*, 1975) and many geriatric osteopenic patients have very low concentrations of the vitamin D biologically active metabolite, 25-hydroxycholecalciferol (Corless *et al.*, 1975).

The pathogenesis of the accelerated bone loss observed in the postmenopausal state is still conjectural at best. Morphometric analyses of biopsied specimens reveal that bone resorption is increased in this form of osteoporosis, whereas bone formation is in general (but not invariably) reduced (Jowsey, 1960; Frost, 1961; Villanueva *et al.*, 1966a,b; Wu *et al.*, 1967). Theories advanced to account for these changes include a failure of osteoblasts to deposit osteoid tissue as a result of decreased estrogen production (Albright *et al.*, 1941), absolute or relative calcium deficiency due to inadequate dietary intakes (Nordin, 1971; Lutwak, 1969; Heaney *et al.*, 1974), imbalance between either the adrenal and gonadal hormones (Smith, 1967; Hollo *et al.*, 1970) or between parathyroid and gonadal hormones (Gallagher and Nordin, 1972; Atkins *et al.*, 1972; Hossain *et al.*, 1970; Ranney, 1959), abnormal adrenal response to corticotropin and defective growth hormone secretion (Smith, 1967), depressed intestinal calcium absorption efficiency (Spencer *et al.*, 1965), acquired defects in amino acid metabolism (Ohata *et al.*, 1970), combination of lean body mass and excessive cigarette smoking (Daniell, 1976), disturbance in the renal handling of calcium (Bhandarkar and Nordin, 1962), and a progressive imbalance between PTH and calcitonin secretion (Bertyne *et al.*, 1975). Of these it appears most likely that both estrogen and calcium deficiencies (Nordin *et al.*, 1976) make significant contributions to the osteopenia of postmenopausal aging females, and in individual cases one or more of the other proposed causes could be operative. In normal men serum calcium and phosphorus both decrease with advancing age; the serum calcium does not fall with age in normal women, and the phosphorus decreases until the age of 40 years, increasing progressively thereafter (Keating *et al.*, 1969). These differences have been attributed to a gradual fall in ovarian estrogen output, since the artificial menopause (i.e., oophorectomy) results in an acute rise in total and ultrafiltrable serum calcium levels and hypercalciuria (Szymendera and Madajewicz, 1967), changes which can be reversed by subsequent administration of estrogen (Parfitt, 1963; Aitken *et al.*, 1971; Young *et al.*, 1968). Estrogens have no direct effect on the renal handling of calcium (Eisenberg, 1969), but do not promote phosphaturia and may inhibit intestinal calcium transport (Samachson, 1966; Lafferty *et al.*, 1964; Finkelstein and Schachter, 1962). Postmenopausal levels of serum calcium and phosphorus could conceivably reflect the additive effects of accelerated bone resorption, decreased renal phosphate clearance, and a gradual loss of the inhibitory effect of estrogens on calcium absorption. This hypothesis must be tempered with the realization that ovarian failure results in a decrease in a number of circulating steroids (Table II), which may also contribute to the maintenance of skeletal and mineral homeostasis.

Evidence advanced in favor of the hypothesis that inadequate ovarian function is the major determinant in relation to bone mineral loss of the postmenopausal female stems primarily from reports of salutary effects of estrogens on preventing height loss and decrease in peripheral bone density (Reifenstein and Albright, 1947; Reifenstein, 1956; Henneman and Wallach, 1957; Wallach and Henneman, 1959; Hernberg, 1960; Davis *et*

TABLE II

Effect of Menopause on Steroid Concentration in Plasma[a]

Steroid	Premenopausal[b] (ng/ml)	Post-menopausal[b] (ng/ml)	Significance (P)
Pregnenolone	2.6 ± 0.3	2.7 ± 0.7	N.S.[d]
17-Hydroxypregnenolone	1.6 ± 0.1	0.45 ± 0.04	<0.001
Progesterone	0.47 ± 0.03	0.17 ± 0.02	<0.01
17-Hydroxyprogesterone	0.40 ± 0.06	0.23 ± 0.03	<0.05
Cortisol	80 ± 10	75 ± 8	N.S.
Corticosterone	4.2 ± 0.8	2.7 ± 0.5	N.S.
Dehydroepiandrosterone	4.2 ± 0.5	1.8 ± 0.2	<0.05
Dehydroepiandrosterone sulfate[c]	1600 ± 350	300 ± 70	<0.01
Androstenedione	1.9 ± 0.1	0.5 ± 0.04	<0.01
Testosterone	0.31 ± 0.02	0.25 ± 0.03	N.S.
Dihydrotestosterone	0.29 ± 0.02	0.15 ± 0.02	<0.05
Estrone (E_1)	0.08 ± 0.01	0.06 ± 0.01	N.S.
17β-Estradiol (E_2)	0.05 ± 0.005	0.013 ± 0.001	<0.001

[a] As described in the *Endocrine Society Program of the Fifty-Sixth Annual Meet., June 12, 13, 14, 1974* p. A-89.

[b] All values represent the mean ±SE.

[c] Estrogen administration leads to threefold increment (300 ± 70 → 990 ± 145 mg/ml).

[d] N.S., not significant.

al., 1966, 1970; Meema and Meema, 1968; Gordan *et al.*, 1973; Meema *et al.*, 1975), although radiologically detectable vertebral remineralization has not been demonstrable *even after 20 years of estrogen replacement* (Howard and Thomas, 1963).

In contrast to these reports, isolated studies of females on long-term estrogen replacement therapy and others defining double-blind trials with randomized codes fail to demonstrate any additional beneficial effects of estrogens when compared to an untreated population or when added to a regimen containing vitamin D and calcium supplements (Solomon *et al.*, 1960; Miller, 1969; Albanese *et al.*, 1975). Some of these discrepancies may be explained by patient selection and the relationship between the time when ovarian function is either artificially or naturally decreased. Aitken *et al.* (1973a), utilizing the radiographic density of the third metacarpal, found that oophorectomy before the age of 45 years resulted in a significantly increased incidence of osteoporosis within 3–6 years after operation, whereas the bone density of women oophorectomized after the age of 45 years was indistinguishable from women with intact ovaries 3–6 years after the operation. These observations are inconsistent with the hypothesis that oophorectomy in *any* premenopausal female carries the same risk of developing osteroporosis irrespective of the age of the patient at the time of oophorectomy. Moreover, when compared to age-matched Caucasian females, the bone density of both American-born and Asiatic-born Chinese and Japanese females is strikingly low (Garn *et al.*, 1964a), even though the estrogen profiles of Oriental women outside of Asia are substantially lower than those of Oriental women in Asia (Dickinson *et al.*, 1974). In addition, patients with congenital 17-hydroxylase deficiencies who lack ovarian estrogens do not develop osteoporosis prematurely (Biglieri *et al.*, 1966; Biglieri, 1968). The principal estrogen formed in either the physiological or postcastration menopause period is estrone (Rader *et al.*, 1973) (Table II), the latter derived from circulating androstenedione. With advancing age, there is, in fact, an increase in the efficiency with which androstenedione is converted to estrone (Hemsell *et al.*, 1974; Grodin *et al.*, 1973) leading in some instances to an actual *increase* in the level of circulating estrogens (Pincus *et al.*, 1954). Since the "estrogen-lack" theory is incompatible with the observations that circulating levels of estradiol and estrone are comparable in postmenopausal females with or without vertebral compression fractures and symptomatic osteoporosis (Riggs *et al.*, 1973b), it has been suggested that the bone cells of osteoporotic females with vertebral collapse have acquired an insensitivity to the normally protective effects of circulating estrogens and an enhanced osseous response to circulating parathyroid hormone. Reports of increased excretion of cyclic AMP in oophorectomized patients on estrogen

replacement therapy suggest that estrogens also enhance the renal respon-
sivity to parathyroid hormone (Lindsay *et al.*, 1976).

Accumulated data derived from isotopic, kinetic, and morphometric
analysis consistently demonstrate that the primary effect of short-term
(2–4 months) estrogen therapy·is to decrease the levels of bone resorption
(Riggs *et al.*, 1969) if they are in fact increased prior to therapy (Riggs *et
al.*, 1972a; Lafferty *et al.*, 1964; Heaney, 1969). This initial short-lived
favorable effect is ultimately negated after longer treatment intervals (9–15
months) by a secondary decrease in bone formation (Riggs *et al.*, 1972a;
Lafferty *et al.*, 1964; Jowsey and Riggs, 1973; Heaney, 1969) (Fig. 16).
Although the cause for this biphasic skeletal response to estrogen therapy
is still uncertain, it may result from the elevations in circulating
parathyroid hormone (Riggs *et al.*, 1972a) and free cortisol observed in
estrogen-treated individuals (Aitken *et al.*, 1974; Wajchenberg *et al.*,
1974). Thus, although estrogen therapy if initiated within 3 years of
oophorectomy may ultimately prove to be prophylactic for the young
castrated female (Aitken *et al.*, 1973c), therapy should not be considered
appropriate for all individuals with a naturally occurring menopause and
symptomatic osteoporosis until controlled prospective long-term thera-

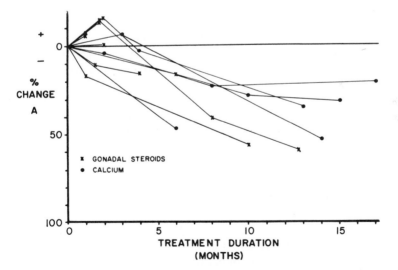

Fig. 16. Percent change in bone accretion (formation) in patients on hormonal or supplemental calcium therapy. The data are plotted as a function of treatment duration. Note that
after 4–6 months of treatment with either gonadal steroids (×) or calcium (●) bone formation falls; the relation between bone formation and bone resorption comes back into equilibrium at a reduced level of turnover, see combination 3 in Fig. 15. (Reprinted from Heaney,
1969: with permission of the author and publisher.)

peutic trials are conducted (Rich *et al.*, 1966). Since estrogen replacement therapy if initiated more than 6 years following cessation of ovarian activity has proved incapable of reversing the progressive fall in bone mass (Aitken *et al.*, 1973c), and since long-term therapy with conjugated estrogens may increase the incidence of endometrial carcinoma (D. C. Smith *et al.*, 1975; Ziel and Finkle, 1975), it would appear inappropriate at this time to subject women arbitrarily in their later postmenopausal years to this form of therapy. Long-term androgen therapy may cause irreversible hepatic injury (Bagheri and Boyer, 1974) and when used alone or in combination with estrogens offers no additional advantage in reversing the osteoporotic process (Melick and Baird, 1970; Lafferty *et al.*, 1964; Heaney, 1969; Dent and Watson, 1966; Solomon *et al.*, 1960). These observations are not surprising, since, in fact, ovarian testosterone secretion is greater in postmenopausal than in premenopausal subjects (Judd *et al.*, 1974).

Experimental calcium deprivation leads to osteoporosis in a variety of animals (Bloom *et al.*, 1960; Harrison and Frazer, 1960; Jowsey and Gershon-Cohen, 1964; Brown *et al.*, 1966; Shah *et al.*, 1967; Saville and Krook, 1968). Evidence that such is the case in man stems primarily from retrospective and epidemiological studies, which are presently controversial. Some reports reveal no significant difference in the incidence of osteoporosis between patients on diets containing less than 500 mg calcium per day and those with intakes greater than 1500 mg per day (Smith and Frame, 1965; Smith and Rizek, 1966; Garn *et al.*, 1967; Garn, 1970; Newton-John and Morgan, 1968; Walker, 1972), whereas others demonstrate a lower calcium intake in symptomatic osteoporotic individuals than in age-matched normal control subjects (Riggs *et al.*, 1967; Hurxthal and Vose, 1969; Owen *et al.*, 1940; Vinther-Paulsen, 1953; Dallas and Nordin, 1962; Lutwak and Whedon, 1963). Epidemiological and dietary survey studies may ultimately prove misleading regardless of the conclusions derived unless more specific emphasis is placed on the dietary habits, the degree of mobilization, the daily intake of minerals other than calcium, the dietary intake of protein and vitamin D, and the extent of sunlight exposure. Modern acid-ash diets that are characteristically rich in animal proteins and phosphorus may prove deleterious to bone, since diets that contain excessive amounts of these ingredients promote hypercalciuria, stimulate the release of parathyroid hormone, and tend toward a metabolic acidosis (Wachmann and Berstein, 1968; Ellis *et al.*, 1972; Reiss *et al.*, 1970; Linkswiler *et al.*, 1974; Anand and Linkswiler, 1974). Immobilization or the relative inactivity that often attends the infirmities of age promotes skeletal demineralization (Deitrick and Whedon, 1948). Peculiar dietary habits may also lead to increased urinary calcium loss and negative calcium balance despite an adequate calcium intake (Phang *et al.*, 1968). Moreover, when phytin is ingested, as may be the case in diets containing an abundance of unpolished rice or unleaven bread, calcium absorption from the intestine may be impaired (McCance and Widdowson, 1942). Elderly populations with adequate calcium intakes may also become deficient in vitamin D (Aaron *et al.*, 1974b; Exton-Smith *et al.*, 1966). Epidemiological studies designed to correlate calcium intake with results obtained from radiological determinants of "osteoporosis" may yield misleading and/or less than adequate conclusions, since, in fact, osteomalacia may prove to be the predominant skeletal histological lesion (Aaron *et al.*, 1974b; Johnson *et al.*, 1971; Anderson *et al.*, 1966).

The calcium requirement for normal adults is still a debatable issue, although it is generally placed between 600 and 1000 mg/day (Irwin and Kienholz, 1973). The majority of young and middle-aged adults are capable of maintaining a positive calcium balance with this intake (Malm, 1958; Irwin and Kienholz, 1973), but higher intakes may be essential to maintain mineral and skeletal homeostasis in elderly individuals, especially those exposed to stressful environments (Malm, 1958; Heaney *et al.*, 1974; Albanese *et al.*, 1975; Roberts *et al.*, 1948; Ackermann and Toro, 1954). The age-related needs for additional dietary calcium may result in part from the observations that absorption as well as the adaptive efficiency of the intestine to fluctuations in calcium intake decrease with age (Alevizaki *et al.*, 1973; Avioli *et al.*, 1965; Bullamore *et al.*, 1970; Ireland and Fordtran, 1973; Berthon *et al.*, 1970). Negative calcium balances observed in osteoporotic patients on low but seemingly adequate calcium intakes have been variously ascribed to slow and noncompensatory adaptation to low calcium intakes (Fig. 6) (Malm, 1963; Spencer *et al.*, 1964), defective renal adaptation and relative hypercalciuria (Bhandarkar and Nordin, 1962; Riggs *et al.*, 1967), and lactose intolerance resulting from intestinal lactase deficiency (Birge *et al.*, 1967; Guller *et al.*, 1973; Rosensweig, 1971; Bayless *et al.*, 1975; Welsh, 1970).

These observations are consistent with the conclusions that the accepted "normal" average adult calcium intake of 400–600 mg/day may ultimately prove inadequate to compensate for the accelerated mineral defects that accompany the senescent postmenopausal state. Therapeutic claims of high dose or intravenous calcium therapy (Pak *et al.*, 1969; Cohn *et al.*, 1968; Whedon, 1969; Shafar, 1973) for osteoporosis have been refuted (Schwartz *et al.*, 1965; Dudl *et al.*, 1973; Jensen *et al.*, 1973; Smith and Frame, 1965; Walton *et al.*, 1973; Garn, 1970) and judged to result in no net benefit, since the documented reductions in bone resorption results in a parallel suppression of bone formation and no apparent gain for the patient (Fig. 16). Although well-documented by appropriate isotopic, kinetic, and metabolic balance studies, these objections to high-dose oral supplementation calcium therapeutic regimens should not be misinterpreted *nor do the objections raised against parenteral calcium therapy necessarily apply to regimens stressing dietary supplementation.* The reported lack of correlation between calcium intake and incidence of osteoporosis (Smith and Frame, 1965; Riggs *et al.,* 1967) represent retrospective analyses. The intestinal adaptation to low calcium diets in man does not only vary considerably but is dependent on vitamin D intake and exercise and most probably a host of additional unknown factors. Variations in adaptive absorption efficiencies and sunlight exposure time, and the habitual ingestion of foods rich in calcium-binding phytin and/or low in vitamin D content may explain the reported increased incidence of "osteoporosis" in certain races and ethnic groups. Chronic restrictive calcium intakes, compiled with inadequate urinary retention and high phosphate intakes, the latter being so characteristic of modern day high protein diets, may ultimately lead to compensated parathyroid overactivity, osteoclastosis, and increased bone resorption (Teitelbaum *et al.,* 1976). Since calcium malabsorption per se normally leads in sequential fashion to a stimulated release of parathyroid hormone, phosphaturia, and osteomalacia, the causal relationship between defective or inadequate intestinal absorption and histological osteoporosis has been considered inappropriate in the past as is the proposed theory that osteoporosis in calcium-deficient states may result from excessively rapid bone resorption secondary to increased parathyroid activity (Harrison and Frazer, 1960; Hossain *et al.,* 1970; Berlyne *et al.,* 1974). In this regard it should be noted that (1) deprivation of dietary calcium in experimental animals results in parathyroid hyperplasia and osteoporosis and not osteomalacia despite decreased vitamin D intake (Jowsey and Gershon-Cohen, 1964); (2) osteoporosis has been identified as the only histological lesion in a young adult with calcium malabsorption (Munck, 1964); (3) serum parathyroid hormone (Riggs *et al.,* 1973a; Berlyne *et al.,* 1974; Joffe *et al.,* 1975; Fujita *et al.,* 1972) and osteoclastic activity may be markedly increased in osteoporotic individuals (Teitelbaum *et al.,* 1976; Frost, 1961; Riggs *et al.,* 1973a); and (4) long-term (2–3 years) calcium supplements of 700 to 800 mg/day leads to detectable increments in skeletal mass in elderly females with long histories of subnormal dietary calcium (Albanese *et al.,* 1975). It, therefore, seems essential to establish an adequate nutritional status for females approaching the fifth decade as well as during the subsequent years of life. Specific emphasis should be placed on maintaining the calcium intake at 1–1.5 gm/day and a dietary calcium : phosphorus ratio of 1 or greater until well-designed, long-term prospective studies of high calcium supplementation become available for scrutiny (Rich *et al.,* 1966; Halperin *et al.,* 1968). Vitamin D supplementation is considered appropriate for those "osteoporotic'' individuals (Riggs et al., 1976) with associated histologically documented osteomalacia (see Chapter 4). Patients resistant to vitamin D may respond favorably to 1,25-dihydroxy-vitamin D_3 [1,25-$(OH)_2D_3$] or its structurally related analogue 1α-hydroxycholecalciferol (Lund et al., 1975b). Vitamin D should not be administered indiscriminately, since preliminary studies of therapy in a small group of osteoporotic patients reveal that a 6-month course of supplementary dietary vitamin D in doses of 50,000 units three times a week neither increased radial bone mass nor decreased circulating parathyroid hormone levels in patients with elevated pretreatment values (Shapiro et al., 1973). Hypercalcemia and its attendant sequelae may also prove hazardous when therapy is not routinely monitored (Gwinup, 1961; Lund et al., 1975b).

Sodium fluoride and calcitonin have also been recommended as therapeutic aids for the postmenopausal osteoporotic individual. Reports of decreased incidence of osteoporosis and collapsed vertebrae in subjects living in areas where the fluoride content of the water supply was greater than 4 ppm (Leone et al., 1955; Korns, 1969; Hodge and Smith, 1968; Bernstein et al., 1966; Alffram et al., 1969) and others citing the potential benefit of sodium fluoride therapy in doses varying from 10 to 175 mg/day (Cohen and Rubini, 1965; Bernstein and Cohen, 1967; Jowsey et al., 1972; Franke et al., 1974; Cass et al., 1966) are consistent with the hypothesis that long-term sodium fluoride may prove therapeutic for symptomatic osteoporosis. This form of therapy must still be regarded as experimental, however, and its use must be tempered by the realization that the chronic ingestion of sodium fluoride leads to osteomalacia and secondary hyperparathyroidism (Jowsey et al., 1972; Franke et al., 1974; Baylink and Bernstein, 1967; Kuhlencordt et al., 1969; Teotia and Teotia, 1973) unless an abundant calcium intake and absorption are well controlled. Moreover optic neuritis, arthritis, chronic gastroenteritis, ulceration, acne, and acute allergic reactions may complicate the treatment (Geall and Beilin, 1964; Waldbott, 1964; Shea et al., 1967). In addition to these complications, it should be noted that fluorine in dosages similar to that suggested for treatment of patients with osteoporosis, when supplied to the drinking water of growing rats over several months, inhibits the synthesis of bone collagen in surviving calvaria in proportion to the concentration of fluoride in bone (Peck et al., 1965). Since the more dense and irregularly structured bone of frank fluorosis is also more brittle, increased bone density observed during fluoride therapy may not be advantageous. Sodium fluoride in a dose of 25 mg/day has the effect of causing active foci of ostosclerosis to become quiescent (Linthicum et al., 1973). Although recommended for individuals with progressive hereditary sensorineural hearing loss and with evidence osteosclerosis by polytomography (Linthicum et al., 1973), elderly osteosclerotic individuals should not also be considered appropriate candidates for fluoride treatment until a safe and effective dose for prolonged use is found. In this regard it should be noted that the results of a recent double-blind trial study in elderly Finnish subjects revealed that fluoride in doses of 25 mg/day for 8 months resulted in an *increased* incidence of fractures and an exacerbation of arthrosis (Inkovaara *et al.*, 1975). When combined with vitamin D and calcium supplementation, the optimum dose of sodium fluoride for therapeutic effectiveness in individuals with axial osteoporosis is reportedly 40–45 mg/day (Jowsey and Riggs, 1973), larger doses (>60 mg/day) producing morphologically abnormal bone (Jowsey *et al.*, 1972) and fluorosis (Singh *et al.*, 1963).

Since in either postmenopausal or senile osteoporosis bone resorption is accelerated and bone formation either normal or suppressed, potentially effective therapeutic modes should be directed toward suppressing bone dissolution while either maintaining or stimulating new bone formation. This ideal biological response is not obtained with either estrogen or supplemental calcium therapy alone, since, because of the poorly understood but well-established cybernetic coupling that occurs between bone formation and bone resorption, the suppression of bone resorption is attended by a "coupled" decrease in bone formation (Harris and Heaney, 1969). Combined treatment with sodium fluoride, calcium, and vitamin D reportedly results in a "uncoupling" of bone formation and bone resorption in osteoporotic subjects, since suppression of bone resorption is attended by stimulated new bone formation and an increase in bone mass (Jowsey *et al.*, 1972; Jowsey and Riggs, 1973). The initial enthusiasm for this therapeutic program must be tempered by reports of paradoxical effects of vitamin D in fluoride-treated osteoporotic patients (Merz *et al.*, 1970), others document abnormal bone marrow cytology in patients receiving as little as 16 mg of sodium fluoride per day for prolonged periods (Duffey *et al.*, 1971) and others demonstrating decreased mechanical strength of bones of fluoride-treated animals in which the bone fluoride content approximated that of humans receiving fluoride, vitamin D, and calcium combinations (Riggins *et al.*, 1974). Rigorous long-term assessment of the effects of prolonged fluoride administration on the structural integrity of bone and extraskeletal tissue metabolism and organ function is essential before an adequate appraisal of therapeutic effectiveness can be made.

Recent studies on the effect of chronic administration of human growth hormone in elderly women with symptomatic osteoporosis revealed that this agent is of no value therapeutically. Complications of therapy included hyperglycemia, hypertension, arthralgia, and the carpal-tunnel syndrome (Aloia *et al.*, 1976).

The therapeutic effects reported to occur with calcitonin in Paget's disease of bone (see Volume II, Chapter 5) have also resulted in limited trials with this agent in patients with senile or postmenopausal osteoporosis. Clacitonin, a peptide hormone normally secreted by the parafollicular or "C" cells of the thyroid gland (see Volume II, Chapter 4), functions primarily to suppress bone resorption (Krane et al., 1973). An accumulating body of evidence is consistent with the hypothesis that progressive osteoporosis in the female may be due in part to calcitonin deficiency. Females have lower basal and stimulated calcitonin levels than males (Heath and Sizemore, 1975). It has also been demonstrated that the basal (Berlyne et al., 1975) and stimulated calcitonin response decreases with age in females and that in pregnancy and in patients on oral contraceptives basal calcitonin levels are higher than normal (Samaan et al., 1975). Favorable therapeutic responses of "osteoporotic" patients to porcine calcitonin for periods ranging from 1 to 29 months have been reported with suppression of bone resorption documented isotopically, biochemically, and histologically (Cohn et al., 1971; Caniggia et al., 1970; Baud et al., 1969; Bloch-Michel et al., 1970; Harrison et al., 1971; Milhaud et al., 1972). Although a likely candidate for suppressing the bone resorption of osteoporotic patients, long-term calcitonin therapy must presently be considered experimental and potentially inappropriate treatment (Jowsey and Riggs, 1973) until more appropriate double-blind placebo study protocols are developed with detailed evaluation of the incidence of fracture rates and the development of secondary hyperparathyroidism and antibodies to nonhuman calcitonin preparations (Van der Sluys Veer et al., 1970).

Potential therapeutic effectiveness of phosphorus supplementation in senile or postmenopausal osteoporosis is suggested by observations that phosphate feeding reverses the hypercalcemia in disorders of bone metabolism characterized by increased bone resorption (see, e.g., Albright et al., 1932; Goldsmith and Ingbar, 1966). Moreover, Asher et al. (1974) have shown that low phosphate concentrations diminish the rate at which bone collagen is synthesized in vitro, observations that are consistent with others demonstrating a stimulating effect of phosphate supplementation on collagen synthesis in in vitro preparations (Raisz, 1969; Flanagan et al., 1969). Although Spencer et al. (1965) have reported that high phosphate feeding in man decreases urinary calcium without suppression of intestinal calcium absorption, Hulley et al. (1971) have demonstrated that high phosphate feeding fails to alter the progressive osteopenia that attends immobilization, despite a significant reduction in urinary calcium. Data regarding the effects of high phosphate feeding on skeletal metabolism are presently limited in man, but it appears to be well established that high phosphate intakes (or low dietary Ca/P ratio) result in progressive bone loss and secondary hyperparathyroidism in horses (Joyce et al., 1971), rats (Draper et al., 1972), dogs (Krook et al., 1971;

Saville *et al.*, 1969), and rabbits (Laflamme and Jowsey, 1972) as well as in metastatic calcification (Jowsey and Balasubramaniam, 1972). Since in the absence of supplemental calcium, high phosphate intake in man (doses of 1 gm/day or greater) leads to significant increments in circulating parathyroid hormone concentrations (Reiss *et al.*, 1970), these latter observations are not surprising. Preliminary studies involving the manipulation of the dietary Ca/P ratio in osteoporotic patients attest to the limited (if any) therapeutic effectiveness of high phosphate feeding in this disorder. Goldsmith *et al.* (1976) noted that after supplementing normal diets with 1.0 gm of phosphate (provided as K_2HPO_4–KH_2PO_4 in a mole ratio of 1.5 : 1), osteoporotic subjects responded with a decrease in active bone formation, and an increase in bone resorption. Moreover, Shapiro *et al.* (1975), having subjected ten osteoporotic women to a diet containing 2200 mg of phosphorus and 2400 mg of calcium for a 2-year period, reported that this regimen not only failed to increase skeletal mass when measured in the radius by photon absorptiometry but also led to a rise in serum parathyroid hormone in four of eight patients. Thus, biological data obtained from studies in animals and humans are presently consistent with the conclusion that diets enriched with phosphate-containing foods or products may prove deleterious to bone and as such should be discouraged in osteoporotic patients with marginal or low calcium intakes.

Within the last decade, diphosphonates, a series of compounds characterized by a molecular backbone of —P—O—P—, have been synthesized because biologically they simulate pyrophosphate, a substance that functions to control bone calcification in man and a variety of animal species (Russell and Fleisch, 1975). Diphosphonate compounds have been effectively utilized in animal models for the prevention of bone resorption (Russell and Fleisch, 1975), and, as detailed in Volume II, Chapter 5, also enjoyed limited success in man in reversing the accelerated bone resorption attending Paget's disease of bone (Smith *et al.*, 1971). Preliminary short-term studies on the effects of one of the diphosphonates, Na_2EHDP, by Saville and Heaney (1972) in osteoporotic patients revealed a tendency toward calcium retention, but more detailed investigations by Jowsey *et al.* (1971) demonstrated that Na_2EHDP produced hyperphosphatemia and histological osteomalacia in osteoporotic patients without histological suppression of bone resorption. Presently the administration of diphosphonates cannot be recommended for senile or postmenopausal osteoporotic patients.

Physical activity that increases both gravitational and muscular stress in bone (Bassett *et al.*, 1964; Friedenberg *et al.*, 1973; Nilsson and Westlin, 1971) has also been suggested as both preventive and rehabilitative therapy for bone loss in the osteoporotic female. The hypothesis that physical activity not only decreases the rate of bone loss but also results in new bone formation has been supported by observations that short-term (8 months) exercise and physical therapy programs lead to 3–8% increments in bone mass in osteoporotic patients with an age range of 55–94 years (Smith and Babcock, 1973). In this regard it seems appropriate to note that the findings of Smith *et al.* (1976) suggest that factors other than decreased physical activity are more important in determining rates of mineral loss.

Obviously, the relentless decrease of bone mass that attends the senescent process will continue until the long sought after "elixir of youth" is discovered. Individuals, either because of race, sex, environmental, dietary, genetic, or activity differences, will be more or less predisposed to symptomatic osteoporosis with increasing age. The careful and knowledgeable physician should, however, make every attempt to rule out potentially remedial subtle forms of demineralizing disorders such as apathetic or T_3 thyrotoxicosis, hyperparathyroidism, malabsorption and osteomalacia, or multiple myeloma, diseases that not only result in an accelerated loss of bone mass and skeletal fractures but also mimic postmenopausal or senile osteoporosis radiologically. Once the metabolic or malignant disorders of bone metabolism have been effectively considered and ruled out, the senescent or postmenopausal osteoporotic state should be approached with the appropriate use of short-term cyclic estrogen therapy in the immediate postmenopausal period, with periodic clinical and histological examination of the breasts, cervix, and uterus; a diet sufficient in vitamin D and calcium; and continued attempts to ensure adequate skeletal mobilization with programmed exercise and physical therapy at a level compatible with age and locomotor activity. Although those processes that lead to progressive bone atrophy in the postmenopausal and senescent years may, in fact, be irreversible, this combined therapeutic approach could result in symptomatic improvement and cessation of further bone mass reduction. Obviously emphasis should be directed toward the prevention of symptomatic "crush fracture" osteoporosis well before the disorder becomes established and/or clinically manifest. Individuals who enjoy an adequate calcium and vitamin D intake and continue to persue a modest but continued physically active program after age 30 should be less subject to symptomatic osteoporosis in the later postmenopausal or senile years.

B. Endocrine Causes of Osteoporosis

1. Thyroid

As described in detail in Volume II, Chapter 4, disturbance in mineral and bone metabolism have been well documented in patients with thyrotoxicosis. The latter include mild and transient hypercalcemia (Farnsworth and Dobyns, 1974; Parfitt and Dent, 1970; Baxter and Bondy, 1966), hypercalciuria, hyperphosphatemia and elevations in circulating alkaline phosphatase (Krane *et al.*, 1956; Cook *et al.*, 1959; Clerkin *et al.*, 1964), hydroxyprolinuria (Georges *et al.*, 1975; Dull and Henneman, 1963), decreased intestinal absorption of calcium (Singhelakis *et al.*, 1974; Shafer and Gregory, 1972), decreased bone mineral content, and increased incidence of fracture (Meema and Meema, 1972; Fraser *et al.*, 1971). These findings are attended by abnormally high increments in bone turnover (e.g., both bone formation and bone resorption are accelerated) (Krane *et al.*, 1956) and histological lesions of osteoclastosis, osteitis fibrosa, wide osteoid seams, and osteoporosis (Follis, 1953).

Radiologically, the skeletal is characteristically indistinguishable from other osteoporotic syndromes (Laake, 1955; Zweymuller and Jesserer, 1973; Meema and Schatz, 1970). This should be emphasized for elderly postmenopausal females in whom the typical hyperkinetic signs and symptoms of the thyrotoxic state are often absent (Ronnov-Jessen and Kirkegaard, 1973; Lazarus and Harden, 1969). Although the catabolism of bone collagen is increased when circulating levels of thyroid hormone are elevated (Fink *et al.*, 1967), the high turnover rate results in an accumulation of osteoid tissue which, unlike the osteomalacia of malabsorption of vitamin D deficiency state, is capable of mineralization. The accumulation of osteoclasts and fibrous tissue is consistent with the rapid bone turnover and stimulated increments in bone resorption (Krane *et al.*, 1956) and the increased skeletal sensitivity of thyrotoxic patients to parathyroid hormone (Castro *et al.*, 1975). The cause for the osteoporotic lesion in bone is still speculative, although it has been attributed to a direct effect of thyroid hormone on bone (Mundy *et al.*, 1976), and the combination of a gradual loss of protein matrix of bone, calcium malabsorption, and hypercalciuria. When the thyroid disease is of short duration, easily recognized clinically, and treated appropriately, the bone disease is a relatively insignificant factor. Bone pain and spontaneous fractures are very late manifestations of thyrotoxicosis. It is, therefore, essential to consider the diagnosis in all asymptomatic osteopenic individuals, especially postmenopausal females who present with radiologically detectable "osteoporosis." Since hypercalciuria and hydroxyprolinuria often accompany the derangements in bone metabolism of hyperthyroid patients (Kivirikko *et al.*, 1965) in contrast to those with either postmenopausal or senile osteoporosis, 24-hour urine collections for calcium and hydroxyproline determinations are of value in establishing the diagnosis. Measurements of urinary hydroxylysyl glycosides may also prove helpful in the differential diagnosis (Askenasi and Demeester-Mirkine, 1975). On the other hand, symptomatic osteoporosis with radiological osteopenia should not be attributed to thyrotoxicosis in all elderly patients with mild elevations in circulating thyroxine. Estimations of total or free triiodotyronine are much more useful in establishing the hyperthyroid state in such cases (Britton et al., 1975). When significant hypercalcemia (>11 mg/dl) is detected in an untreated hyperthyroid subject or if the hypercalcemia persists after control of the thyrotoxicosis, primary hyperparathyroidism should be excluded, since 1–2% of patients with hyperparathyroidism have coexisting hyperthyroidism (Parfitt and Dent, 1970; Heimann, 1970).

2. Hypercortisolism

In 1932, Harvey Cushing described the classical syndrome of obesity, hypertension, weakness, amenorrhea, and impotence with "basophilic pituitary adenomas" and noted a "spinal osteoporosis" in six of eight autopsied subjects (Cushing, 1932). It has subsequently been well documented that skeletal mass is decreased in varying degrees in patients with hyperactive adrenal glands or others subjected to long-term corticosteroid therapy (Ruder et al., 1974; Follis, 1951; Sissons, 1956; Howland et al., 1958; Murray, 1960, 1961; Innaccone et al., 1960; Aloia et al., 1974). Although radiographic evidence of skeletal rarefraction is noted in 40–50% of patients with the complete clinical expression of Cushing's disease syndrome (Innaccone et al., 1960; Howland et al., 1958; Ross et al., 1966), it should be emphasized that severe bone loss may also obtain in patients (usually young adults) with micronodular adrenal disease with minimal clinical manifestations of hypercortisolism (Ruder et al., 1974).

The relationship between dosage and duration of therapy and either the clinical expression or radiological detection of osteoporosis in patients on steroid therapy is still conjectural (McConkey et al., 1962; Hosking and Chamberlain, 1973; David et al., 1970; Saville and Kharmosh, 1967). Postmenopausal females with accelerated rates of bone loss, immobilized subjects, and actively growing children appear more susceptible to the adverse skeletal effects of glucocorticoid medication (Saville and Kharmosh, 1967; Blodgett et al., 1956; Arnoldsson, 1958). Moreover, growth rates are retarded in children exposed to high levels of circulating glucocorticoids (Blodgett et al., 1956; Mosier et al., 1972), and the degree of catch-up growth following normalization of blood steroid levels is dependent both on duration and intensity of glucocorticoid exposure and on the age of the patient (Mosier et al., 1972). Using routine radiological detection devices, Saville and Kharmosh (1967) noted no difference in the incidence in vertebral fractures, in adults younger than 50 years of age treated daily for more than 5 years with 5–10 mg of prednisone or its

TABLE III

Dose Equivalents of Cortisol

Steroid	Trade name	Half-life[a]	Dose equivalent (× cortisol)
Cortisol	Solu-cortef	90	1.0
Cortisone	Cortone	30	0.8
Prednisone	Metacorten	60	4.0
Prednisolone	Metacortelone	200	5.0
Dexamethazone	Decadron	200	25–40
α-Fluorocortisol	Florinef	90	15

[a] Plasma half-life in minutes as published in *Ann. N.Y. Acad. Sci.* **82,** 846 (1959).

equivalent (see Table III). Hahn *et al.* (1974), utilizing more sensitive monochromatic photon densitometric measurements of forearm bone mass, were unable to correlate corticosteroid dosage and degree of bone loss in 48 adult subjects on prednisone—equivalent doses of 10–45 mg/day (Table III) for periods varying from one to 20 years. A definite relationship was demonstrated, however, between the duration of therapy and the decrease in bone mass (Fig. 17).

Although the entire skeleton is effected by chronic elevations in plasma

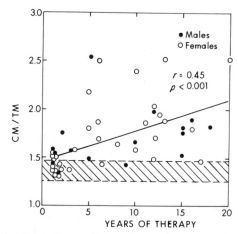

Fig. 17. Correlation of cortical mass (CM) and trabecular mass (TM) ratios of the forearm with duration of corticosteroid therapy in 48 adults. The hatched area indicate the normal mean ± S.D. Photon absorption technique of Cameron and Sorenson (1963) was used to quantitate bone mass. (Reprinted from Hahn *et al.*, 1974; with permission from the author and publisher.)

glucocorticoids, the distribution of the osteoporosis appears to be greater in the axial than in the appendicular portion. The osteoporosis is usually detected first in the vertebrae with accentuation of the vertical trabeculae and prominence of the vertebral plates (Fig. 10). Gradual progressive loss of vertebral mass usually results in generalized expansion of the intervertebral discs (Fig. 10) and vertebral collapse, with the lower dorsal and upper lumbar vertebrae particularly susceptible in this regard. Cortical and subcortical microfractures may result in localized areas of compression and compaction or "marginal condensation" (Howland et al., 1958) and increased density radiologically. Unlike senile osteoporosis or that associated with diseases other than hypercortisolism, osteoporosis may be quite severe in the skull. The decrease in cranial bone mass may be manifested either by a diffuse decalcification or a "metastatic decalcification" (most evident in the frontal or parental regions), the latter consisting of irregular zones of rarefaction separated by areas of bone of relatively normal appearance (Sussman and Copleman, 1942; Howland et al., 1958; Murray, 1961). Generalized rarefaction is also noted in the ribs and pelvis, and asymptomatic fractures are not infrequent in these areas even in the absence of marked vertebral osteoporosis. Characteristically, fractures heal with abundant callus formation often imparting a "cotton-wool" appearance radiologically (Sosman, 1949; Wang and Robbins, 1956). This incomplete fracture healing has been attributed to inhibition of osteoblastic activity (Murray, 1960, 1961).

Chemical testing in patients with hypercortisolism reveals a tendency toward hypocalcemia, hypophosphatemia with a decrease in the tubular reabsorption of phosphate, and hypercalciuria (Gallagher et al., 1973; Caniggia and Gennari, 1972a). Circulating alkaline phosphatase may be elevated in patients with Cushing's syndrome (Iannaccove et al., 1960; Gallagher et al., 1973), although decreases in alkaline phosphatase (Avioli et al., 1963) and urinary hydroxyproline (Smith et al., 1968) have been noted in growing children when subjected to high-dose prednisone therapy. In adults, urinary hydroxyproline is either normal or elevated in selected instances (Gallagher et al., 1973; Caniggia and Gennari, 1972a). Blood levels of the vitamin D metabolite, 25-hydroxycholecalciferol, are either normal (Aloia et al., 1974) or low (Bayard et al., 1974). In some instances, plasma parathyroid hormone levels are also elevated (Fucik et al., 1975). Histologically, the skeletal defect is classically that of osteoporosis and characterized by an increase in bone resorption and a decrease in total bone formation (Frost, 1962; Heaney and Whedon, 1958; Rich et al., 1966; Jowsey and Riggs, 1970). These changes are often associated with abnormally high osteoclastic activity and an increase in the number of active osteoblasts in trabecular bone (Birkenhager et al., 1967).

Hypercortisolism in man also results in a malabsorption of calcium (Miravet et al., 1966; Caniggia and Gennari, 1972a; Gallagher et al., 1973), and alterations in the biological activation of vitamin D (Avioli et al., 1968). Animals treated with cortisone or a variety of its synthetic analogues also respond with a decrease in calcium absorption (Collins et al., 1962; Harrison and Harrison, 1960; Kimberg et al., 1971), increased bone resorption (Jee et al., 1970; Thompson et al., 1972; Jowsey and Riggs, 1970), inhibition of epiphyseal cartilage growth (Mosier et al., 1972; Balogh and Kunin, 1971), and an accelerated metabolism of the very potent vitamin D metabolite 1,25-dihydroxy-vitamin D_3 [1,25-$(OH)_2D_3$] (Carré et al., 1974) (see Chapter 5 and Volume II, Chapter 2). An excess of glucocorticoids not only produces growth failure and decreased calcium absorption from the intestine but also leads to deficient synthesis of bone matrix (Cruess and Hong, 1975; Sobel and Feinberg, 1970; Peck et al., 1967; Cruess and Sakai, 1972) and delays the initiation of fracture repair and the remodeling response (Hellewell et al., 1974).

When the glucocorticoid-excess syndrome has been alleviated, either by successful surgical intervention or by the termination of cortisone-like drug medication, the progression of the osteoporosis is halted. In adults radiological improvement in the osteoporosis is rarely observed thereafter (Innaccone et al., 1960; Skeels, 1958), although marked increments in bone formation rates have been demonstrated histologically (Riggs et al., 1966). In selected instances, recalcification of the "metastatic" skull lesions and disappearance of the vertebral "marginal condensation" deformities (Howland et al., 1958) have been demonstrated. In growing children with the capacity of endochrondral new bone formation, amelioration of the hypercortisolism often results in an accentuation of linear growth rates and marked improvement in the osteoporosis with new bone deposited in the less dense osteoporotic old bone (Albright and Reifenstein, 1948b; Mosier et al., 1972; Blodgett et al., 1956; Kenney, 1972).

In those circumstances where high dose adrenocorticoid therapy is essential, the osteoporosis is usually progressive. Although anabolic steroids and fluoride have been advocated in the past, they have proved to be of limited practical value in halting the osteoporotic process. In children, the growth retardation may be minimized by alternate day administration of glucocorticoids (Soyka and Saxena, 1965). Vitamin D in doses of 20,000–50,000 units/day corrects the intestinal absorptive defect in adults (Gallagher et al., 1973), and, when supplemented with calcium, corrects the rate of bone loss in children (Harnapp, 1967) and adults (T. H. Hahn, personal observation). Vitamin D metabolites, 25-hydroxy-vitamin D_3 [25-$(OH)D_3$] and 1,25-$(OH_2D_3$, have also proved effective in reversing the defect in calcium absorption in both man (Caniggia and Gennari, 1972a) and animals (Carré *et al.*, 1973) during periods of induced hypercortisolism. Reports of the beneficial effects of calcitonin in retarding the progression of steroid-induced osteoporosis in man (Palmieri *et al.*, 1974) and animals (Thompson *et al.*, 1972) await further documentation, although they confirm earlier histological studies defining opposing action of calcitonin and cortisone on osteogenesis (Thompson and Urist, 1973). The most practical approach for adults appear to be one in which steroid dosage is minimized to levels of 15 mg of prednisone or its equivalent (Table III) per day in order to minimize the deleterious effects on calcium absorption and bone metabolism (Lekkerkerker *et al.*, 1972).

3. Acromegaly

Growth hormone normally stimulates endochondral bone growth at epiphyseal cartilaginous plates and excessive amounts lead to accelerated rates of longitudinal growth and ''giantism'' in children. In the adult skeleton where normal endochondral bone growth has terminated, elevations in circulating growth hormone lead to a reactivation of endochondral bone growth at certain existing cartilage–bone junctions, resulting in an overgrowth of ''acral'' bones as well as a variety of spinal and peripheral joint abnormalities (Bluestone *et al.*, 1971). Although osteoporosis has often been considered to result from growth hormone-excess syndromes (Scriver *et al.*, 1935; Bell and Bartter, 1967; Molinatti *et al.*, 1961), the incidence of osteoporosis or fractures does not, in fact, appear to be increased in individuals with acromegaly (Nadarajah *et al.*, 1968; Aloia *et al.*, 1972; Doyle *et al.*, 1970; Riggs *et al.*, 1972b). Cortical bone content is either normal or increased in acromegalic individuals (Aloia *et al.*, 1972; Riggs *et al.*, 1972b), trabecular bone may be normal (Aloia *et al.*, 1972) or reduced in content (Riggs *et al.*, 1972b), and the overall rates of bone formation and mesenchymal proliferation increased (Ramser *et al.*, 1966a; Villanueva *et al.*, 1966a). Increased size of the vertebral bodies (Fig. 18) resulting from endosteal and subperiosteal new bone formation (Harris *et al.*, 1972; Heaney *et al.*, 1972) reflects the net increase in skeletal mass which characterizes the acromegalic patient.

Elevations in plasma growth hormone also lead to hyperphosphatemia and a reversal of the normal diurnal variation of serum inorganic phosphate (Corvilain and Abramov, 1962; McMillan *et al.*, 1968). Although serum calcium is usually normal, hypercalciuria (Scriver *et al.*, 1935; Henneman *et al.*, 1960; Hanna *et al.*, 1961; Bell and Bartter, 1967; Maymovitz and Horwith, 1964; Molinatti *et al.*, 1961) is not infrequent, probably reflecting an increase in both bone turnover (Bell and Bartter, 1967; Aloia *et al.*, 1972) and glomerular filtration rates (Corvilain and Abramov, 1962). Hypercalcemia and elevations in plasma alkaline phosphatase although

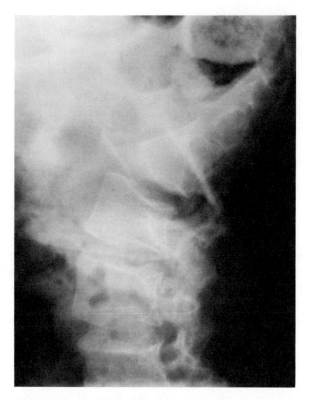

Fig. 18. Lumbar spine in a 26-year-old man with acromegaly of 5 years duration. There is no evidence of osteopenia radiologically. Increased vertebral size is due to subperiosteal new bone deposition primarily in the anteroposterior vertebral plane.

rare (Nadarajah *et al.*, 1968) have been attributed to parathyroid hyperplastic response to growth hormone (Summers *et al.*, 1966; Hartog and Joplin, 1967). The persistence of hypercalcemia following successful pituitary surgery or irradiation suggests autonomous parathyroid activity and/or a pluriglandular syndrome (Perlman, 1944; Axon *et al.*, 1973; Boey *et al.*, 1975), and demands careful follow-ups with appropriate sequential biological testing.

4. Hypogonadism

Osteoporosis has been associated with panhypopituitarism (Fraser and Smith, 1941), Klinefelter's syndrome (Dent, 1971; Klinefelter *et al.*, 1943; Garn and Poznanski, 1972), and ovarian agenesis (Turner's syndrome).

The last syndrome, observed in individuals with XO chromosome complements and characterized by short stature, cubitus valgus, and congenital webbing of the neck occurs with a frequency of about 1:2500 births. Although shortness of stature and a delay in skeletal maturation are characteristic features of the syndrome, radiologically detectable osteoporosis is not a universal finding, occurring with a frequency ranging from 31 to 86% (Engel and Forbes, 1965; Finby and Archibald, 1963; Preger *et al.*, 1968; Lemli and Smith, 1963; Beals, 1973). The osteoporosis is characteristically asymptomatic in children and most easily detected in the vertebrae. Although the loss of bone mass has been ascribed in the past to estrogen deficiency (Albright and Reifenstein, 1948c), it (along with the growth failure) most probably results from an inherited abnormality in skeletal development (Brook *et al.*, 1974; Smith *et al.*, 1973). The occurrence of osteoporosis in young prepubertal children with ovarian agenesis (most obvious in the hands, feet, and elbows) is also consistent with the hypothesis that its cause is unrelated to defective gonadal function (Beals, 1973). The osteoporosis progresses with increasing age, often resulting in mild scoliosis, vertebral collapse, and protrusio acetabuli (Finby and Archibald, 1963; Preger *et al.*, 1968). Estrogen therapy offers little advantage in reversing growth failure and osteoporosis in children (Brook *et al.*, 1974), but may prove effective in decreasing the rate of bone loss in adults with this disorder.

C. Osteoporosis and Inherited Disorders of Bone and/or Connective Tissue

1. Osteogenesis Imperfecta

This is an inherited disorder characterized by a variety of phenotypic abnormalities, the most significant being osseous fragility and fractures (Fig. 19). It is usually inherited as an autosomal dominant, although autosomal recessive patterns have been documented (McKusick, 1972a). Clinically, patients are usually divided into two groups: "congenita" and "tarda," the former defined by the presence of fractures at birth, blue sclerae, "wormian bones," and severe skeletal deformities; the latter by the absence of fractures at birth, with deformities resulting from recurrent fractures in later life. Although the disease has been described in the medical literature for almost 200 years, the pathogenesis is still ill-defined. Abnormalities in the molecular organization of skin (Pentinnen *et al.*, 1975; Stevenson *et al.*, 1970) and bone (Teitelbaum *et al.*, 1974; Lindenfelser *et al.*, 1972) collagen have been documented as well as changes in the metabolism of noncollagenous bone proteins (Dickson *et al.*, 1975).

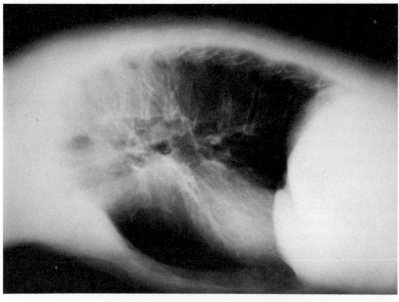

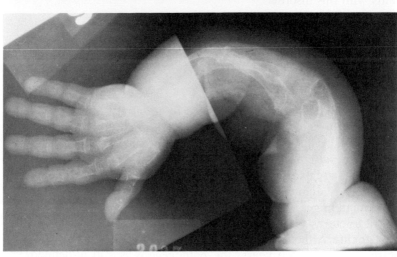

Fig. 19. Skeletal abnormalities in a 6-year-old child (left) with osteogenesis imperfecta congenita and a 30-year-old man (right) with osteogenesis imperfecta tarda. The patient with the "tarda" form was considered to have "idiopathic spinal osteoporosis" until the specific skeletal abnormality was established by scanning electron microscopic analysis of an iliac crest biopsy.

The skeletal lesion is characterized by an accumulation of stainable glycosoaminoglycans, an abnormal orientation of collagen fibers (Fig. 20), and an increase in bone resorption (Ramser *et al.*, 1966b; Jett *et al.*, 1966; Robichon and Germain, 1968). Alterations in bone metabolism in osteogenesis imperfecta often result in elevations in plasma alkaline and acid phosphatases, and in urinary hydroxyproline and glycosoaminoglycans (Rosenberg *et al.*, 1977). The "congenita" form of the disease is often complicated by recurrent fractures and prolonged periods of immobilization, the latter often contributing most dramatically to the osteoporosis and increased bone fragility (Fig. 19). Proposed regimens for the management of the progressive osteopenia that invariably occurs in the majority of young adults with this disorder include therapy with sodium fluoride (Pierog *et al.*, 1969; Aeschlimann *et al.*, 1966), androgens (Hernberg, 1952a; Muldowney *et al.*, 1964), and magnesium oxide (Solomons and Styner, 1969), but the clinical response to these agents has been less than adequate (Cattell and Clayton, 1968; Riley and Jowsey, 1973; Shoenfeld *et al.*, 1975). Favorable responses in the "tarda" variety have been reported with calcitonin (Goldfield *et al.*, 1972; Castells *et al.*, 1972, 1974; Caniggia and Gennari, 1972b; Rosenberg *et al.*, 1977). In the "tarda" form of the disease, a decreased incidence of fractures is also observed after puberty

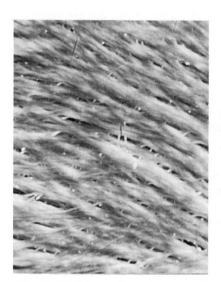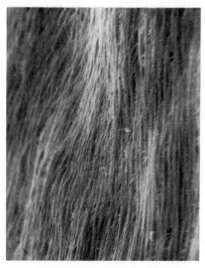

Fig. 20. Scanning electron microscope view of bone collagen in an iliac crest biopsy of a normal child (left) and an age-matched individual with osteogenesis imperfecta congenita (right). In contrast to the normal, the collagen fibrils of the patients with osteogenesis imperfecta exhibit no compaction into fibers and the mean fiber width is $^1\!/_5$ normal ($\times$ 870). (Reprinted from Teitelbaum *et al.*, 1974; with permission from authors and publisher.)

(Bryan *et al.*, 1956), whereas increased incidence occurs after menopause. The disease may be confused with "idiopathic juvenile osteoporosis." However, in this latter skeletal disorder, the sclera are normal in color, the osteoporosis is typically localized to the vertebral column, and the family history for fractures and resulting deformities is negative. Osteogenesis imperfecta in children may also mimic the juvenile form of "hypophosphatasia" (Rathbun, 1943), although the low circulating alkaline phosphatase, rachitic skeletal changes, and phosphorylethanolaminuria which accompany the hypophosphatasia syndrome should make the disorder readily identifiable (see Volume II, Chapter 7). Because of an exceedingly wide range of phenotypic expressivity of the inherited connective tissue defect in osteogenesis imperfecta, the disease may often be misdiagnosed in the adult as a routine case of "postmenopausal" or "idiopathic" osteoporosis (Fig. 19). A detailed historical family survey and bone biopsy evaluation may often prove quite helpful in establishing the correct diagnosis.

2. Hypophosphatasia

This is a hereditary, generalized skeletal disorder that follows an autosomal recessive pattern and has been categorized into four types according to the age of onset and the severity of the clinical and radiological manifestations (Fraser, 1957). Childhood forms of the disease resemble rickets radiologically and are discussed in Volume II, Chapter 7. The adult form, although relatively rare (Eisenberg and Pimstone, 1967; Bethune and Dent, 1960), should be considered in individuals who present with fractures following minimal trauma or localized arthropathy (Beisel *et al.*, 1960; O'Duffy, 1970). Adults with the mild form of the disease characteristically give a history of renal stones, dentition difficulties, delayed growth, and/or childhood "rickets." Radiologically, the disorder is characterized by radiolucent bones and pseudofractures (see Chapter 5). The biochemical hallmarks of the disease are an abnormally low tissue and circulating levels of alkaline phosphatase activity (Goldfischer *et al.*, 1976) and an increased excretion of phosphoethanolamine. Although phosphoethanolamine is normally undetected in urine, it is also found in vitamin C deficiency, hypothyroidism, coeliac disease, and magnesium deficiency (Fraser, 1957; Hanna *et al.*, 1960). Elevations in urinary phosphocholine (Eisenberg and Pimstone, 1967) and phosphoserine (personal observations) may also occur. When the diagnosis is clinically suspected in a patient with elevations in urinary phosphoethanolamine, a "normal" alkaline phosphatase as described by Scriver and Cameron (1969) in patients with "pseudohypophosphatasia" need not be considered inappropriate for the disease entity. In certain nutritional states the intestinal isoenzyme alkaline phosphatase may prove to be the primary circulating form of alkaline phosphatase (Warshaw *et al.,* 1971) in contrast to the pattern identified in normal individuals (see Chapter 3). Attempts to reverse the skeletal calcification defect with vitamin D, cortisone or structurally related synthetic analogues, and phosphate supplements have been unsuccessful; fractures usually heal normally with conventional forms of orthopedic management.

3. Homocystinuria and Other Inherited Diseases

This is a metabolic disease inherited as an autosomal recessive and is characterized clinically by mental retardation, chronic back pain, kyphoscoliosis, anterior chest deformities in adults, (either pectus carinatum or pectus excavatum) genu valgum, joint laxity, ectopic lentis, vascular dilatation and thrombotic diatheses, and a marked osteoporosis. Fractures occur with relatively minor trauma with severe vertebral osteopenia and concavity of the vertebral end-plates (Westerman *et al.,* 1974; McKusick, 1972b) contributing to the associated kyphoscoliotic deformities. Other skeletal findings include punctate or linear longitudinal radiological densities in the distal ulna and radius, microencephaly, and large paranasal sinuses with abnormally thick calvaria. The basic defect in homocystinuria is a deficiency in the enzyme, cystathionine synthetase, the latter resulting in elevations in plasma homocysteine, homocystine, and methionine and an "overflow" homocystinuria (Mudd *et al.,* 1964). Homocysteine interferes with the formation of intermolecular cross-links, which normally stabilize the collagen macromolecular network (see Chapter 1), by binding to the aldehydic functional groups on the collagen molecule (Kang and Trelstad, 1973). Since the administration of lathyrogens such as β-aminopropionitrile to animals leads to disturbances in collagen cross-linking and connective tissue and bone abnormalities not unlike those seen in homocystinuria (Ponseti and Shepard, 1954; Levine and Gross, 1959), the osteoporosis of homocystinuria is presently attributed to the homocysteine effect on bone collagen maturation (Kang and Trelstad, 1973). Vitamin B_6 (a cofactor for cystathionine synthetase) deficiency also leads to osteoporosis in the rat (Benke *et al.,* 1972). When vitamin B_6 is administered to homocystinuric patients in pharmacologic doses of 50 to 300 mg/day, the level of urinary homocystine, an oxidation product of homocysteine, falls (Mudd *et al.,* 1970). Since the reported homocysteine effect on the collagen molecule is also reversible (Kang and Trelstad, 1973), continued high dose vitamin B_6 therapy may ultimately prove therapeutic for the osteopenia seen in patients with homocystinuria.

Although the incidence is much less than that seen with homocystinuria, increased radiolucency of the vertebrae and exaggeration of the normal concavity of the dorsal aspect of the vertebral bodies has also been reported in Marfan's syndrome and Ehlers–Danlos syndrome (Mitchell *et al.*, 1967). Whereas the fundamental defect in Marfan's syndrome is still unknown, the connective tissue and bone defects of Ehlers–Danlos syndrome may be related to the faulty conversion of procollagen to collagen (see Chapter 1) (Lichtenstein *et al.*, 1973).

Osteoporosis is also observed in children with Menkes syndrome (Menkes *et al.*, 1962; Danks *et al.*, 1972a), an X-linked recessive inherited disorder of connective tissue characterized by an intestinal malabsorption of copper, low serum copper ceruloplasmin concentration, severe copper deficiency, growth retardation, and kinky or "steely" hair (Danks *et al.*, 1972b). The skeletal pathology may also result from maturational defects in bone collagen, since the lysine oxidase enzyme essential for collagen cross-link formation is copper-dependent (see Chapter 1). The observation that experimental copper deficiency results in severe osteoporosis is most consistent with this hypothesis (Baxter and Van Wyk, 1953). Cultured human fibroblasts may ultimately prove valuable in establishing this diagnosis, since they continually exhibit elevated copper concentrations in patients with this disorder (Yoka *et al.*, 1970).

Decreased bone density and radiologically detectable osteoporosis has also been reported in an inherited disorder characterized by hypercalciuria, hypouricemia, increased uric acid clearance (Sperling *et al.*, 1974), and in the Riley–Day syndrome (familial dysautonomia) a rare autosomal recessive disorder found mostly in Jewish children of Eastern European extraction. Other distinctive features of the Riley–Day syndrome include scoliosis, hyperhydrosis, disordered swallowing, dysarthria, motor incoordination, relative insensitivity to pain, episodic hypertension, postural hypotension, and transient blotching of the skin (Yoslow *et al.*, 1971). Although inherited forms of vitamin D-resistant rickets classically present with richitic deformities (children) or pseudofractures (adults) (see Chapter 5), severe osteopenia without distinct alterations in epiphyseal bone maturation may also occur (Fig. 21).

D. Juvenile Osteoporosis

Juvenile (idiopathic) osteoporosis is a rare disorder of prepubertal children between the ages of 8 and 14 years which is characterized by an abrupt onset of bone pains, (usually close to the metaphysis of long bones), fractures following minimal trauma, and osteoporosis of the entire skeleton including the hands and feet (Dent and Friedman, 1965; Gooding and Ball, 1969; Fanconi *et al.*, 1966; Lapatsanis *et al.*, 1971). When uncomplicated by the sequellae of recurrent fracture diathesis, the disease is self-

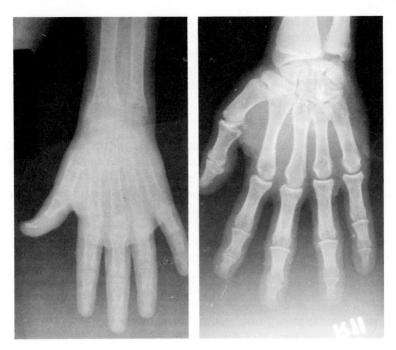

Fig. 21. Radiographs of the hands of a 12-year-old boy with vitamin D-resistant rickets before (left) and after (right) therapy with vitamin D and phosphate. Note severe osteopenia of metacarpal, carpal, and phalangeal bones despite mineral rachitic epiphyseal deformities (left).

limited with most patients recovering completely within 4 or 5 years. As noted in children successfully treated for Cushing's syndrome, endochondral new bone is deposited around less dense permanently altered bone during the recovery phase. Histologically, haversian bone remodeling is severely impaired, osteoid content is decreased, bone formation rates are either normal or low, and bone resorption is strikingly increased (Cloutier *et al.*, 1967; Gooding and Ball, 1969; Jowsey and Johnson, 1972). Serum calcium and phosphate are usually at the upper limits; serum alkaline phosphatase and urinary hydroxyproline may be abnormally high for the patient's age (Jowsey and Johnson, 1972). Transient hypercalciuria (Fanconi *et al.*, 1966) and calcium malabsorption (Dent and Friedman, 1965) have been observed. Detailed family history and iliac crest bone biopsy may be essential to differentiate juvenile osteoporosis from osteogenesis imperfecta, since both disorders may present with a history of fractures and slender bones with thin cortices. The juvenile form of osteoporosis may also mimic the bone disease associated with childhood leukemic syndromes (Dent and Friedman, 1965). Because of the self-limited course of the disorder, therapy beyond minimizing immobilization and excessive weight gain is unwarranted.

E. Immobilization Osteoporosis

Immobilization or disuse osteoporosis may be generalized or confined to specific immobilized skeletal segments. It has been associated with the immobilization resulting from disuse (Jenkins and Cochran, 1969), traumatic fractures, spinal cord fusions (Lawrence et al., 1973; Millard et al., 1970), paralytic states following either cerebral vascular accidents (Panin et al., 1971), traumatic cord lesions (Claus-Walker et al., 1975; Minaire et al., 1974), attacks of poliomyelitis (Dunning and Plum, 1957; Whedon and Shorr, 1957), and with the hypodynamic environment of orbital space flights (Mack and Vogt, 1971; Mack et al., 1967; Whedon et al., 1974). The loss of skeletal mass results from a combination of moderate decreases in osteoblastic bone formation and marked increments in the osteoclastic resorption of trabecular bone (Minaire et al., 1974; Heaney, 1962). The rate of bone loss is greater in young (<20 years) than old (>50 years) individuals (Jones, 1969) and in weight-bearing bones (Donaldson et al., 1970). It appears that the skeletal demineralization is also a function of the amount of bone present prior to the immobilization insult (Lockwood et al., 1973). Calcium malabsorption (Deitrick and Whedon, 1948; Lockwood et al., 1973), hypercalcemia, hypercalciuria, and hydroxyprolinuria frequently attend disuse osteoporosis and, rarely, elevations in plasma alkaline phosphatase activity (Claus-Walker et al., 1975; Klein et al., 1966; Dunning and Plum, 1957; Lawrence et al., 1973; Moore Ede et al., 1972; Donaldson et al., 1970; Moore et al., 1972; Minaire et al., 1974; Millard et al., 1970; Heath et al., 1972; Deitrick and Whedon, 1948). Abnormally high levels of circulating alkaline phosphatase have been consistently noted, however, in immobilized paraplegic patients coincident with the development of ectopic bone formation (Furman et al., 1970). Whereas vertebral osteopenia may be undetectable by routine radiographic analysis for periods as long as 6 months in immobilized patients with severe hypercalciuria (Deitrick and Whedon, 1948; Whedon and Shorr, 1957), localized osteoporosis may be evident in the long bones radiographically within 3 months in paraplegic patients (Whedon and Shorr, 1957), and the bone loss is primarily trabecular (Griffiths et al., 1972). More sensitive γ-ray transmission analyses reveal 25–45% decrements in bone mass of the os calcis during periods of total body immobilization that span 30–36 weeks (Hulley *et al.*, 1971; Donaldson *et al.*, 1970) and losses approximating 20% in some astronauts during short-term orbital space flights (Mack and Vogt, 1971).

The radiological manifestations of skeletal immobilization vary, although generalized osteopenia with subperiosteal scalloping of cortical bone are frequent findings (Fig. 22). "Speckled" or "spotty" osteoporosis in the carpal, tarsal, or tubular bones of the hands and feet and horizontal linear translucent bands involving the long and short tubular bones of the extremities are early changes usually seen in the younger age group (Jones, 1969). Although the changes are usually reversible with appropriate mobilization of the involved skeletal segment, immobilization osteoporosis may lead to irretrivable bone loss in the elderly postmenopausal patient with significant osteopenia prior to the immobilization period. Hormonal imbalance (Burkhart and Jowsey, 1967) and vascular stasis (Deitrick and Whedon, 1948) may contribute to the development and progression of the osteoporotic process which attends skeletal immobilization. The most widely accepted theory, however, is that which attributes the osteopenia to a loss of muscular tone and mass, and the disruption of the normal muscle–bone interplay which regulates bone remodeling and formation (Friedenberg *et al.*, 1973; Kenner *et al.*, 1975; Rodan *et al.*, 1975; Doyle *et al.*, 1970; McCally and Lawton, 1963; Ragan and Briscoe, 1964).

Continued hydration is essential in the hypercalciuric, immobilized patient in order to prevent the dreaded sequence of

Recurrent renal calculi → urinary stasis → infection → renal insufficiency

Low sodium diets, thiazide diuretics, anabolic steroid hormones, and sodium fluoride offer limited effectiveness in reducing the rate of bone loss and calciuria (Griffith, 1971; Whedon and Shorr, 1957; Plum and Dunning, 1958a; Keele and Vose, 1969, 1971). Attempts to increase muscle tone and mass using mobilization with crutch walking, skeletal compression and oscillating beds have also enjoyed limited success (Whedon *et al.*, 1949; Hantman *et al.*, 1973; Plum and Dunning, 1958b). Although calcitonin (Hantmann *et al.*, 1973; Chiroff and Jowsey, 1970; Singh and Jowsey, 1970) and inorganic phosphate therapy (Keele and Vose, 1971; Hulley *et al.*, 1971) are of no value in retarding the progressive skeletal demineralization of immobilized patients, phosphate supplementation (Hulley *et al.*, 1971) and glucocorticoids (Lawrence *et al.*, 1973) may prove effective in reversing the hypercalcemia and hypercalciuria. Alkali (Barzel, 1971) and diets supplemented with both calcium and phosphate (Hantman *et al.*, 1973) have been reported to suppress the fecal and urinary losses of calcium, but these measures should be attempted with caution in im-

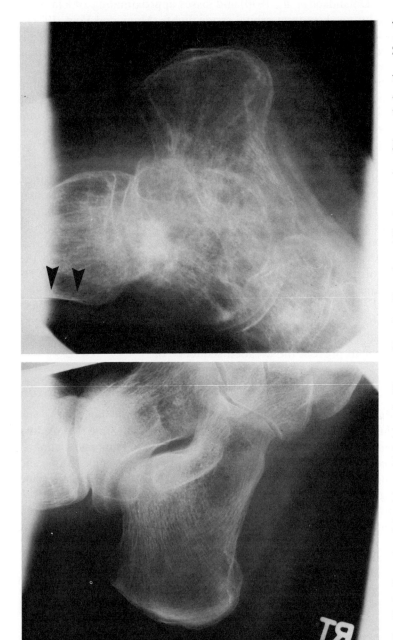

Fig. 22. Radiographs of the right and left foot of a 27-year-old male with an immobilized extremity of 6-month duration. Note the irregularities of the endosteal surface of the tibia (arrowheads), and "patchy" decreases in density in the tarsal bones. Cortical bone, although thin, is dense when contrasted with the diffuse trabecular osteopenia.

mobilized patients until definite improvement in bone mass is documented and the propensity toward recurrent calculi formation assessed.

Regional forms of osteoporosis also include in the Sudeck's atrophy of patients with reflex sympathetic dystrophy which is commonly localized to the hands and feet (Drucker *et al.*, 1959) and *transient osteoporosis,* a disease of unknown etiology reportedly associated with type IV hyper-lipoproteinemia (Pinals and Jabbs, 1972), which has a predelection for the knees, ankles, and hips (Duncan *et al.*, 1969; Langloh *et al.*, 1973). Lo-calized pain or discomfort (which may be severe on occasion) occurs in both forms of osteoporosis; atrophic, glossy, tight skin with persistent restriction of joint movements is more characteristic of Sudeck's atrophy, however. The pain of Sudeck's atrophy is often dramatically relieved by paravertebral lumbar or stellate ganglion sympathetic block. Both disor-ders are treated conservatively with gradual ambulation and physical therapy. Glucocorticoids, in a dosage equivalent to 30–40 mg prednisone per day (Table III), may prove effective in alternating the pain which often precludes programmed ambulation and skeletal mobilization (Curtiss and Kincaid, 1959; Lequense, 1968; Arnstein, 1972; Miller and DeTakats, 1942; DeTakats, 1965).

The course of the transient osteoporosis syndrome is usually self-limited with no residual skeletal deformities (Langloh *et al.*, 1973), whereas Sudeck's atrophy may be recurrent and episodic, often terminating in permanent skeletal injury (Plewes, 1956). In transient osteoporosis early disease or recovery is associated with increased skeletal turnover and can be detected early by isotopic scanning of the involved skeletal segment (Swezey, 1970; Hunder and Kelly, 1971).

F. Miscellaneous Causes of Osteoporosis

Although relatively rare, hypertrophic osteoarthropathy (Han and Col-lins, 1968) and avascular necrosis (Leach and Baskies, 1973) are often cited as the skeletal complications of chronic hepatic insufficiency. There are, however, reports of demineralization of the dorsum sellae (Albert and LeMay, 1968), radiologically detectable vertebral "osteoporosis" (Heuck, 1970; Huguenin *et al.*, 1960; Lichtwitz *et al.*, 1959), an increased incidence of severe alcoholism in men with femoral neck fractures (Nilsson, 1970a,b), and other observations demonstrating that the skeletal mass of patients with excessive alcoholic intake is significantly less than that of age- and sex-matched control populations (Nilsson and Westlin, 1973; Saville, 1965), (Table IV). Osteoporosis is also seen in nonalcoholic subjects with biliary cirrhosis (Kehayoglou *et al.*, 1968), siderotic cirrhosis (Seftel *et al.*, 1966; Lynch *et al.*, 1967), and hemochromatosis (Delbarre,

TABLE IV

Bone Mineral Parameters in Chronic Alcoholism[a]

	No. of subjects	Age (years)	CM^b (gm/cm^2)	TM^b (gm/cm^2)	CM/TM
White males					
Control	27	46 ± 7	0.88 ± 0.05	0.67 ± 0.06	1.34 ± 0.11
Chronic alcoholism	14	50 ± 7	0.81 ± 0.06^c	0.53 ± 0.06^c	1.58 ± 0.12^c
Black males					
Control	10	46 ± 6	0.92 ± 0.05	0.67 ± 0.06	1.40 ± 0.17
Chronic alcoholism	13	51 ± 6	0.83 ± 0.10^d	0.50 ± 0.08^c	1.69 ± 0.29^d

[a] Bone mass quantitated (mean ± SD) according to ^{125}I-photon densinometric methodology as described in *Invest. Radiol.* **3,** 141 (1968).

[b] CM and TM represent measurements made at radial midshaft and distal radius, respectively.

[c] $P < 0.001$.

[d] $P < 0.025$.

1960). The underlying cause(s) for the decreased skeletal mass of alcoholic individuals with hepatic insufficiency is still conjectural at best. Poor correlation between either the amount of ingested alcohol or the duration of the alcoholism, and other observations demonstrating less bone loss in socially acceptable nourished alcoholics (Dalen and Feldreich, 1974) suggest that the events leading to and perpetuating the skeletal demineralization are multifactorial. Chronic pancreatitis and small intestinal dysfunction commonly associated with hepatic insufficiency (Losowsky and Walker, 1969) results in the malabsorption of calcium (Whelton *et al.,* 1971; D'Souza and Gloch, 1973) and amino acids essential to the maintenance of the integrity of skeletal tissue; elevations in plasma free cortisol (McCann and Fulton, 1975; Merry and Marks, 1972), gastrectomy (Nilsson and Westlin, 1972a), magnesium deficiency (Lim and Jacob, 1972), decreased levels of ionized calcium in serum (Moore, 1971), ethanol-induced structural alterations in the intestinal mucosa (Rubin *et al.,* 1972), metabolic acidosis due to elevations in blood lactic or pyruvic acids (Mulhausen *et al.,* 1967), defective hepatic metabolism of vitamin D to its 25-hydroxylated metabolite (Darnis, 1973; Avioli *et al.,* 1967), and secondary hyperparathyroidism (Loeper *et al.,* 1939; Boisseau *et al.,* 1974) probably all contribute to the loss of bone mass. Reports of a direct inhibition of both bone collagen maturation (Walker and Shand, 1972) and the intestinal absorption of calcium (Krawitt, 1975) by ethanol in experimental animal models also warrant attention. Clinical testing of patients

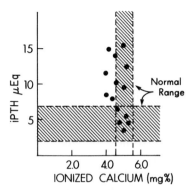

Fig. 23. Circulating parathyroid hormone (iPTH) and ionized calcium in 14 adult patients with nonicteric alcoholic cirrhosis (established by hepatic biopsy). The horizontal and vertical hatched areas denote normal ranges for iPTH and ionized calcium, respectively.

with chronic hepatic insufficiency often reveals hypophosphatemia (Territo and Tanaka, 1974), hydroxyprolinuria (Kratzch, 1969), hypocalcemia, and elevations in circulating immunoreactive parathyroid hormone (Figs. 23 and 24). Hypophosphatemia and hypocalcemia, however, commonly reflect the patients poor nutritional status and hypoalbuminemia, respectively. Circulating alkaline phosphatase may be normal or high depending on the extent and activity of hepatic dysfunction and the degree of stimulated skeletal osteoblastic activity. Differentiation of the various alkaline phosphatase isoenzymes by heat inactivation technique often proves of value in delineating relative degrees of hepatic and skeletal disease in cirrhotic patients with elevations in total alkaline phosphatase (see Chapter 3).

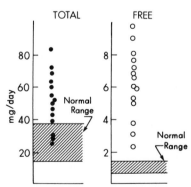

Fig. 24. Twenty-four hour total and free hydroxyproline excretion in 14 adult patients (see Fig. 23) with nonicteric alcoholic cirrhosis obtained following 3-day dietary preparational period on a hydroxyproline-free diet. The shaded areas represent the normal adult ranges for total and free hydroxyproline.

The coexistence of "osteoporosis" and diabetes mellitus has been reported in the past (Albright and Reifenstein, 1948a; Hernberg, 1952b; Berney, 1952; Menczel et al., 1972) as well as the increased incidence of hip fractures in a diabetic population (Menczel et al., 1972). When compared to age- and sex-matched control populations, decreased forearm mineral content has also been observed in patients with either juvenile and adult onset of diabetes using resonant frequency (Jurist, 1970) or direct photon absorptiometric (Levin et al., 1976) techniques. The demonstration of a decrease in bone mass at the time when the diabetes becomes clinically overt in either juvenile or adult onset of diabetics suggests that the basic defect is not one of accelerated bone resorption, but rather a decrease in bone formation intrinsic to the inherited disorder. The increased incidence of skeletal abnormalities in the fetuses of diabetic mothers (Pedersen, 1967) is also consistent with the hypothesis that the osteopenia noted in children or adults with diabetes mellitus represents an inherited abnormality in bone formation and remodeling (Wu et al., 1970; Klein and Frost, 1964). Although the size of the average skeletal osteon is normal in diabetic subjects, the rate of osteon formation is decreased to approximately 36% of normal so that in individuals thus affected two to eight times longer than normal is required to form an osteon (Klein and Frost, 1964). Factors contributing to the osteopenia of diabetic patients may be related to experimental observations that insulin stimulates the uptake of amino acids (Hahn et al., 1971) and collagen synthesis (Wettenhall et al., 1969) of bone cells and also reverses the malabsorption of calcium in the alloxan-diabetic rat (Schneider and Schedl, 1972). Whereas insulin therapy appears to exert a protective effect on the skeleton, oral hypoglycemic agents tend to accelerate the osteopenic process (Levin et al., 1976).

Osteopenia and alterations in bone remodeling have been reported in Down's syndrome (Garn et al., 1972b). Characteristically, subjects with this disorder have small bones that are relatively deficient in cortical mass during infancy and childhood with diffuse osteopenia evident radiologically during the first year of life. However, during the period of adolescence and accelerated sexual maturation, the osteopenia is dramatically reversed, a phenomenon that should be contrasted with the irreversible osteoporosis of adolescents with ovarian agenesis. This pubertal "bone recovery" phenomenon observed in children with Down's syndrome has been ascribed to accelerated rates of subperiosteal and endosteal bone formation in response to gonadal steroid stimulation (Garn and Poznanski, 1970).

Heparin in doses ranging from 15,000–40,000 units/day induces an osteopenia that radiologically also mimic osteoporosis (Avioli, 1975; Sackler and Liu, 1973; Kher *et al.,* 1973). Clinically, patients with heparin-induced osteopenia complain of back pain, sustain spontaneous vertebral and rib fractures with minimal trauma (Avioli, 1975), and respond favorably to heparin withdrawal and coumarin therapy. In experimental animals diphosphonates also inhibit heparin-induced osteoporosis (Hahnel *et al.,* 1974). The underlying skeletal defect that results in the osteopenia is still unknown, although osteoblastic inhibition, osteoclastic stimulation, altered glycosoaminoglycan synthesis, and (in children) impaired endochondral ossification have all been implicated in this regard (Avioli, 1975). It has also been suggested that, inasmuch as systemic mastocytosis is associated with skeletal demineralization (Prost *et al.,* 1974; Sirois, 1963; Griffith *et al.,* 1965; Poppel *et al.,* 1959; Sagher and Even-Paz, 1967), a direct relationship exists between the osteopenia and the heparin-containing mast cell. Moreover, the documented increments in the bone marrow mast cell population of elderly osteoporotic individuals (Kruse *et al.,* 1974; Frame and Nixon, 1968) has been considered to be of pathogenetic importance in the development of senile or postmenopausal osteoporosis (Frame and Nixon, 1968). Although potentially contributing to the osteopenia of systemic mastocytosis and age-related decreases in bone mass, heparin of mast cells may not be the sole circulating or local bone toxin, since mast cells also contain a variety of proteolytic enzymes (Langunoff and Benditt, 1963) and histamine (Riley and West, 1953). At least one of these (histamine) can also inhibit bone remodeling and maturation (Norton *et al.,* 1969).

Diffuse skeletal osteopenia has also been reported in patients with chronic pulmonary disease (Harris, 1967), Waldenström's macroglobulinemia (Vermess *et al.,* 1972; Renner *et al.,* 1971; Welton *et al.,* 1968), untreated leukemia (Baty and Vogt, 1935; Kalayjian *et al.,* 1946; Willson, 1959), and during methotrexate therapy of acute leukemia in remission (Ragab *et al.,* 1970). The combined cytotoxic and calciuric effects of methotrexate (Nevinny and Hall, 1962; Nevinny *et al.,* 1965) may explain this latter finding as well as the observation that progressive osteopenia can occur in patients with psoriasis treated with methotrexate (L. V. Avioli, personal observations, 1976).

A generalized osteopenia and spontaneous fractures also develop in untreated patients with active rheumatoid arthritis (Duncan *et al.,* 1965; McConkey *et al.,* 1962; Bjelle and Nilsson, 1970; Saville and Kharmosh, 1967; Badley and Ansell, 1960). The incidence is higher in the elderly and in female patients in whom the disease becomes clinically manifest before 5 years of age (Badley and Ansell, 1960). The basic etiology is still conjectural, although immobilization (Duncan, 1972) and vitamin D deficiency (Maddison and Bacon, 1974) appear to be significant contributing factors.

REFERENCES

Aaron, J. E., Stasiak, L., Gallagher, J. C., Longton, E. B., Nicholson, M., Anderson, J., and Nordin, B. E. C. (1974a). *Lancet* **1**, 29.

Aaron, J. E., Gallagher, J. C., and Nordin, B. E. C. (1974b). *Lancet* **2**, 84.

Ackermann, P. G., and Toro, G. (1954). *J. Gerontol.* **9**, 446.

Adams, P., Davies, G. T., and Sweetnam, P. (1970). *Q. J. Med.* **39**, 601.

Adler, S., Lindeman, R. D., Yiengst, M. J., Beard, E., and Shock, N. W. (1968). *J. Lab. Clin. Med.* **72**, 278.

Aeschlimann, M. I., Grunt, J. A., and Crigler, J. E., Jr. (1966). *Metab. Clin. Exp.* **15**, 905.

Aitken, J. M., Hart, D. M., and Smith, D. A. (1971). *Clin. Sci.* **41**, 233.

Aitken, J. M., Hart, D. M., Anderson, J. B., Lindsay, R., Smith, D. A., and Speirs, C. F. (1973a). *Br. Med. J.* **1**, 325.

Aitken, J. M., Anderson, J. B., and Horton, P. W. (1973b). *Nature (London)* **241**, 59.

Aitken, J. M., Hart, D. M., and Lindsay, R. (1973c). *Br. Med. J.* **2**, 515.

Aitken, J. M., Hall, P. E., Rao, L. G. S., Hart, D. M., and Lindsay, R. (1974). *Clin. Endocrinol.* **3**, 167.

Albanese, A. A., Edelson, A. H., Lorenze, E. J., Jr., Woodhull, M. L., and Wein, E. H. (1975). *N.Y. State J. Med.* **75**, 326.

Albert, M., and LeMay, M. (1968). *Br. J. Radiol.* **41**, 331.

Albright, F., and Reifenstein, E. D., Jr. (1948a). *In* "Parathyroid Glands and Metabolic Bone Disease; Selected Studies," Chapter 6, p. 150. Williams & Wilkins, Baltimore, Maryland.

Albright, F., and Reifenstein, E. C., Jr. (1948b). *In* "Parathyroid Glands and Metabolic Bone Disease; Selected Studies," Chapter 6, pp. 165–182. Williams & Wilkins, Baltimore, Maryland.

Albright, F., and Reifenstein, E. C. (1948c). *In* "Parathyroid Gland and Metabolic Bone Disease; Selected Studies," Chapter 6, p. 161. Williams & Wilkins, Baltimore, Maryland.

Albright, F., Bauer, W., Claffin, D., and Cockrill, J. R. (1932). *J. Clin. Invest.* **11**, 411.

Albright, F., Smith, P. H., and Richardson, A. M. (1941). *J. Am. Med. Assoc.* **116**, 2465.

Alevizaki, C. C., Ikkos, D. G., and Singhelakis, P. (1973). *J. Nucl. Med.* **14**, 760.

Alffram, P. A., Hernborg, J., and Nilsson, B. E. R. (1969). *Acta Orthop. Scand.* **40**, 137.

Alhava, E. M., and Puittinen, J. (1973). *Ann. Clin. Res.* **5**, 398.

Allen, T. H., Anderson, E. C., and Langham, W. H. (1960). *J. Gerontol.* **15**, 348.

Alioa, J. F., Roginsky, M. S., Jowsey, J., Dombrowski, C. S., Shukla, K. K., and Cohn, S. H. (1972). *J. Clin. Endocrinol. Metab.* **35**, 543.

Aloia, J. F., Roginsky, M., Ellis, K., Shukla, K., and Cohn, S. (1974). *J. Clin. Endocrinol. Metab.* **39**, 981.

Aloia, J. F., Zanzi, I., Ellis, K., Jowsey, J., Roginsky, M., Wallach, S. and Cohn, S. H. (1976). *J. Clin. Endocrinol. Metab.* **43**, 992.

Anand, C. R., and Linkswiler, H. M. (1974). *J. Nutr.* **104**, 695.

Anderson, I., Campbell, A. E. R., Dunn, A., and Runciman, E. (1966). *Scott. Med. J.* **11**, 429.

Anttinen, H., Orava, S., Ryhanen, L., and Kivirikko, K. I. (1973). *Clin. Chim. Acta* **47**, 289.

Arnold, J. S. (1964). *In* "Dynamic Studies of Metabolic Bone Disease" (O. H. Pearson and G. F. Joplin, eds.), pp. 59–76. Blackwell, Oxford.

Arnoldsson, H. (1958). *Acta Allergol., Suppl.* **6**, 134.

Arnstein, A. R. (1972). *Orthop. Clin. N. Am.* **3**, 585.

Asher, M. A., Sledge, C. B., and Glimcher, M. J. (1973). *J. Clin. Endocrinol. Metab.* **38**, 376.

Askenasi, R., and Demeester-Mirkine, N. (1975). *J. Clin. Endocrinol. Metab.* **40**, 342.

Atkins, D., Zannelli, J. M., Peacock, M., and Nordin, B. E. C. (1972). *J. Endocrinol.* **54**, 107.

Atkinson, P. J. (1967). *Calcif. Tissue Res.* **1**, 24.

Avioli, L. V. (1975). *In* "Heparin" (R. A. Bradshaw and S. Wessler, eds.), pp. 375–387. Plenum, New York.

Avioli, L. V., Lasersohn, J. T., and Lopresti, J. M. (1963). *Medicine (Baltimore)* **42**, 119.

Avioli, L. V., McDonald, J. E., and Lee, S. W. (1965). *J. Clin. Invest.* **44**, 1960.

Avioli, L. V., Lee, S. W., McDonald, J. E., Lund, J., and DeLuca, H. F. (1967). *J. Clin. Invest.* **46**, 983.

Avioli, L. V., Birge, S. J., and Lee, S. W. (1968). *J. Clin. Endocrinol. Metab.* **28**, 1341.

Axon, A. T. R., West, T. E. T., and Sonksen, P. H. (1973). *Proc. R. Soc. Med.* **66**, 444.

Badley, B. W. D., and Ansell, B. M. (1960). *Ann. Rheum. Dis.* **19**, 135.

Bagheri, S. A., and Boyer, J. L. (1974). *Ann. Intern. Med.* **81**, 610.

Balogh, K., Jr., and Kunin, A. S. (1971). *Clin. Orthop. Relat. Res.* **80**, 208.

Barnett, E., and Nordin, B. E. C. (1960). *Clin. Radiol.* **11**, 166.

Barnett, E., and Nordin, B. E. C. (1961). *Br. J. Radiol.* **34**, 683.

Barzel, U. S. (1971). *Isr. J. Med. Sci.* **7**, 499.

Bassett, C. A. L., Pawluk, R. J., and Becker, R. O. (1964). *Nature (London)* **204**, 652.

Baty, J. M., and Vogt, E. C. (1935). *Am. J. Roentgenol. Radium Ther.* [N.S.] **34**, 310.

Baud, C. A., de Siebenthal, J., Langer, B., Tupling, M. R., and Mach, R. S. (1969). *Schweiz. Med. Wochenschr.* **99**, 657.

Bauer, G. C. H. (1960). *In* "Bone as a Tissue" (K. Rodahl, J. T. Nicholson, and E. M. Brown, Jr., eds.), pp. 118–127. McGraw-Hill, New York.

Bayard, F., Bec, P., Louvet, J. P., and Boulard, C. (1974). *Prog. Endocrinol., Proc. Int. Cong. Endocrinol., 4th, 1972* Excerpta Med. Found. Int. Cong. Congr. Ser. No. 184, p. 238.

Baxter, J. D., and Bondy, P. K. (1966). *Ann. Intern. Med.* **65**, 429.

Baxter, J. H., and Van Wyk, J. J. (1953). *Bull. Johns Hopkins Hosp.* **93**, 1.

Bayless, T. M., Rothfeld, B., Massa, C., Wise, L., Paige, D., and Bedine, M. S. (1975). *N. Engl. J. Med.* **292**, 1156.

Baylink, D. J., and Bernstein, D. S. (1967). *Clin. Orthop. Relat. Res.* **55**, 53.

Beals, R. K. (1973). *Clin. Orthop. Relat. Res.* **97**, 19.

Beisel, W. R., Austen, K. F., Rosen, H., and Herndon, E. G., Jr. (1960). *Am. J. Med.* **29**, 369.

Bell, N. H., and Bartter, F. C. (1967). *J. Clin. Endocrinol. Metab.* **27**, 178.

Benke, P. J., Fleshood, H. L., and Pitot, H. C. (1972). *Biochem. Med.* **6**, 526.

Berg, E. (1972). *Clin. Orthop. Relat. Res.* **82**, 263.

Berlyne, G. M., Ben-Ari, J., Galinsky, D., Hirsch, M., Kushelevsky, A., and Shainkin, R. (1974). *J. Am. Med. Assoc.* **229**, 1904.

Berlyne, G. M., Ben-Ari, J., Kushelevsky, A., Idelman, A., Galinsky, D., Hirsch, M., Shaikin, R., Yagil, R., and Zlotnik, M. (1975). *Q. J. Med.* **44**, 505.

Berney, P. W. (1952). *J. Iowa Med. Soc.* **42**, 10.

Bernstein, D. S., and Cohen, P. (1967). *J. Clin. Endocrinol Metab.* **27**, 197.

Bernstein, D. S., Sadowsky, N., Hegsted, D. M., Guri, C. D., and Stare, F. J. (1966). *J. Am. Med. Assoc.* **198**, 499.

Berthon, M. P., Carrat, S., Cabanel, G., and Rinaldi, R. (1970). *Rev. Rhum. Mal. Osteo-Articularies* **37**, 705.

Bethune, J. E., and Dent, C. E. (1960). *Am. J. Med.* **28**, 615.

Bhandarkar, S. D., and Nordin, B. E. C. (1962). *Br. Med. J.* **1,** 145.

Biglieri, E. G. (1968). *Calif. Med.* **108,** 295.

Biglieri, E. G., Herron, M. A., and Brust, N. (1966). *J. Clin. Invest.* **45,** 1946.

Birkenhager, J. C., Van der Heul, R. O., Smeenk, D., Van der Sluys Veer, J., and Van Seters, A. P. (1967). *Pro. R. Soc. Med.* **60,** 1134.

Birge, S. J., Jr., Keutmann, H. T., Cuatrecasas, P., and Whedon, G. D. (1967). *N. Engl. J. Med.* **276,** 445.

Bjelle, A. O., and Nilsson, B. E. (1970). *Calcif. Tissue Res.* **5,** 327.

Bloch-Michel, H., Milhaud, G., Coutris, G., Waltzing, P., Charret, A., Morin, Y., Verger, D., and Dussart, N. (1970). *Rev. Rhum. Mal. Osteo-Articulaires* **37,** 629.

Blodgett, F. M., Burgin, L., Iezzoni, D., Gribetz, D., and Talbot, N. B. (1956). *N. Engl. J. Med.* **254,** 636.

Bloom, W., Nalbandov, A. V., and Bloom, M. A. (1960). *Clin. Orthop. Relat. Res.* **17,** 206.

Bluestone, R., Bywaters, E. G. L., Hartog, M., Holt, P. J. L., and Hyde, S. (1971). *Ann. Rheum. Dis.* **30,** 243.

Boey, J. H., Gilbert, J. M., Cooke, T. J. C., Sweeney, E. C., and Taylor, S. (1975). *Lancet* **2,** 781.

Boisseau, V. C., Teitelbaum, S. J., and Avioli, L. V. (1974). *Clin. Res.* **22,** 567A.

Bollet, A. J., Engh, G., and Parson, W. (1965). *Arch. Intern. Med.* **116,** 191.

Boukhris, R., and Becker, K. L. (1972). *J. Am. Med. Assoc.* **219,** 1307.

Boukhris, R., and Becker, K. L. (1973). *Clin. Orthop. Relat. Res.* **90,** 209.

Boukhris, R., and Becker, K. L. (1974). *Clin. Orthop. Relat. Res.* **104,** 275.

Britton, K. E., Ellis, S. M., Miralles, J. M., Quinn, V., Cayley, A. C. D., Brown, B. L., and Ekins, R. P. (1975). *Lancet* **2,** 141.

Brook, C. G. D., Murset, G., Zachmann, M., and Prader, A. (1974). *Arch. Dis. Child.* **49,** 789.

Brown, R. W., Krook, L., and Pond, W. C. (1966). *Cornell Vet.* **54,** 1.

Bryan, R. S., Cain, J. C., and Lipscomb, P. R. (1972). *Mayo Clin. Proc.* **31,** 475.

Bullamore, J. R., Wilkinson, R., Gallagher, J. C., Nordin, B. E. C., and Marshall, D. H. (1970). *Lancet* **2,** 535.

Burkhart, J. M., and Jowsey, J. (1967). *Endocrinology* **81,** 1053.

Cahill, G. F. (1974). *J. Am. Med. Assoc.* **227,** 448.

Cameron, J. R., and Sorenson, J. A. (1963). *Science* **142,** 230.

Cameron, J. R., Mazess, R. B., and Sorenson, J. A. (1968). *Invest. Radiol.* **3,** 141.

Caniggia, A., and Gennari, C. (1972a). *Helv. Med. Acta* **37,** 221.

Caniggia, A., and Gennari, C. (1972b). *Calcif. Tissue Res.* **9,** 243.

Caniggia, A., Gennari, C., Bencini, M., Cesari, L., and Borrello, G. (1970). *Clin Sci.* **38,** 397.

Carré, M., Miravet, L., and Hioco, D. (1973). *Int. Res. Commun. Syst.*

Carré, M., Ayigbede, O., Miravet, L., and Rasmussen, H. (1974). *Proc. Natl. Acad. Sci. U.S.A.* **71,** 2996.

Cass, R. M., Croft, J. D., Perkins, P., Nye, W., Waterhouse, C., and Terry, R. (1966). *Arch. Intern. Med.* **118,** 111.

Castells, S., Inamdar, S., Baker, R. K., and Wallach, S. (1972). *Pediatrics* **80,** 757.

Castells, S., Lu, C., Baker, R. K., and Wallach, S. (1974). *Curr. Ther. Res.* **16,** 1.

Castro, J. H., Genuth, S. M., and Klein, L. (1975). *Metab., Clin. Exp.* **24,** 839.

Cattell, H. S., and Clayton, B. (1968). *J. Bone Joint Surg., Am. Vol.* **50,** 123.

Chatterji, S., Wall, J. C., and Jeffery, J. W. (1972). *Experientia* **28,** 156.

Chiroff, R. T., and Jowsey, J. (1970). *J. Bone Joint Surg., Am. Vol.* **52,** 1138.

Claus-Walker, J., Carter, R. E., Campos, R. J., and Spencer, W. A. (1975). *J. Chronic Dis.* **28,** 81.

Clerkin, E. P., Haas, H. G., Mintz, D. H., Meloni, C. R., and Canary, J. J. (1964). *Metab., Clin. Exp.* **13**, 161.

Cloutier, M. D., Hayles, A. B., Riggs, B. L., Jowsey, J., Phil, D., and Bickel, W. H. (1967). *Pediatrics* **40**, 649.

Cohen, M. B., and Rubini, M. E. (1965). *Clin. Orthop. Relat. Res.* **40**, 147.

Cohn, S. G., Dombrowski, C. S., Hauser, W., and Atkins, H. L. (1968). *Am. J. Clin. Nutr.* **21**, 1246.

Cohn, S. H., Dombrowski, C. S., Hauser, W., Klopper, J., and Atkins, H. L. (1971). *J. Clin. Endocrinol. Metab.* **33**, 719.

Collins, E. J., Garrett, E. R., and Johnston, R. L. (1962). *Metab., Clin. Exp.* **11**, 716.

Cook, P. B., Nassim, J. R., and Collins, J. (1959). *Q. J. Med.* **28**, 505.

Corless, D., Boucher, B. J., Beer, M., Gupta, S. P., and Cohen, R. D. (1975). *Lancet* **1**, 1404.

Corvilain, J., and Abramov, M. (1962). *J. Clin. Invest.* **41**, 1230.

Courpron, P., Meunier, P., Edouard, C., Bernard, J., Bringuier, J. P., and Vignon, B. G. (1973). *Rev. Rhum. Mal. Osteo-Articulaires* **40**, 469.

Cruess, R. L., and Hong, K. C. (1975). *Proc. Soc. Exp. Biol. Med.* **148**, 887.

Cruess, R. L., and Sakai, T. (1972). *Clin. Orthop. Relat. Res.* **86**, 253.

Curtiss, P. J., Jr., and Kincaid, W. E. (1959). *J. Bone Joint Surg., Am. Vol.* **41**, 1327.

Cushing, H. (1932). *Bull. Johns Hopkins Hosp.* **50**, 137.

Dalen, N., and Feldreich, A. L. (1974). *Clin. Orthop. Relat. Res.* **99**, 201.

Dalen, N., and Lamke, B. (1974). *Acta Radiol. Diagn.* **15**, 177.

Dalen, N., Lamke, B., and Wallgren, A. (1974). *J. Bone Joint Surg., Am. Vol.* **56**, 1235.

Dallas, I., and Nordin, B. E. C. (1962). *Am. J. Clin. Nutr.* **11**, 263.

Daniell, H. W. (1976). *Arch. Intern. Med.* **136**, 298.

Danks, D. M., Campbell, P. E., Stevens, B. J., Mayne, V., and Cartwright, E. (1972a). *Pediatrics* **50**, 188.

Danks, D. M., Campbell, P. E., Walker-Smith, J., Stevens, B. J., Gillespie, J. M., Bloomfield, J., and Turner, B. (1972b). *Lancet* **1**, 1100.

Dantzig, P. I. (1975) *Arch. Intern. Med.* **135**, 1514.

Darnis, F. (1973). *Nouv. Presse Med.* **2**, 2443,

Dauphine, R. T., Riggs, B. L., and Scholz, D. A. (1975). *Ann. Intern Med.* **83**, 365.

David, D. S., Grieco, N. H., and Cushman, P., Jr. (1970). *J. Chronic Dis.* **22**, 637.

Davis, M. E., Strandjord, N. M., and Lanzl, L. H. (1966). *J. Am. Med. Assoc.* **196**, 129.

Davis, M. E., Lanzl, L. H., and Cox, A. B. (1970). *J. Obstet. Gynecol.* **36**, 187.

Deitrick, J. E., and Whedon, G. D. (1948). *Am. J. Med.* **4**, 3.

Delbarre, F. (1960). *Sem. Hop.* **36**, 575.

Dent, C. E. (1971). *Practitioner* **206**, 793.

Dent, C. E., and Friedman, M. (1965). *Q. J. Med.* **34**, 177.

Dent, C. E., and Hodson, C. J. (1954). *Br. J. Radiol.* **27**, 605.

Dent, C. E., and Watson, L. (1966). *Postgrad. Med. J.* **42**, Suppl., 583.

Dequeker, J., and Merlevede, W. (1971). *Biochim. Biophys. Acta* **244**, 410.

Dequeker, J., Heylen, H., Van Steenkiste, J., and Vroninkx, R. (1972). *Pharmacology* **7**, 321.

DeTakats, G. (1965). *Med. Clin. N. Am.* **49**, 117.

Dewey, J. R., Bartley, M. H. Jr., and Armelagos, G. J. (1969). *Clin. Orthop. Relat. Res.* **65**, 61.

Dickinson, L. E., MacMahon, B., Cole, P., and Brown, J. B. (1974). *N. Engl. J. Med.* **291**, 1211.

Dickson, I. R., Millar, E. A., and Veis, A. (1975). *Lancet* **2**, 586.

Donaldson, C. L., Hulley, S. B., Vogel, J. M., Hattner, R. S., Bayers, J. H., and McMillan, D. E. (1970). *Metab., Clin. Exp.* **19**, 1071.

Donaldson, I. A., and Nassim, J. R. (1954). *Br. Med. J.* **1**, 1228.

Doyle, F. H. (1967). *Proc. R. Soc. Med.* **60**, 1131.

Doyle, F. H., Gutteridge, D. H., Joplin, G. F., and Fraser, R. (1967). *Br. J. Radiol.* **40**, 241.

Doyle, F., Brown, J., and Lachance, C. (1970). *Lancet* **1**, 391.

Draper, H. H., Sie, T. L., and Bergan, J. G. (1972). *J. Nutr.* **102**, 1133.

Drucker, W. R., Hubay, C. A., Holden, W. D., and Bukovnic. J. A. (1959). *Am. J. Surg.* **97**, 454.

D'Souza, A., and Gloch, M. H. (1973). *Am. J. Clin. Nutr.* **26**, 352.

Dudl, R. J., Ensinck, J. W., Bayling, D., Chesnut, C. H., Sherrard, D., and Nelp, W. B. (1973). *Am. J. Med.* **55**, 631.

Duffey, P. H., Tretbar, H. C., and Jarkowski, T. L. (1971). *Ann Intern. Med.* **74**, 745.

Dull, T. A., and Henneman, P. H. (1963). *N. Engl. J. Med.* **268**, 132.

Duncan, H. (1972). *Orthop. Clin. N. Am.* **3**, 571.

Duncan, H., Frost, H., Villanueva, A. R., and Sigler, J. W. (1965). *Arth. Rheum.* **8**, 943.

Duncan, H., Frame, B., Frost, H., and Arnstein, A. R. (1969). *South. Med. J.* **62**, 41.

Dunning, M. F., and Plum, F. (1957). *Arch. Intern. Med.* **99**, 716.

Eisenberg, E. (1969). *In* "Metabolic Effects of Gonad Hormones and Contraceptive Steroids" (H. A. Salhanick, D. M. Kipnis, and R. L. Vande Wiele, eds.), pp. 503–518. Plenum, New York.

Eisenberg, E., and Pimstone, B. (1967). *Clin. Orthop. Relat. Res.* **52**, 199.

Ellis, F. R., Holesh, S., and Ellis, J. W. (1972). *Am. J. Clin. Nutr.* **25**, 555.

Engel, E., and Forbes, A. P. (1965). *Medicine (Baltimore)* **44**, 135.

Epstein, S., Van Mieghem, W., Sagel, J., and Jackson, W. P. U. (1973). *Metab., Clin. Exp.* **22**, 1163.

Exton-Smith, A. N., Hodkinson, H. M., and Stanton, B. R. (1966). *Lancet* **2**, 999.

Exton-Smith, A. N., Millard, P. H., Payne, P. R., and Wheeler, E. F. (1969). *Lancet* **2**, 1154.

Faccini, J. M., Exton-Smith, A. N., and Boyde, A. (1976) *Lancet* **1**, 1089.

Fanconi, A., Illig, R., Poley, J. R., Prader, A., Francillon, M., Labhart, A., and Uehlinger, E. (1966). *Helv. Paediatr. Acta* **21**, 531.

Farnsworth, A. E., and Dobyns, B. M. (1974). *Med. J. Aust.* **2**, 782.

Finby, N., and Archibald, R. M. (1963). *Am. J. Roentgenol., Radium Ther. Nucl. Med.* [N.S.] **89**, 1222.

Fink, C. W., Ferguson, J. L., and Smiley, J. D. (1967). *J. Lab. Clin. Med.* **69**, 950.

Finkelstein, J. D., and Schachter, D. (1962). *Am. J. Physiol.* **203**, 873.

Flanagan, B., Ault, S., and Nichols, G., Jr. (1970). *In* "Osteoporosis" (U.S. Barzel, ed.), pp. 217–238. Grune & Stratton, New York.

Follis, R. H., Jr. (1951). *Bull. Johns Hopkins Hosp.* **88**, 440.

Follis, R. H., Jr. (1953). *Bull. Johns Hopkins Hosp.* **92**, 405.

Forbes, G. B., and Reina, J. C. (1970). *Metab. Clin. Exp.* **19**, 653.

Foss, M. V. L., and Byers, P. D. (1972). *Ann. Rheum. Dis.* **31**, 259.

Frame, B., and Nixon, R. K. (1968). *N. Engl. J. Med.* **279**, 626.

Franke, J., Rempel, H., and Franke, M. (1974). *Acta Orthop. Scand.* **45**, 1.

Fraser, D. (1957). *Am. J. Med.* **22**, 730.

Fraser, R. W., and Smith, P. H. (1941). *Q. J. Med.* **10**, 297.

Fraser, S. A., Anderson, J. B., Smith, D. A., and Wilson, G. M. (1971). *Lancet* **1**, 981.

Friedenberg, Z. B., Harlow, M. C., Heppenstall, R. B., and Brighton, C. T. (1973). *Calcif. Tissue Res.* **13**, 53.

Friedman, S. A., Raizner, A. E., Rosen, H., Solomon, N. A., and Syn, W. (1972). *Ann. Intern. Med.* **76**, 41.

Frost, H. M. (1961). *J. Am. Geriatr. Soc.* **9**, 1078.

Frost, H. M. (1962). *J. Clin. Endocrinol. Metab.* **22**, 631.

Fucik, R. F., Kukreja, S. C., Hargis, G. K., Bowser, E. N., Henderson, W. J., and Williams, G. A. (1975). *J. Clin. Endocrinol. Metab.* **40**, 152.

Fujita, T., Orimo, H., Okano, K., Yoshikawa, M., Shimo, R., Inoue, T., and Itami, Y. (1972). *Endocrinol. Jpn.* **19**, 571.

Furman, R., Nicholas, J. J., and Jivoff, L. (1970). *J. Bone Joint Surg., Am. Vol.* **52**, 1131.

Gallagher, J. C., and Nordin, B. E. C. (1972). *Lancet* **1**, 7749.

Gallagher, J. C., Aaron, J., Horsman, A., Wilkinson, R., and Nordin, B. E. C. (1973). *Clin. Endocrinol. Metab.* **2**, 355.

Garn, S. M. (1970). *Am. J. Clin. Nutr.* **23**, 1149.

Garn, S. M. (1972). *Orthop. Clin. N. Am.* **3**, 503.

Garn, S. M., and Hull, E. J. (1966). *Invest. Radiol.* **1**, 255.

Garn, S. M., and Poznanski, A. K. (1970). *In* "Osteoporosis" (U.S. Barzel, ed.), pp. 114–123. Grune & Stratton, New York.

Garn, S. M., Pao, E. M., and Rihl, M. E. (1964a). *Science* **143**, 1439.

Garn, S. M., Rohmann, C. G., Behar, M., Viteri, F., and Guzman, M. A. (1964b). *Science* **145**, 1444.

Garn, S. M., Rohmann, C. G., and Wagner, B. (1967). *Fed. Proc., Fed. Am. Soc. Exp. Biol.* **26**, 1729.

Garn, S. M., Rohmann, C. G., Wagner, B., Davila, H. G., and Ascoli, W. (1969). *Clin. Orthop. Relat. Res.* **65**, 51.

Garn, S. M., Poznanski, A. K., and Nagy, J. M. (1971). *Diagn. Radiol.* **100**, 509.

Garn, S. M., Sandusky, S. T., Nagy, J. M., and McCann, M. B. (1972a). *J. Pediatr.* **80**, 965.

Garn, S. M., Gall, J. C., Jr., and Nagy, J. M. (1972b). *Invest. Radiol.* **7**, 97.

Geall, M. G., and Beilin, L. J. (1964). *Br. Med. J.* **2**, 255.

Georges, L. P., Santangelo, R. P., Mackin, J. F., and Canary, J. J. (1975). *Metab. Clin. Exp.* **24**, 11.

Goka, T. J., Stevenson, R. E., Hefferan, P. M. and Howell, R. R. (1976). *Proc. Natl. Acad. Sci. U.S.A.* **73**, 604.

Goldfischer, S., Johnson, A. B., and Morecki, R. (1976). *Lab. Invest.* **35**, 55.

Goldfield, E. B., Braiker, B. M., Predergast, J. J., and Kolb, F. O. (1972). *J. Am. Med. Assoc.* **221**, 1127.

Goldsmith, M. F., Johnston, J. O., Ury, H., Vose, G., and Colbert, C. (1971). *J. Bone Joint Surg., Am. Vol.* **53**, 83.

Goldsmith, R. S., and Ingbar, S. H. (1966). *N. Engl. J. Med.* **274**, 1.

Goldsmith, R. S., Jowsey, J., Dube, W. J., Riggs, B. L., Arnaud, C. D., and Kelly, P. J. (1976). *J. Clin. Endocrinol. Metab.* **43**, 523.

Goldsmith, R. S., and Ingbar, S. H. (1966). *N. Engl. J. Med.* **274**, 1.

Gooding, C. A., and Ball, J. H. (1969). *Radiology* **93**, 1349.

Gordan, G. S., Picchi, J., and Roof, B. S. (1973). *Trans. Assoc. Am. Physicians* **86**, 326.

Greenberg, R. A., Winters, R. W., and Graham, J. B. (1960). *J. Clin. Endocrinol. Metab.* **20**, 364.

Griffith, D. P. (1971). *Aerosp. Med.* **42**, 1322.

Griffith, G. C., Nichols, G., Asher, J. D., and Flannagan, B. (1965). *J. Am. Med. Assoc.* **193**, 85.

Griffiths, J. H., D'Orsi, C. J., and Zimmerman, R. E. (1972). *Invest. Radiol.* **7**, 107.

Grodin, J. M., Siiteri, P. K., and MacDonald, P. C. (1973). *J. Clin. Endocrinol. Metab.* **36**, 207.

Gryfe, C. I., Exton-Smith, A. N., Payne, P. R., and Wheeler, E. F. (1971). *Lancet* **1**, 523.

Guggenheim, K., Menczel, J., Reshef, A., Schwartz, A., Ben-Menachem, Y. Bernstein, D. S., Hegsted, M., and Stare, F. J. (1971). *Arch. Environ. Health* **22**, 259.

Guller, R., Kayasseh, L., and Haas, H. G. (1973). *Schweiz. Med. Wochensschr.* **103**, 107.

Gwinup, G. (1961). *J. Clin. Endocrinol. Metab.* **21**, 101.

Haas, H. G., Canary, J. J., Kyle, L. H., Meyer, R. J., and Schaaf, M. (1963). *J. Clin. Endocr. Metab.* **23**, 605.

Hahn, T. J., Downing, S. J., and Phang, J. M. (1971). *Am. J. Physiol.* **220**, 1717.

Hahn, T. J., Boisseau, V. C., and Avioli, L. V. (1974). *J. Clin. Endocrinol. Metab.* **39**, 274.

Hahnel, H., Muhlbach, R., Lindenhayn, K., Schaetz, P., Schmidt, U. J., and Alternsforsch, Z. (1974). *Calcif. Tissue Abstr.* **6**, 61.

Halperin, M., Rogot, E., Gurian, J., and Ederer, F. (1968). *J. Chronic Dis.* **21**, 13.

Hamlin, C. R., Kohn, R. R., and Luschin, J. H. (1975). *Diabetes* **24**, 902.

Han, S. Y., and Collins, L. C. (1968). *Radiology* **91**, 795.

Hanna, S., Harrison, M., MacIntyre, I., and Fraser, R. (1960). *Lancet* **2**, 172.

Hanna, S., Harrison, M. T., MacIntyre, I., and Fraser, R. (1961). *Br. Med. J.* **2**, 12.

Hantman, D. A., Vogel, J. M., Donaldson, C. L., Friedman, R., Goldsmith, R. S., and Hulley, S. B. (1973). *J. Clin. Endocrinol. Metab.* **36**, 845.

Harden, R., Harrison, M. T., Alexander, W. D., and Nordin, B. E. C. (1964). *J. Endocrinol.* **28**, 281.

Harnapp, G. O. (1967). *Ger. Med. Mon.* **12**, 544.

Harris, F. (1967). *Proc. R. Soc. Med.* **60**, 46.

Harris, W. H., and Heaney, R. P. (1969). *N. Engl. J. Med.* **280**, 253.

Harris, W. H., Heaney, R. P., Jowsey, J., Cockin, J., Akins, C., Graham, J., and Weinberg, E. H. (1972). *Calcif. Tissue Res.* **10**, 1.

Harrison, H. E., and Harrison, H. C. (1960). *Am. J. Physiol.* **199**, 265.

Harrison, H. E., Hitchman, A. J. W., Finlay, J. M., Fraser, D., Yendt, E. R., Bayley, T. A., and McNeill, K. G. (1971). *Metab., Clin. Exp.* **20**, 1107.

Harrison, M., and Frazer, R. (1960). *J. Endocrinol.* **21**, 197.

Hartog, M. and Joplin, G. F. (1967). *Proc. R. Soc. Med.* **60**, 477.

Heaney, R. P. (1962). *Am. J. Med.* **33**, 188.

Heaney, R. P. (1969). *In* "Metabolic Effects of Gonadal Hormones and Contraceptive Steriods" (H. A. Salhanick, H. A., D. M. Kipnis, and R. L. Vande Wiele, eds.), pp. 493–503. Plenum, New York.

Heaney, R. P., and Whedon, G. D. (1958). *J. Clin. Endocrinol. Metab.* **18**, 1246.

Heaney, R. P., Harris, W. H., Cockin, J., and Weinberg, E. H. (1972). *Calcif. Tissue Res.* **10**, 14.

Heaney, R. P., Recker, R. R., and Saville, P. D. (1974). *Clin. Res.* **22**, 649A.

Heath, H., III, and Sizemore, G. W. (1975). *Endocrine Soc. Program 57th Annu. Meet.* p. 77.

Heath, H., III, Earll, J. M., Schaat, M., Peichocki, J. T., and Li, T. K. (1972). *Metab. Clin. Exp.* **21**, 633.

Heimann, P. (1970). *Acta Chir. Scand.* **136**, 143.

Hellewell, A. B., Beljan, J. R., and Goldman, M. (1974). *Clin. Orthop. Relat. Res.* **100**, 349.

Hemsell, D. L., Grodin, J. M., Brenner, P. F., Siiteri, P. K., and MacDonald, P. C. (1974). *J. Clin. Endocrinol. Metab.* **38**, 476.

Henneman, P. H., and Wallach, S. (1957). *Arch. Intern. Med.* **100**, 715.

Henneman, P. H., Forbes, A. P., Moldawer, M., Dempsey, E. F., and Carroll, E. L. (1960). *J. Clin. Invest.* **39**, 1223.

Hernberg, C. A. (1952a). *Acta Med. Scand.* **141**, 309.

Hernberg, C. A. (1952b). *Acta Med. Scand.* **143**, 1.

Hernberg, C. A. (1960). *Acta Endocrinol. (Copenhagen)* **34**, 51.

Heuck, F. (1970). *Radiologe* **6**, 234.

Hockaday, T. D. R., and Keynes, W. M. (1966). *J. Endocrinol.* **34**, 413.

Hodge, H. C., and Smith, F. A. (1968). *Annu. Rev. Pharmacol.* **8**, 395.

Hollo, I., Feher, T., and Szucs, J. (1970). *Acta Med. Acad. Sci. Hung.* **27**, 155.

Hosking, D. J., and Chamberlain, M. J. (1973). *Br. Med. J.* **3**, 125.

Hossain, M., Smith, D. A., and Nordin, B. E. C. (1970). *Lancet* **1**, 809.

Howard, J. E., and Thomas, W. C., Jr. (1963). *Medicine (Baltimore)* **42**, 25.

Howland, W. J., Jr., Pugh, D. G., and Sprague, R. G. (1958). *Radiology* **71**, 69.

Huguenin, A., Sudaka, P., Monier, J. G., and Mme. Monier, (1960). *Alger. Med.* **64**, 711.

Hulley, S. B., Vogel, J. M., Donaldson, C. L., Bayers, J. H., Friedman, R. J., and Rosen, S. N. (1971). *J. Clin. Invest.* **50**, 2506.

Hunder, G. G., and Kelly, P. J. (1971). *Ann Intern. Med.* **75**, 134.

Hurxthal, L. M., and Vose, G. P. (1969). *Calcif. Tissue Res.* **4**, 245.

Iannaccone, A., Gabrilove, J. L., Brahms, S. A., and Soffer, L. J. (1960). *Ann Intern. Med.* **52**, 570.

Inkovaara, J., Heikinheimo, R., Jarvinen, K., Kasurinen, U., Hanhijarvi, H., and Iisalo, E. (1975). *Br. Med. J.* **3**, 73.

Ireland, P., and Fordtran, J. S. (1973). *J. Clin. Invest.* **52**, 2672.

Irwin, M. I., and Kienholz, E. W. (1973). *J. Nutr.* **103**, 1019.

Iskrant, A. P. (1968). *Am. J. Public Health* **58**, 485.

Iskrant, A. P., and Smith, R. W., Jr. (1969). *Public Health Rep.* **84**, 33.

Israel, H. (1967). *Fed. Proc., Fed. Am. Soc. Exp. Biol.* **26**, 1723.

Jee, W. S., Park, H. Z., Roberts, W. E., and Kenner, G. H. (1970). *Am. J. Anat.* **129**, 477.

Jenkins, D. P., and Cochran, T. H. (1969). *Clin. Orthop. Relat. Res.* **63**, 128.

Jensen, H., Christiansen, C., Munck, O., and Toft, H. (1973). *Scand. J. Clin. Lab. Invest.* **32**, 94.

Jett, S., Ramser, J. R., Frost, H. M., and Villanueva, A. R. (1966). *Arch. Pathol.* **81**, 112.

Joffe, B. I., Seftel, H. C., Goldberg, R. C., Bersohn, I., and Hackeng, W. H. L. (1975). *S. Afr. Med. J.* **49**, 965.

Johnson, K. A., Riggs, B. L., Kelly, P. J., and Jowsey, J. (1971). *J. Clin. Endocrinol. Metab.* **33**, 745.

Jones, G. (1969). *Clin. Radiol.* **20**, 345.

Jowsey, J. (1960). *Clin. Orthop. Relat. Res.* **17**, 210.

Jowsey, J., and Balasubramaniam, P. (1972). *Clin. Sci.* **42**, 289.

Jowsey, J., and Gershon-Cohen, J. (1964). *Proc. Soc. Exp. Biol. Med.* **116**, 437.

Jowsey, J., and Johnson, K. A. (1972). *J. Pediatr.* **81**, 511.

Jowsey, J., and Riggs, B. L. (1970). *Acta Endocrinol. (Copenhagen)* **63**, 21.

Jowsey, J., and Riggs, B. L. (1973). *Mod. Med. Australia,* (Aug.) p. 6.

Jowsey, J., Riggs, B. L., Kelly, P. J., Hoffman, D. L., and Bordier, P. (1971). *J. Lab. Clin. Med.* **78**, 574.

Jowsey, J., Riggs, B., Kelly, P. J., and Hoffman, D. L. (1972). *Am. J. Med.* **54**, 43.

Joyce, J. R., Pierce, K. R., Romane, W. M., and Baker, J. M. (1971). *J. Am. Vet. Med. Assoc.* **158**, 2033.

Judd, H. L., Judd, G. E., Luca, W. E., and Yen, S. S. C. (1974). *J. Clin. Endocrinol. Metab.* **39**, 1020.

Jurist, J. M. (1970). *Phys. Med. & Biol.* **15**, 427.

Kalayjian, B. S., Nerbut, P. A., and Erf, L. A. (1946). *Radiology* **47**, 223.

Kang, A. H., and Trelstad, R. L. (1973). *J. Clin. Invest.* **52**, 2571.

Keating, F. R., Jr., Jones, J. D., Elveback, L. R., and Randall, R. V. (1969). *J. Lab. Clin. Med.* **73**, 825.

Keats, T. E., and Bruns, T. W. (1964). *Radiol. Clin. N. Am.* **2**, 297.

Keele, D. K., and Vose, G. P. (1969). *Am. J. Dis. Child.* **118**, 759.

Keele, D. K., and Vose, G. P. (1971). *Am. J. Dis. Child.* **121**, 204.

Kehayoglou, A. K., Agnew, J. E., Holdsworth, C. D., Whelton, M. J., and Sherlock, S. (1968). *Lancet* **1**, 715.

Kelly, P. J., Jowsey, J., Riggs, B. L., and Elveback, L. R. (1967). *J. Lab. Clin. Med.* **69**, 110.

Kenner, G. H., Gabrielson, E. W., Lovell, J. E., Marshall, A. E., and Williams, W. S. (1975). *Calcif. Tissue Res.* **18**, 111.

Kenny, F. M. (1972). *Clin. Pediatr.* **11**, 395.

Khanna, P., and Bhargava, S. (1971). *Indian J. Med. Res.* **59**, 1599.

Kher, A., Toulemonde, F., and Raby, C. (1973). *Nouv. Presse Med.* **2**, 1585.

Kimberg, D. V., Baerg, R. D., Gershon, E., and Graudusius, R. T. (1971). *J. Clin. Invest.* **50**, 1309.

Kivirikko, K. I. (1970). *Int. Rev. Connect. Tissue Res.* **5**, 93.

Kivirikko, K. I., Laitinen, O., and Lamberg, B. A. (1965). *J. Clin. Endocrinol. Metab.* **25**, 1347.

Klein, L., Van der Noort, S., and DeJak, J. J. (1966). *Med. Serv. J., Can.* (Jul.–Aug.), 524.

Klein, M., and Frost, H. M. (1964). *Henry Ford Hosp. Med. Bull.* **12**, 527.

Klinefelter, H. F., Jr., Albright, F., and Griswold, G. C. (1943). *J. Clin. Endocrinol. Metab.* **3**, 529.

Korns, R. F. (1969). *Public Health Rep.* **84**, 815.

Krane, S. M., Grownell, G. L., Stanbury, J. B., and Corrigan, H. (1956). *J. Clin. Invest.* **35**, 874.

Krane, S. M., Harris, E. D., Jr., Singer, F. R., and Potts, J. T., Jr. (1973). *Metab., Clin. Exp.* **22**, 51.

Kratzsch, K. H. (1969). *Ger. Med. Mon.* **14**, 457.

Krawitt, E. L. (1975). *J. Clin. Lab. Med.* **85**, 665.

Krokowski, E. (1973). *Radiologe* **13**, 97.

Krook, L., Lutwak, L., Henrikson, P. A., Kallfelz, F., Hirsch, C., Romanus, B., Bélanger, L. F., Marier, J. R., and Sheffy, B. E. (1971). *J. Nutr.* **101**, 233.

Kruse, H. P., and Kuhlencordt, F. (1975). *Horm. Metab. Res.* **7**, 488.

Kruse, H. P., Kyhlencordt, F., and Wernecke, Y. (1974). *Calcif. Tissue Res.* **6**, 88.

Kuhlencordt, F., Kruse, H. P., Lozano-Tonkin, C., and Eckermeier, L. (1969). *Dtsch. Med. Wochenschr.* **94**, 1730.

Laake, H. (1955). *Acta Med. Scand.* **151**, 229.

Lachman, E. (1955). *Am. J. Roentgenol. Radium Ther.* [N.S.] **74**, 712.

Lachman, E., and Whilan, M. (1936). *Radiology* **26**, 165.

Lafferty, F. W., Spencer, G. E., Jr., and Pearson, O. H. (1964). *Am. J. Med.* **36**, 514.

Laflamme, G. H., and Jowsey, J. (1972). *J. Clin. Invest.* **51**, 2834.

Lagunoff, D., and Benditt, E. P. (1936). *Ann. N.Y. Acad. Sci.* **103**, 185.

Langloh, N. D., Hunder, G. G., Riggs, B. L., and Kelly, P. J. (1973). *J. Bone Joint Surg., Am. Vol.* **55**, 1188.

Lapatsanis, P., Kavadias, A., and Vretos, K. (1971). *Arch. Dis. Child.* **46**, 66.

Lawrence, G. D., Loeffler, R. G., Martin, L. G., and Connor, T. B. (1973). *J. Bone Joint Surg., Am. Vol.* **55**, 87.

Lazarus, J. H., and Harden, R. McG. (1969). *Gerontol. Clin.* **11**, 371.

Leach, R. E., and Baskies, A. (1973). *Clin. Orthop. Relat. Res.* **90**, 95.

Lee, C. A., and Lloyd, H. M. (1964). *Med. J. Aust.* **1**, 992.

Lekkerkerker, J. F. F., van Woudenberg, F., and Doorenbos, H. (1972). *Acta Endocrinol. (Copenhagen)* **69**, 488.

LeMay, M., and Blunt, J. W., Jr. (1949). *J. Clin. Invest.* **28**, 521.

Lemli, L., and Smith, D. (1963). *J. Pediatr.* **63**, 577.

Leone, N. C., Stevenson, C. A., Hilbish, T. F., and Sosman, M. C. (1955). *Am. J. Roentgenol.* **74**, 847.

Lequesne, M. (1968). *Ann. Rheum. Dis.* **27**, 463.

Levin, J., and Kupperman, H. S. (1961). *Arch. Intern. Med.* **113**, 730.

Levin, M. E., Boisseau, V. C., and Avioli, L. V. (1976). *N. Engl. J. Med.* **294**, 241.

Levine, C. I., and Gross, J. (1959). *J. Exp. Med.* **100**, 771.

Lichtenstein, J. R., Martin, G. R., Kohn, L. D., Byers, P. H., and McKusick, V. A. (1973). *Science* **182**, 298.

Lichtwitz, A., Cachin, M., Hioco, D., Tutin, M., and Seze, S. (1959). *Sem. Hop.* **35**, 2399.

Lim, P., and Jacob, E. (1972). *Q. J. Med.* **41**, 291.

Lindenfelser, R., Hasselkus, W., Haubert, P., and Kronert, W. (1972). *Virchows Arch. B* **11**, 80.

Lindsay, R., Sweeney, A., and Hart, D. M. (1976a). *Lancet* **1**, 417.

Lindsay, R., Aitken, J. M., Anderson, J. B., Hart, D. M., MacDonald, E. B., and Clark, A. C. (1976b). *Lancet* **1**, 1038.

Linkswiler, H. M., Joyce, C. L., and Anad, C. R. (1974). *Trans. N.Y. Acad. Sci.* [2] **36**, 333.

Linthicum, F. H., Jr., House, H. P., and Althaus, S. R. (1973). *Ann. Otol., Rhinol., & Laryngol.* **82**, 609.

Little, K., Kelly, M., and Courts, A. (1962). *J. Bone Joint Surg., Br. Vol.* **44**, 503.

Lockwood, D. R., Lammert, J. E., Vogel, J. M., and Hulley, S. B. (1973). *In* "Clinical Aspects of Metabolic Bone Disease" (B. Frame, A. M. Parfitt, and H. Duncan, eds.), pp. 261–265. Excerpta Med. Found., Amsterdam.

Loeper, M., Lemaire, A., and Lesobre, R. (1939). *Arch. Mal. Appar. Dig. Mal. Nutr.* **29**, 577.

Losowsky, M. S., and Walker, B. E. (1969). *Gastroenterology* **56**, 589.

Lund, B., Sorensen, O. H., and Christensen, A. B. (1975a). *Lancet* **2**, 300.

Lund, B., Kjaer, I., Friis, T., Hjorth, L., Reimann, I., Andersen, R. B., and Sorensen, O. H. (1975b). *Lancet* **2**, 1168.

Lutwak, L. (1969). *J. Am. Geriatr. Soc.* **17**, 115.

Lutwak, L., and Whedon, G. D. (1963). *Dis. Mon.* p. 1.

Lynch, S. R., Berelowtiz, I., Seftel, H. C., Miller, G. B., Krawitz, P., Charlton, R. W., and Bothwell, T. H. (1967). *Am. J. Nutr.* **20**, 799.

McCally, M., and Lawton, R. W. (1963). Tech. Doc. Rep. No. AMRL-TDR-63-3. Wright-Patterson Air Force Base, Ohio.

McCance, R. A., and Widdowson, E. M. (1942). *J. Physiol. (London)* **101**, 44.

McCann, V. J., and Fulton, T. T. (1975). *J. Clin. Endocrinol Metab.* **40**, 1038.

McConkey, B., Fraser, G. M., and Bligh, A. S. (1962). *Q. J. Med.* **31**, 419.

McConkey, B., Fraser, G. M., and Bligh, A. S. (1963). *Lancet* **1**, 693.

McFarland, W. (1954). *Science* **119**, 810.

Mack, P. B., and Vogt, F. B. (1971). *Am. J. Roentgenol., Radium Ther. Nucl. Med.* [N.S.] **113**, 621.

Mack, P. B., LaChance, P. A., Vose, G. P., and Vogt, F. B. (1967). *Am. J. Roentgenol., Radium Ther. Nucl. Med.* [N.S.] **100**, 503.

McKusick, V. A. (1972a). *In* "Heritable Disorders of Connective Tissue," 4th ed., pp. 390–455. Mosby, St. Louis, Missouri.

McKusick, V. A. (1972b). *In* "Heritable Disorders of Connective Tissue," 4th ed., pp. 224–282. Mosby, St. Louis, Missouri.

McMillan, D. E., Deller, J. J., Grodsky, G. M., and Forsham, P. H. (1968). *Metab. Clin. Exp.* **17**, 966.

Maddison, P. J., and Bacon, P. A. (1974). *Br. Med. J.* **4**, 433.

Malm, O. J. (1958). *J. Clin. Lab. Invest.* **10,** Suppl., 1.

Malm, O. J. (1963). *In* "The Transfer of Calcium and Strontium Across Biological Membranes" (R. H. Wasserman, ed.), pp. 143–173. Academic Press, New York.

Manzke, E., Chesnut, C. H., III, Wergedal, J. E., Baylink, D. J., and Nelp, W. B. (1975). *Metab. Clin. Exp.* **24,** 605.

Maymovitz, A., and Horwith, M. (1964). *J. Clin. Endocrinol. Metab.* **24,** 4.

Mazess, R. B. (1970). *Arct. Anthropol.* **7,** 114.

Mazess, R. B., and Cameron, J. R. (1971). *Am. J. Phys. Anthropol.* **35,** 399.

Mazess, R. B., and Cameron, J. R. (1973). *In* "International Conference on Bone Mineral Measurement," NIH No. 75-683, pp. 228–238. U.S. Dept. of Health, Education and Welfare, Washington, D.C.

Meema, H. E. (1966). *J. Bone Joint Surg., Am. Vol.* **48,** 1138.

Meema, H. E., and Meema, S. (1968). *Can. Med. Assoc. J.* **99,** 248.

Meema, H. E., and Meema, S. (1969). *J. Am. Geriatr. Soc.* **17,** 120.

Meema, H. E., and Meema, S. (1972). *Invest. Radiol.* **7,** 88.

Meema, H. E., and Reid, D. B. W. (1969). *J. Gerontol.* **24,** 28.

Meema, H. E., and Schatz, D. L. (1970). *Radiology* **97,** 9.

Meema, S., Reid, D. B. W., and Meema, H. E. (1973). *Calcif. Tissue Res.* **12,** 101.

Meema, S., Bunker, M. L., and Meema, H. E. (1975). *Arch. Intern. Med.* **135,** 1436.

Melick, R. A., and Baird, C. W. (1970). *Med. J. Aust.* **2,** 960.

Melsen, F., Mosekilde, L., and Beck-Nielsen, H. (1975). *Ugeskr. Laeg.* **137,** 933.

Menczel, J., Makin, M., Robin, G., Jaye, I., and Naor, E. (1972). *Isr. J. Med. Sci.* **8,** 918.

Menkes, J. H., Alter, M., Steigleder, G. K., Weakly, D. K., and Sung, J. H. (1962). *Pediatrics* **29,** 764.

Merry, J., and Marks, V. (1972). *Lancet* **2,** 990.

Merz, W. A., Schenk, R. K., and Reutter, F. W. (1970). *Calcif. Tissue Res.* **4,** 49.

Milhaud, G., Calmettes, C., Jullienne, A., Tharaud, D, Bloch-Michel, H., Cavaillon, J. P., Colin, R., and Moukhtar, M. S. (1972). *In* "Calcium, Parathyroid Hormone and the Calcitonins" (R. V. Talmage and P. L. Munson), Int. Congr. Ser. No. 243, pp. 56–70. Excerpta Med. Found., Amsterdam.

Millard, F. J. C., Nassim, J. R., and Woolen, J. W. (1970). *Arch. Dis. Child.* **45,** 399.

Miller, D. S., and DeTakats, G. (1942). *Surg., Gynecol. Obstet.* **75,** 558.

Miller, R. G. (1969). *Gerontol. Clin.* **11,** 244.

Minaire, P., Meunier, P., Edouard, C., Barnard, J., Courpron, P., and Bourret, J. (1974). *Calcif. Tissue Res.* **17,** 57.

Miravet, L., Hioco, D., Debeyre, N., Dryll, A., Ryckewaert, A., and de Seze, S. (1966). *Sem. Hop.* (Nov.) p. 60.

Mitchell, G. E., Lourie, H., and Berne, A. S. (1967). *Radiology* **89,** 67.

Molinatti, G. M., Caminni, F., Losana, O., and Olivetti, M. (1961). *Acta Endocrinol. (Copenhagen)* **36,** 161.

Moore, E. W. (1971). *Gastroenterology* **60,** 43.

Moore Ede., M. C., Faulkner, M. H., and Tredre, B. E. (1972). *Clin. Sci.* **42,** 433.

Morgan, D. B., and Newton-John, H. F. (1969). *Gerontologia* **15,** 140.

Moseley, J. E. (1965). *Am. J. Roentgenol., Radium Ther. Nucl. Med.* [N.S.] **95,** 135.

Mosier, H. D., Jr., Smith, F. G., Jr., and Schultz, M. A. (1972). *Am. J. Dis. Child.* **124,** 251.

Moskowitz, R. W., Klein, L., and Katz, D. (1965). *Arthritis Rheum.* **8,** 61.

Mudd, S. H., Finkelstein, J. D., Irreverre, F., and Laster, L. (1964). *Science* **143,** 1443.

Mudd, S. H., Edwards, W. A., Loeb, P. M., Brown, M. S., and Lasfer, L. (1970). *J. Clin. Invest.* **49,** 1762.

Muldowney, F. P., O'Donovan, D. K., and Gallangher, J. E. (1964). *J. Ir. Med. Assoc.* **54,** 132.

Mulhausen, R., Eichenholz, A., and Blumentals, A. (1967). *Medicine (Baltimore)* **46**, 185.
Munck, O. (1964). *Q. J. Med.* **33**, 209.
Mundy, G. R., Shapiro, J. L., Bandelin, J. G., Canalis, E. M., and Raisz, L. G. (1976). *J. Clin. Invest.* **58**, 529.
Murata, K. (1973). *Experientia* **15**, 1219.
Murray, R. O. (1960). *Br. J. Radiol.* **33**, 1.
Murray, R. O. (1961). *Radiology* **77**, 729.
Myhre, L. G., and Kessler, W. V. (1966). *J. Appl. Physiol.* **21**, 1251.
Nadarajah, A., Hartog, M., Redfern, B., Thalassinos, N., Wright, A. D., Joplin, G. F., and Fraser, T. R. (1968). *Br. Med. J.* **4**, 797.
Neuhauser, G., Kaveggia, E. G., and Opitz, J. M. (1976). *Clin. Genetics* **9**, 324.
Nevinny, H. B., and Hall, T. C. (1962). *Cancer Chemother. Rep.* **16**, 305.
Nevinny, H. B., Krant, M. J., and Moore, E. W. (1965). *Metab., Clin. Exp.* **14**, 135.
Newton-John, H. F., and Morgan, D. B. (1968). *Lancet* **1**, 232.
Newton-John, H. F., and Morgan, D. B. (1970). *Clin. Orthop. Relat. Res.* **71**, 229.
Nilsson, B. E. (1970a). *Clin. Orthop. Relat. Res.* **68**, 93.
Nilsson, B. E. (1970b). *Acta Chir. Scand.* **136**, 383.
Nilsson, B. E., and Westlin, N. E. (1971). *Clin. Orthop. Relat. Res.* **77**, 179.
Nilsson, B. E., and Westlin, N. E. (1972a). *Acta Orthop. Scand.* **43**, 504.
Nilsson, B. E., and Westlin, N. E. (1972b). *Calcif. Tissue Res.* **10**, 167.
Nilsson, B. E., and Westlin, N. E. (1973). *Clin. Orthop. Relat. Res.* **90**, 229.
Nordin, B. E. C. (1971). *Br. Med. J.* **1**, 571.
Nordin, B. E. C. (1976). *Clin. Endocrinol.* (Suppl.) **5**, 3535.

Norton, L. A., Proffit, W. R., and Moore, R. R. (1969). *Nature (London)* **221**, 469.
O'Duffy, J. D. (1970). *Arthritis Rheum.* **13**, 381.
Ohata, M., Fujita, T., Orimo, H., and Yoshitakawa, M. (1970). *Am. Geriatr. Soc.* **18**, 295.
Owen, E. C., Irving, J. T., and Lyall, A. (1940). *Acta Med. Scand.* **103**, 235.
Pak, C. Y. C., Zisman, E., Evens, R., Jowsey, J., Delea, C. S., and Bartter, F. C. (1969). *Am. J. Med.* **47**, 7.
Palmieri, M. A., Dvorak, J., and Bottomley, R. (1974). *N. Engl. J. Med.* **290**, 1490.
Panin, N., Gorday, W. J., and Paul, B. J. (1971). *Stroke* **2**, 41.
Parfitt, A. M. (1963). *J. Bone Joint Surg.* **45**, 137.
Parfitt, A. M., and Dent, C. E. (1970). *Q. J. Med.* **39**, 171.
Peck, W. A., Zypkin, L., and Whedon, G. D. (1965). *Clin. Res.* **13**, 330.
Peck, W. A., Brandt, J., and Miller, I. (1967). *Proc. Natl. Acad. Sci. U.S.A.* **57**, 1599.
Pedersen, J. (1967). *In* "The Pregnant Diabetic and her New Born: Problems and Management," p. 60. Williams & Wilkins, Baltimore, Maryland.
Pedrini-Mille, A., Pedrini, A., and Ponseti, I. (1974). *J. Lab. Clin. Med.* **84**, 465.
Pentinnen, R. P., Lichtenstein, J. R., Martin, G. R., and McKusick, V. A. (1975). *Proc. Natl. Acad. Sci. U.S.A.* **72**, 586.
Perlman, R. M. (1944). *J. Clin. Endocrinol. Metab.* **4**, 483.
Perzigian, A. J. (1973). *J. Am. Geriatr. Soc.* **21**, 100.
Phang, J. M., Kales, A. N., and Hahn, T. J. (1968). *Lancet* **1**, 84.
Pierog, S. H., Fontana, V. J., and Ferrara, A. (1969). *N.Y. State J. Med.* **69**, 310.
Pinals, R. S., and Jabbs, J. M. (1972). *Lancet* **2**, 929.
Pincus, C., Romanoff, L. P., and Carlo, J. (1954). *J. Gerontol.* **9**, 113.
Plewes, L. W. (1956). *J. Bone Joint Surg., Br. Vol.* **38**, 195.
Plum, F., and Dunning, M. F. (1958a). *Am. J. Med.* **18**, 860.
Plum, F., and Dunning, M. F. (1958b). *Arch. Intern. Med.* **101**, 528.
Pommer, G. (1885). "Rachitis and Osteomalacie." Vogel, Leipzig.
Pommer, G. (1925). *Arch. Klin. Chir.* **136**, 1.

Ponseti, I. V., and Shepard, R. S. (1954). *J. Bone Joint Surg., Am. Vol.* **36**, 1031.
Poppel, M. H., Gruber, W. F., Silber, R., Holder, A. K., and Christman, R. O. (1959). *Am. J. Roentgenol., Radium Ther. Nucl. Med.* [N.S.] **82**, 239.
Preger, L., Steinbach, H. L., Moskowitz, P., Scully, A. L., and Goldberg, M. B. (1968). *Am. J. Roentgenol., Radium Ther. Nucl. Med.* [N.S.] **104**, 899.
Prockop, D. J., and Kivirikko, K. I. (1967). *Ann. Intern. Med.* **66**, 1243.
Prost, A., Cottin, S., Malkani, K., Bureau, B., Le Bodic, L., and Rebel, A. (1974). *Calcif. Tissue Abstr.* **6**, 63.
Rader, M. D., Flickinger, G. L., DeVilla, G. O., Jr., Mikuta, J. J., and Mikhail, G. (1973). *Am. J. Obstet. Gynecol.* **116**, 1069.
Ragab, A. H., Frech, R. S., and Vietti, T. J. (1970). *Cancer* **25**, 580.
Ragan, C., and Briscoe, A. M. (1964). *J. Clin. Endocrinol. Metab.* **24**, 385.
Raisz, L. G. (1970). *In* "Osteoporosis" (U. S. Barzel, ed.), pp. 174–187. Grune & Stratton, New York.
Ramser, J. R., Frost, H. M., and Smith, R. (1966a). *Clin. Orthop. Relat. Res.* **49**, 169.
Ramser, J. R., Villanueva, A. R., Frost, H. M., and Pirok, D. (1966b). *Clin. Orthop. Relat. Res.* **49**, 1515.
Rathbun, J. C. (1943). *Am. J. Dis. Child.* **75**, 822.
Reifenstein, E. C., Jr. (1956). *South. Med. J.* **49**, 993.
Reifenstein, E. C., Jr., and Albright, F. (1947). *J. Clin. Invest.* **24**, 24.
Reiss, E., Canterbury, J. M., Bercovitz, M. A., and Kaplan, E. L. (1970). *J. Clin. Invest.* **49**, 2146.
Renner, R. R., Nelson, D. A., and Lozner, E. L. (1971). *Am. J. Roentgenol., Radium Ther. Nucl. Med.* [N.S.] **113**, 499.
Rich, C., Bernstein, D. S., Gates, S., Heaney, R. P., Johnston, C. C., Jr., Rosenberg, C. A., Schnape, E., Tewkbury, R. B., and Williams, G. A. (1966). *Clin. Orthop. Relat. Res.* **45**, 63.
Riggins, R. S., Zeman, F., and Moon, D. (1974). *Calcif. Tissue Res.* **14**, 283.
Riggs, L. B., Jowsey, J., and Kelly, P. J. (1966). *Metab., Clin. Exp.* **15**, 773.
Riggs, B. L., Kelly, P. J., Kinney, V. R., Scholz, D. A., and Bianco, A. J., Jr. (1967). *J. Bone Joint Surg., Am. Vol.* **49**, 915.
Riggs, B. L., Jowsey, J., Kelly, P. J., Jones, J. D., and Maher, F. T. (1969). *J. Clin. Invest.* **48**, 1065.
Riggs, B. L., Jowsey, J., Goldsmith, R. S., Kelly, P. J., Hoffman, D. L., and Arnaud, C. D. (1972a). *J. Clin. Invest.* **51**, 1659.
Riggs, B. L., Randall, R. V., Wahner, H. W., Jowsey, J., Kelly, P. J., and Singh, M. (1972b). *J. Clin. Endocrinol. Metab.* **34**, 911.
Riggs, B. L., Arnaud, C. D., Jowsey, J., Goldsmith, R. S., and Kelly, P. J. (1973a). *J. Clin. Invest.* **52**, 181.
Riggs, B. L., Ryan, R. J., Wahner, H. W., Jiang, N., and Mattox, V. R. (1973b). *J. Clin. Endocrinol. Metab.* **36**, 1097.
Riggs, L., Jowsey, J., Kelly, P. J., Hoffman, D. L., and Arnaud, C. D. (1976). *J. Clin. Endocr. Metab.* **42**, 1139.
Riley, F. C., and Jowsey, J. (1973). *Pediatr. Res.* **9**, 757.
Riley, J. F., and West, G. B. (1953). *J. Physiol. (London)* **120**, 528.
Roberts, P. H., Kerr, C. H., and Ohlson, A. (1948). *J. Am. Diet. Assoc.* **24**, 292.
Robichon, J., and Germain, J. P. (1968). *Can. Med. Assoc. J.* **99**, 975.
Ronnov-Jessen, V., and Kirkegaard, C. (1973). *Br. Med. J.* **1**, 41.
Rose, G. A. (1964). *Clin. Radiol.* **15**, 75.
Rose, G. A. (1967). *Clin. Orthop. Relat. Res.* **55**, 17.

Rosenberg, E. M., Boissesu, V. C., Lang, R., and Avioli, L. V. (1976). *J. Clin. Endocrinol. Metab.* **42,** 346.

Rosensweig, N. S. (1971). *Gastroenterology* **60,** 464.

Ross, E. J., Marshall-Jones, P., and Friedman, M. (1966). *Q. J. Med.* **35,** 149.

Rubin, E., Rybak, B. J., Lindenbaum, J., Gerson, C. D., Walker, G., and Lieber, C. S. (1972). *Gastroenterology* **63,** 801.

Ruder, J. H., Loriaux, D. L., and Lipsett, M. B. (1974). *J. Clin. Endocrinol. Metab.* **39,** 1138.

Ruikka, I., Gronroos, M., Bourander, L. B., and Virtama, P. (1968). *Geriatrics* **23,** 165.

Russell, R. G. G., and Fleisch, H. (1975). *Clin. Orthop. Relat. Res.* **108,** 241.

Sackler, J. P., and Liu, L. (1973). *Br. J. Radiol.* **46,** 548.

Sagher, F., and Even-Paz, Z. (1967). *In* ''Mastocytosis and the Mast Cell,'' p. 107. Yearbook Publ., Chicago, Illinois.

Samaan, N. A., Anderson, G. D., and Adam-Mayne, M. E. (1975). *Am. J. Obstet, Gynecol.* **212,** 622.

Samachson, J. (1966). *Radiat. Res.* **27,** 64.

Saville, P. D. (1965). *J. Bone Joint Surg., Am. Vol.* **47,** 492.

Saville, P. D. (1967). *Clin. Orthop. Relat. Res.* **55,** 43.

Saville, P. D., and Heaney, R. (1972). *Stud. Drug Treat.* **2,** 47.

Saville, P. D., and Kharmosh, O. (1967). *Arthritis Rheum.* **10,** 423.

Saville, P. D., and Krook, L. (1968). *Proc. Symp. Calcif. Tissue Res., 6th,* Suppl. 2, p. 24.

Saville, P. D., Krook, L., Gustafsson, P., Marshall, J. L., and Figarola, F. (1969). *Cornell Vet.* **59,** 155.

Schartum, S., and Nichols, G., Jr. (1961). *Proc. Soc. Biol. Med.* **108,** 228.

Schlenker, R. A., and Von Seggen, W. W. (1976). *Calc. Tiss. Res.* **20,** 41.

Schneider, L. E., and Schedl, H. P. (1972). *Am. J. Physiol.* **223,** 1319.

Schwartz, E., Panariello, V. A., and Saeli, J. (1965). *J. Clin. Invest.* **44,** 1547.

Scriver, C. R., and Cameron, D. (1969). *N. Engl. J. Med.* **281,** 604.

Scriver, W. de M., and Bryan, A. H. (1935). *J. Clin. Invest.* **14,** 212.

Seftel, H. C., Malkin, C., Schmaman, A., Abrahams, C., Lynch, S. R., Charlton, R. W., and Bothwell, T. H. (1966). *Br. Med. J.* **1,** 642.

Selle, W. A., and Jurist, J. M. (1966a). *J. Am. Geriatr. Soc.* **14,** 930.

Selle, W. A., and Jurist, J. M. (1966b). *Proc. Soc. Exp. Biol. Med.* **121,** 150.

Shafar, J. (1973). *Br. J. Clin. Pract.* **27,** 405.

Shafer, R. B., and Gregory, D. H. (1972). *Gastroenterology* **63,** 235.

Shah, B. G., Krishnarao, G. V. G., and Draper, H. H. (1967). *J. Nutr.* **92,** 30.

Shamos, M. H., and Lavine, L. S. (1964). *Clin. Orthop. Relat. Res.* **35,** 177.

Shapiro, J. R., Moore, W. T., Jorgensen, H., Epps, C., Reid, J., and Whedon, G. D. (1973). *Int. Conf. Bone Mineral Meas., 1973* October 12–13 p. 222.

Shapiro, J. R., Moore, W. T., Jorgensen, H., Reid, J., Epps, C. H., and Whedon, D. (1975). *Arch. Intern. Med.* **135,** 563.

Shea, J. J., Gillespie, S. M., and Waldbott, G. L. (1967). *Ann. Allergy* **25,** 388.

Shoenfeld, Y., Fried, A., and Ehrenfeld, N. E. (1975). *Am. J. Dis. Child.* **129,** 679.

Siemon, N. J., and Moodie, E. W. (1973). *Nature (London)* **243,** 541.

Singh, A., Jolly, S. S., Bansal, B. C., and Mathur, C. C. (1963). *Medicine (Baltimore)* **42,** 229.

Singh, M., and Jowsey, J. (1970). *Endocrinology* **87,** 183.

Singh, M., Nagrath, A. R., and Maini, R. S. (1970). *J. Bone Joint Surg.* **52,** 457.

Singhelakis, P., Alevizaki, C. C., and Ikkos, D. G. (1974). *Metab., Clin. Exp.* **23,** 311.

Sirois, J. (1963). *Can Med. Assoc. J.* **89,** 1043.

Sissons, H. A. (1956). *J. Bone Joint Surg., Br. Vol.* **38**, 418.

Skeels, R. F. (1958). *J. Clin. Endocrinol. Metab.* **18**, 61.

Smith, D. A., and Nordin, B. E. C. (1964). *Proc. Roy. Soc. Med.* **57**, 368.

Smith, D. C., Prentice, R., Thompson, D. J., and Herrmann, W. L. (1975). *N. Engl. J. Med.* **293**, 1164.

Smith, D. M., Johnston, C. C., and Yu, P. L. (1972). *J. Am. Med. Assoc.* **219**, 325.

Smith, D. M., Nance, W. E., Kang, K. W., Christian, J. C., and Johnston, C. C., Jr. (1973). *J. Clin. Invest.* **52**, 2800.

Smith, D. M., Khairi, M. R. A., and Johnston, C. C., Jr. (1975). *J. Clin. Invest.* **56**, 311.

Smith, D. M., Norton, J. A., Jr. Khairi, R., and Johnston, C. C., Jr., (1976a). *J. Lab. Clin. Med.* **87**, 882.

Smith, D. M., Khairi, M. R. A., Norton, J., and Johnston, C. C., Jr. (1976b). *J. Clin. Invest.* **58**, 716.

Smith, E. L., and Babcock, S. W. (1973). Annual Project Report No. COO-1422-159. Bone Mineral Laboratory, University of Wisconsin, Madison.

Smith, M., Ansell, B. M., and Bywaters, E. G. L. (1968). *J. Pediatr.* **73**, 875.

Smith, R., Russell, R. G. G., and Bishop, M. (1971). *Lancet* **1**, 945.

Smith, R. W., Jr. (1967). *Fed. Proc., Fed. Am. Soc. Exp. Biol.* **26**, 1737.

Smith, R. W., Jr., and Frame, B. (1965). *N. Engl. J. Med.* **273**, 73.

Smith, R. W., Jr., and Rizek, J. (1966). *Clin. Orthop. Relat. Res.* **45**, 31.

Smith, R. W., Jr., Eyler, W. R., and Mellinger, R. C. (1960). *Ann. Intern. Med.* **52**, 773.

Smith, R. W., Jr., Frame, B., Mansour, J., and Rizek, J. (1962). *J. Lab. Clin. Med.* **60**, 1019.

Smith, R. W., Jr., Rizek, J., and Frame, B. (1964). *Am. J. Clin. Nutr.* **14**, 98.

Sobel, H., and Feinberg, S. (1970). *Calcif. Tissue. Res.* **5**, 39.

Solomon, G. F., Dickerson, W. J., and Eisenberg, E. (1960). *Geriatrics* **15**, 46.

Solomons, C. C., and Styner, J. (1969). *Calcif. Tissue Res.* **3**, 318.

Sosman, M. C. (1949). *Am. J. Roentgenol. Radium Ther.* [N.S.] **62**, 1.

Soyka, L. F., and Saxena, K. M. (1965). *J. Am. Med. Assoc.* **192**, 225.

Spencer, H., Menczel, J., and Lewin, I. (1964). *Clin. Orthop. Relat. Res.* **35**, 202.

Spencer, H., Menczel, J., Lewin, I., and Samachson, J. (1965). *J. Nutr.* **86**, 125.

Sperling, O., Weinberger, A., Oliver, I., Liberman, U. S., and DeVries, A. (1974). *Ann. Intern. Med.* **80**, 482.

Steinbach, H. L., and Obata, W. G. (1957). *Am. J. Roentgenol., Radium. Ther. Nucl. Med.* [N.S.] **78**, 39.

Steinbach, H. L., Kolb, F. O., and Crane, J. T. (1959). *Am. J. Roentgenol., Radium Ther. Nucl. Med.* [N.S.] **82**, 875.

Steinberg, M. E., Boxch, A., Schwan, A., Jr., and Glazer, R. (1968). *Clin. Orthop. Relat. Res.* **61**, 294.

Stevenson, C. J., Bottoms, V., and Shuster, S. (1970). *Lancet* **1**, 860.

Summers, V. K., Hunter, W. R., Hipkin, L. J., and Davis, J. C. (1966). *Lancet* **1**, 601.

Sussman, M. L., and Copleman, B. (1942). *Radiology* **39**, 288.

Swezey, R. L. (1970). *Arthritis Rheum.* **13**, 858.

Szymendera, J., and Madajewicz, S. (1967). *Lancet* **1**, 1091.

Teitelbaum, S. L., Kraft, W. J., Lang, R., and Avioli, L. V. (1974). *Calcif. Tissue Res.* **17**, 75.

Teitelbaum, S. L., Rosenberg, E. M., Richardson, C. A., and Avioli, L. V. (1976). *J. Clin. Endocrinol. Metab.* **42**, 537.

Teotia, S. P. S., and Teotia, M. (1973). *Br. Med. J.* **1**, 637.

Territo, M. C., and Tanaka, K. R. (1974). *Arch. Intern. Med.* **134**, 445.

Thompson, J. S., and Urist, M. R. (1973). *Clin. Orthop. Relat. Res.* **90**, 201.

Thompson, J. S., Palmieri, G. M. A., Eliel, L. P., and Crawford, R. L. (1972). *J. Bone Joint Surg., Am. Vol.* **54**, 1490.
Trotter, M., Broman, G. E., and Peterson, R. R. (1960). *J. Bone Joint Surg., Am. Vol.* **42**, 50.
Urist, M. R. (1960). *In* "Bone as a Tissue" (P. Fourman, ed.), pp. 18–45. McGraw-Hill, New York.
Van der Sluys Veer, J., Bijvoet, O. L. M., and Smeenk, D. (1970). *Calcif. Tissue Res.* **4**, 88.
Vermess, M., Pearson, K. D., Einstein, A. B., and Fahey, J. I. (1972). *Radiology* **102**, 497.
Vernon-Roberts, B., and Pirie, C. J. (1973). *Ann. Rheum. Dis.* **32**, 406.
Villanueva, A. R., Ilnicki, L., Duncan, H., and Frost, H. M. (1966a). *Clin. Orthop. Relat. Res.* **49**, 135.
Villanueva, A. R., Frost, H. M., Ilnicki, L., Frame, B., Smith, R., and Arnstein, R. (1966b). *J. Lab. Clin. Med.* **68**, 599.
Vinther-Paulsen, N. (1953). *Geriatrics* **8**, 76.
Wachmann, A., and Bernstein, D. S. (1968). *Lancet* **1**, 958.
Wajchenberg, B. L., Fazia, A. I. M., Costa, A. A., Borges, R., and Nagueira, O. (1974). *Metab., Clin. Exp.* **23**, 337.
Waldbott, G. L. (1964). *Br. Med. J.* **2**, 945.
Walker, A. R. P. (1972). *Am. J. Clin. Nutr.* **25**, 518.
Walker, F., and Shand, J. (1972). *Lancet* **1**, 233.
Wallach, S., and Henneman, P. H. (1959). *J. Am. Med. Assoc.* **171**, 1637.
Walton, J., Dominguez, M., and Bartter, F. C. (1973). *Metab., Clin. Exp.* **24**, 849.
Wang, C. C., and Robbins, L. L. (1956). *Radiology* **67**, 17.
Warshaw, J. B., Littlefield, J. W., Fishman, W. H., Inglis, N. R., and Stolbach, L. L. (1971). *J. Clin. Invest.* **50**, 2137.
Weaver, J. K., and Chalmers, J. (1966). *J. Bone Joint Surg., Am. Vol.* **48**, 289.
Welsh, J. D. (1970). *Medicine (Baltimore)* **49**, 257.
Welton, J., Walker, S. R., Sharp, G. C., Herzenberg, L. A., Wistar, R., Jr., and Creger, W. P. (1968). *Am. J. Med.* **44**, 280.
Westerman, M. P., Greenfield, G. B., and Wong, P. W. K. (1974). *J. Am. Med. Assoc.* **230**, 261.
Wettenhall, R. E. H., Schwartz, P. L., and Bornstein, J. (1969). *Diabetes* **18**, 280.
Whedon, G. D. (1969). *J. Am. Geriatr. Soc.* **17**, 167.
Whedon, G. D., and Shorr, E. (1957). *J. Clin. Invest.* **36**, 966.
Whedon, G. D., Deitrick, J. E., and Shorr, E. (1949). *Am. J. Med.* **6**, 684.
Whedon, G. D., Lutwak, L., Reid, J., Rambaut, P., Whittle, M., Smith, M., and Leach, C. (1974). *Trans. Assoc. Am. Physicians* **87**, 95.
Whelton, J. M., Kehayoglou, A. K., Agnew, J. E., Trunbert, L. A., and Sherlock, S. (1971). *Gut* **12**, 978.
Willson, J. K. V. (1959). *Radiology* **72**, 672.
Wray, J. B., Sugarman, E. D., and Schneider, A. J. (1963). *J. Am. Med. Assoc.* **182**, 118.
Wu, K., Jett, S., and Frost, H. M. (1967). *J. Lab. Clin. Med.* **69**, 810.
Wu, K., Schubeck, K., Frost, H. M., and Villanueva, A. (1970). *Calcif. Tissue Res.* **6**, 204.
Yoslow, W., Becker, M. H., Bartels, J., and Thompson, W. A. L. (1971). *J. Bone Joint Surg., Am. Vol.* **53**, 1541.
Young, M. M., Jansani, C., Smith, D. A., and Nordin, E. C. (1968). *Clin. Sci.* **34**, 411.
Ziel, H. K., and Finkle, W. D. (1975). *N. Engl. J. Med.* **293**, 1167.
Zimmerman, R. E., Griffiths, H. J., and D'Orsi, C. (1973). *Radiology* **106**, 561.
Zweymuller, K., and Jesserer, H. (1973). *Cah. Med.* **14**, 1117.

7

Nephrolithiasis

HIBBARD E. WILLIAMS AND EDWIN L. PRIEN, JR.

I. INTRODUCTION

A discourse on nephrolithiasis in a text dealing with bone disease seems, at first, dubious or at best, tenuous. In fact, since most renal stones are composed of calcium, often in the form of hydroxyapatite, and since many bone diseases are complicated by nephrolithiasis, this chapter does not seem entirely inimical to the major focus of this text. From a historical viewpoint, perhaps because of the obvious nature of the afflictions, both nephrolithiasis and bone disease have shared a great deal of notoriety. Stone disease holds a remarkable place in antiquity with substantial evidence to prove that this problem plagued the pharoahs of ancient Egypt and the patients of Galen and Hippocrates. Despite this notable background, renal stone disease remains today one of the more poorly understood phenomena of clinical medicine, perhaps another point of overlap between nephrolithiasis and bone disease. This somewhat harsh indictment is intended only to stimulate the search for greater understanding of pathogenetic mechanisms and therapeutic approaches to nephrolithiasis.

II. TYPES OF STONES FOUND IN THE URINARY TRACT

A knowledge of stone composition is fundamental to the understanding of stone pathogenesis and allows the selection of proper therapy. Furthermore, it seems inescapable that the composition of the stone's nucleus or at least its central portion must bear an even more direct relationship to its ultimate cause. Yet, there is no consensus as to what method(s) of analysis is best suited for urinary stones, especially for routine analyses. It is a fundamental principle of all analytical work that no single method can answer all of the questions that might be asked about the composition and structure of calculi. However, it should be self-evident that for urinary stones and especially for routine analyses, the method should fulfill the following criteria. It should be accurate and identify substances as compounds and not simply as radicals. It should be sensitive enough to allow the analysis of tiny amounts of material from many areas of the stone including its macroscopic nucleus if evident. It should be semiquantitative and be able to deal with mixtures of two or more substances. It should be rapid, simple, and convenient. Finally, it should be inexpensive.

The chemical methods of analysis employed so widely by clinical laboratories meet few, if any, of these criteria. Often the task of analysis is assigned to a technician with little experience in the method and with no independent means of corroborating the analysis. The result is frequently uninterpretable and discouraging to both technician and physicians involved. The methods of X-ray diffraction (either by powder camera or diffractometer) and infrared spectroscopy are more exact and rigorous and meet more of the criteria. They are especially suited for the analysis of new substances of unknown composition. However, they are rather time consuming (and therefore expensive), requiring from 30 to 120 minutes for analysis. In addition, they are not well suited for resolving mixtures of compounds or for dealing with small samples (Sutor, 1968; Sutor et al., 1971; Tsay, 1961). The only method that meets all of these criteria is optical crystallography combining the use of the dissecting and polarizing microscopes (Prien and Frondel, 1947). Small samples can be handled with great facility. Analysis time is generally 1 minute or less. Mixtures are immediately appreciated and resolved. However, since some subjective interpretation is necessary, the method requires more experience and a rather practiced eye on the part of the technician. This feature has deterred the wider acceptance of the method. Failure to appreciate this requirement has led to an unfavorable review of the use of optical crystallography for urinary stones (Beeler et al., 1964). With the proper training, the optical techniques represent the ideal primary method for routine stone analysis. It should be stated that for new substances and for the occasional stone composed of very thin crystals, X-ray diffraction is indispensable as a secondary method.

In the United States, the majority of stones recovered from patients with stone disease are composed of calcium oxalate with or without variable amounts of admixed apatite (Table I). As a group they are referred to loosely as "calcium stones," all of which are radio-opaque. About half of these stones are pure calcium oxalate composed either entirely of the monohydrate or with a nucleus of monohydrate with the dihydrate occurring peripherally to the more central portions. The physiochemical basis for this constant relationship between the two hydrates of calcium oxalate is not understood. In the remaining 50% of calcium stones, varying amounts of calcium phosphate are admixed with the calcium oxalate. This calcium phosphate occurs almost exclusively as hydroxyapatite or carbonate–apatite. It is the latter that accounts for the erroneous reporting of calcium carbonate urinary stones when analyses are performed by chemical methods. Brushite ($CaHPO_4$) is also found, but it is distinctly uncommon. The frequency with which apatite or brushite forms the original crystal nidus of a renal stone continues to be debated.

Magnesium ammonium phosphate (struvite) or "triple" phosphate stones are more frequently found in women, sometimes forming staghorn calculi, and are usually associated with both persistent urinary alkalinity and frequent infections with urea-splitting microorganisms. They are usually mixed with varying amounts of calcium phosphate (apatite). The

TABLE I

**The Relative Incidence of Various
Kinds of Stones**[a,b]

Calcium oxalate (mono- and dihydrate)	33%
Calcium oxalate and apatite, mixed	34%
Apatite, pure	4%
Brushite $CaHPO_4$, pure or mixed	2%
Struvite $MgNH_4PO_4$ and apatite, mixed	15%
Uric acid	8%
Cystine	3%
Artifacts	1%
	100%

[a] The varieties of "calcium stones" appear as a group.

[b] The composition of urinary stones is classified by 97% polycrystalline conglomerate and 3% matrix.

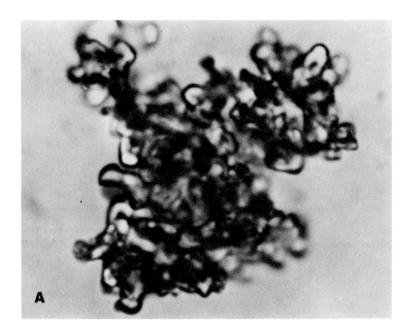

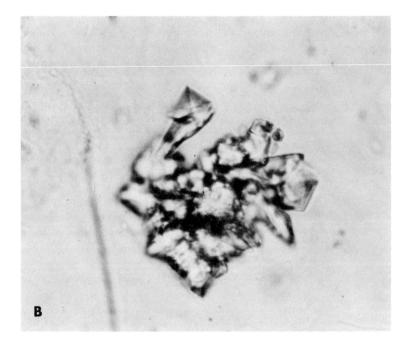

calcium found in the stones by chemical methods is from the apatite and is not a component of the struvite crystal lattice. Hence, the term "triple phosphate," if it refers to three different cations in the struvite crystal, is incorrect.

Approximately 8% of renal stones recovered in the United States are composed of uric acid, usually present as crystals of the free acid. Ammonium and sodium acid urate crystals are much less common but may be found as minor components of some calcium oxalate and calcium phosphate calculi. The unusually high incidence of urate calculi in bladder stones from children in southeast Asia, particularly Thailand, remains for the most part unexplained. Differences in climate, diet, and activity have been pointed out, but no clear-cut factor can be identified.

Cystine stones account for 2–3% of urinary calculi and are always associated with the genetic metabolic disorder cystinuria. Rarer components of urinary calculi include xanthine, silicates, ochronotic pigments, and matrix protein. The last component is of particular importance because of its constancy in all urinary calculi, forming about 3% of the dry weight of the stone. Its chemical composition has been investigated extensively by Boyce (1968). This macromolecular organic matrix is composed of approximately two-thirds protein and one-third carbohydrate. Analytic studies suggest that it is a mucoprotein, although sialic acid is rarely found. It contains both hexosamine and nonamino sugars together with small amounts of albumin, γ-globulins, α-globulins, and Tamm–Horsfall mucoprotein. An interesting component is matrix substance A, representing the most potent antigenic substance in stone matrix. It has a molecular weight of 30,000–40,000 with an isoelectric point near pH 4.5. It is apparently of renal origin, as it has not been detectable in plasma. Its role in the nucleation of stones or in stone growth has not been determined with certainty, since it has been found in urine from both stone formers and from patients with noncalculous renal disease (Keutel and King, 1964). Matrix, uric acid, and xanthine stones are radiolucent.

Finally, it should be mentioned that artifacts are occasionally submitted by a patient either as an honest mistake or by deceit. Their recognition is facilitated if all stones are carefully examined by eye with a 10× lens.

Stones vary considerably in both size and structure. The smallest is probably represented by the tiny crystal aggregates or "microliths" seen frequently in the fresh urine sediments examined at body temperature of calcium oxalate stone formers (Fig. 1). Normal urine may contain much

Fig. 1. Crystal aggregates in urinary sediments maintained at 37°C in recurrent calcium oxalate stone formers. (A) Calcium oxalate monohydrate as dumbbell shapes (greatest diameter in 100 μm). (B) Calcium oxalate dihydrate as envelope crystals (greatest diameter is 75 μm).

smaller crystals without aggregation that are not appreciated under the light microscope (Lemann *et al.,* 1971; Robertson *et al.,* 1969). It is not clear what critical size must be attained before stones are retained in the urinary passages and assume clinical significance. A diameter of 200 μm has been suggested (Finlayson, 1972). By the time these crystals become recognizable as gravel (300 to 500 μm), their appearance is typical of larger calculi, and this polycrystalline conglomerate presumably already contains mucoprotein matrix, which is a constant feature of all calculi (Boyce, 1968).

While some larger stones may appear as formless masses, the majority have an internal structure with varying degrees of macroscopic organization. Cross sections frequently reveal concentric laminations and radial striations. The basis for these macroscopic features resides in variations in crystal size, density, and orientation rather than in variations in composition; the lighter the color, the smaller the grain size. These structural features are similarly represented in the matrix organization and suggest the considerable intimacy of the crystal–matrix relationship. Occasionally, cross sections reveal alternating layers of different composition. This is especially well demonstrated, in the extreme case, in stones composed of a mixture of calcium oxalate and apatite in which there are innumerable alternating layers (Fig. 2). In many stones a macroscopic

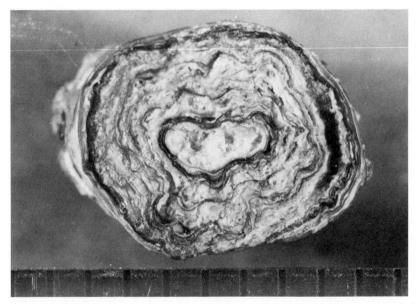

Fig. 2.   Calculus composed of calcium oxalate and apatite in alternating layers. Scale in millimeters.

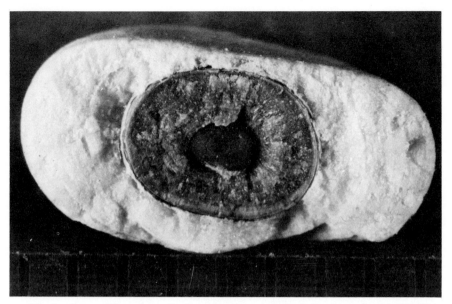

Fig. 3. Stone with nucleus of uric acid and outer shell of mixed struvite ($MgNH_4PO_4$) and apatite indicating superimposed urea-splitting infection. Scale in millimeters.

nucleus is clearly seen. It is frequently central and of the same composition as the rest of the stone. The significance of such a nucleus is unknown. Clearly, it is far too large to function as the ultimate nucleus in the physicochemical sense. However, in some stones this nucleus is of a different composition and no doubt reflects historical events in the genesis of the stone. This is most eloquently portrayed when small nuclei of different composition are found in stones composed of a mixture of apatite and struvite following infection with urea-splitting organisms (Fig. 3). Presumably, these stones and central nuclei were formed and grown while free somewhere in the urinary passages.

There is another structural variant in which the nucleus and any associated concentric laminations are eccentrically located. Such a nucleus generally occurs at the bottom of a cavity in the external surface of the stone and is frequently composed of apatite while the remainder of the stone is typically calcium oxalate monohydrate (Fig. 4). This structure suggests that nucleation and growth of the stone occurred while attached to the summit of a renal papilla (Fig. 5) and that the apatite nucleus corresponds to the subepithelial plaques of calcium phosphate, which were well described by Randall (1939). Such microscopic plaques are frequently found in the normal urinary tract (Haggitt and Pitcock, 1971). Nucleation may occur when such plaques erode through the urinary tract

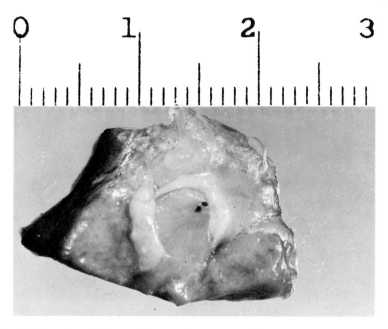

Fig. 4. Two tiny calcium oxalate monohydrate calculi adherent to the summit of an excised human renal papilla. Scale in millimeters. From E. L. Prien, Sr. (1955). *J. Urol.* **73,** 627–652. Copyright 1955 The Williams & Wilkin Co., Baltimore.

epithelium and are exposed to urine, which is conducive to stone growth. As a testimony to this relationship, small pieces of organic material are occasionally seen associated with the apatite nucleus in the papillary cavity and may well represent bits of epithelium that are torn off when the stone is shed. In a study of small ureteral calcium stones, Elliot (1973) found evidence for this mechanism of stone formation in 60% of the patients studied. These findings with their implications and paradoxes have recently been reviewed (Prien, 1975).

    Among "calcium stones," there are several riddles that remain to be solved. In pure calcium oxalate stones when both the monohydrate and dihydrate occur together, the dihydrate is almost universally found peripheral to the more central portions (or nucleus), which are composed entirely of monohydrate. In calculi that appear to be composed entirely of dihydrate, it is a simple matter to demonstrate monohydrate crystals in the central portions using polarized light (Prien, 1949). Some investigators have suggested that it is monohydrate that functions as the nucleator for all calcium oxalate stones. Yet, in fresh urinary sediment examinations performed at body temperature, crystal aggregates consisting entirely of the dihydrate (envelope crystals) are, if anything, more frequent than aggregates of monohydrate (dumbbells). An alternative theory suggests that the dihydrate transforms into the monohydrate after the initial formation of the calculus while still in the urine (Jensen, 1941). This would account for the absence of dihydrate in the more central (earlier) portions of the stones. Indeed, "pseudomorphs" (crystals retaining the shapes of dihydrate crystals but with the optical behavior of monohydrate) are occasionally found in the transitional zone between the two hydrates of calcium oxalate. Aside from this circumstantial evidence, there are little other data to solve this riddle of structure at the present time.

A second point of contention has revolved around the significance of finding apatite as a nucleus, in scattered nests, or in alternating layers in a calcium oxalate stone. The simplest explanation is that its occurrence is indicative of nothing more than a period of more alkaline urine. Indeed, pure apatite is the usual type of stone found in renal tubular acidosis. A more complex theory suggests that it is the presence of apatite crystals (having transformed from brushite) in the urine that nucleates and governs the growth of a calcium oxalate stone (Pak, 1969). Although the applicabil-

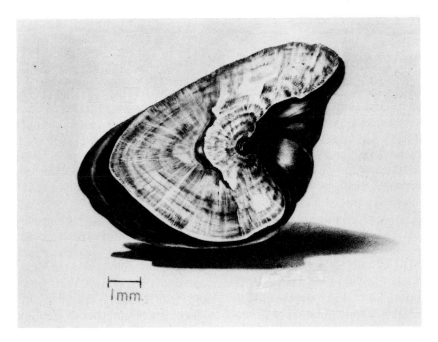

Fig. 5. Drawing of the cross section of a calcium oxalate monohydrate calculus with concentric laminations oriented about an eccentric nucleus situated at the bottom of a concavity probably representing the point of attachment to the renal papilla. From E. L. Prien, Sr. (1949). *J. Urol.* **73**, 825. Copyright 1949 The Williams & Wilkin Co., Baltimore.

ity of this theory of pathogenesis is debated, the ready transformation of brushite to apatite is widely accepted and probably accounts for the rarity of this substance in urinary calculi. It has also been clearly shown that hydroxyapatite crystals can nucleate supersaturated solutions of calcium oxalate (Meyer *et al.*, 1975). In scrutinizing small calcium oxalate stones for structure and composition, the results vary according to the methods used (Elliot 1973; Chambers *et al.* 1972). Pure calcium oxalate is found in 20–50%. Calcium oxalate with areas of apatite intermixed is found in 50–80% of stones. However, a clear demonstration that the apatite is in a nuclear position is distinctly less common, perhaps 10–20%. In future studies of the presence and significance of small amounts of other substances, such as apatite, uric acid, and sodium acid urate that might be found in calcium oxalate stones, it will be important to study the smallest stones, less than 0.5 cm in diameter. The larger a stone becomes, the greater the likelihood of finding mixtures and the less likely these additional substances have a possible "nucleating" role in calcium oxalate stone disease.

Table I outlines the relative incidence of various types of stones.

III. STONE FORMATION AND GROWTH

The events leading to stone genesis and growth remain an enigma that has fascinated investigators since the original description of stones. Several theories have been proposed, but none fully satisfies all the requirements posed by known facts. Part of this problem is related to the heterogeneous physicochemical events that control the entire formation and modeling of the final calculus. No one theory can explain each of these events, particularly when so many different types of stones form within the urinary tract.

The "precipitation–crystallization" theory has, perhaps, received the most attention. It seems particularly applicable to stones made up predominantly of cystine, uric acid, xanthine, and mixed magnesium ammonium phosphate and apatite. In conditions associated with recurrent formation of these types of stones, excessive excretion of each of the constituents frequently exceeds the solubility of each crystalloid in urine and leads to precipitation of crystals. Subsequent crystal growth results in a macroscopic calculus. Such a theory is more difficult to apply to the more common condition of recurrent calcium oxalate stones, particularly when both calcium and oxalate excretion are within the normal range.

The "matrix nucleation" theory has been invoked to explain stone growth in this circumstance. Here matrix mucoprotein is thought to play a primary role in the initial nidus for stone growth, with subsequent stone formation by crystallization within the interstices of this organic matrix substance. As emphasized by Boyce (1968), there are a number of objections to assigning a primary role to the organic matrix in stone formation. These include the fact that "every crystalline component of native calculi can be induced to homogeneous nucleation and growth from metastable or supersaturated solutions without the presence of organic molecules" and "the very diversity of clinical situations in which concretions are formed of the most concentrated and precipitable components of urine (oxaluria, cystinuria, etc.) argues against the assumption of a 'special' macromolecule essential to concrement formation." Spector *et al.* (1976) have recently reexamined the matrix proteins in urinary calculi. They confirmed Boyce's work but emphasized the highly acidic nature of these proteins which are rich in both aspartic and glutamic acids accounting for over 650 residues per 1000 amino acid residues. Similar highly acidic matrix proteins are associated with other mineralized tissues such as bone, dentin, enamel, mollusk shells, and hen egg shells. They further noted that when stones of different chemical composition were examined, there were differences in the amino acid composition of certain matrix protein fractions. These findings again raise the possibility that a unique matrix protein is present and possibly confers the template specificity required for the nucleation of the different stone types: calcium oxalate, apatite–struvite, and uric acid. Others have shown that the newly discovered amino acid, γ-carboxyglutamic acid (Gla), is present in the extractable matrix proteins of bone (Hauschka *et al.,* 1975), ectopic calcifications, and renal calculi. The Gla content is especially enriched in the matrix proteins of the calcium-containing stones (calcium oxalate, apatite, and apatite–struvite) and is practically absent from uric acid and pure struvite (canine) stones (Lian and Prien, 1976). In calcium oxalate stone matrix protein, Gla accounts for 25 residues per 1000. In the peak 2 fraction it is enriched to 45 residues per 1000. Since it is known that Gla confers the essential calcium-binding property to prothrombin which is required for the homeostatic conversion to thrombin, it is conceivable that Gla operates in other calcium-binding processes either physiologically as in bone or pathologically as in stone. Whether the highly acidic proteins mentioned above or the Gla-containing proteins serve as templates to promote nucleation or as inhibitors to retard nucleation or as passive coprecipitants can only be speculated upon at this point. However, there is evidence to suggest that matrix may well serve to retard the dissolution of concretions during periods of urine undersaturation (Vermeulen *et al.* 1966).

This should not discount the important investigations of Vermeulen and Lyon (1968), which emphasize the important role of the renal papilla in calculus formation. Using oxamide-induced stone disease in rats, these investigators demonstrated in elegant fashion the sequential intraluminal crystallization of calcium oxamide in renal-collecting ducts leading to the eventual appearance of a stone nidus protruding from the papillary tip. As this sloughs, the fragments formed offer a fertile nidus for subsequent crystallization and stone growth, and eventually generalized oxalate stone disease appears in these experimental animals. These experiments have suggested by analogy that human stone disease may be caused by the "triggering" of stone formation during a brief episode of highly concentrated urine excretion setting off papillary embryogenesis. Once this stone nidus forms, continued stone growth may occur despite the presence of urine that is no longer propitious for spontaneous crystallization.

In any discussion of stone formation and growth, the state of saturation of the common urinary crystalloids must receive serious consideration. In the urine of many nonstone formers as well as in many stone formers (particularly those who are hypercalciuric), both calcium oxalate and calcium phosphate exist in a state of supersaturation (Pak, 1969). Although some controversy exists, there now seems to be evidence that urine of stone formers has higher concentrations of both calcium and oxalate than that of non-stone-formers (Robertson *et al.*, 1971). These studies have led to differing theories concerning the genesis of stone formation. The studies of Pak *et al.* (1971) have suggested that precipitation of calcium phosphate in the form of brushite may govern the formation of calcium-containing stones. Such a theory is supported by the finding of areas of brushite commonly found in calcium-containing renal stones. This may, however, represent nothing more than the intermittent precipitation of calcium phosphate on a calcium oxalate stone during periods of more alkaline urine. In addition, this theory presupposes that urine of stone formers alone contains preformed nuclei for stone growth and that such nuclei are not found in urine from non-stone-formers—a supposition that is not supported by fact.

The findings of the Leeds group support the alternate view that stone formation is related more to transient periods of supersaturation of the urine with calcium oxalate, a theory supported strongly by their recent data (Robertson and Peacock, 1973). Their findings also suggest that small changes in urinary oxalate may be of much greater importance than large changes in urinary calcium in promoting supersaturation of the urine and, thereby, stone formation. If such a theory is true, then maneuvers to lower urinary oxalate excretion require much greater emphasis than they have received in the past. They have also shown that dietary calcium restriction will cause a modest elevation of urinary oxalate excretion. Here may be the clue to stone recurrence in patients on low calcium diets.

If urine is saturated with the components that often form stones, why then is stone disease not a much more common event? The explanation for this phenomenon undoubtedly relates to the presence of a number of substances in urine that are capable of holding these salts in solution. These include protective colloids (Pinto, 1973), polyphosphates (Lewis *et al.*, 1966), small peptides (Howard and Thomas, 1968), and other inorganic components of urine (Fleisch, 1973a). The studies of Fleisch and his colleagues (Yendt and Gagne, 1968) have demonstrated that pyrophosphate, in concentrations normally present in urine, is capable of preventing crystallization of both calcium phosphate and calcium oxalate *in vitro*. Although the excretion of pyrophosphate has been shown to be reduced in some stone formers, no consistent reduction in this inorganic phosphate compound has been found in large groups of patients with recurrent stone disease. Initial enthusiasm over the finding that the urine of stone formers is often deficient in a low molecular weight polypeptide that is a potent *in vitro* inhibitor of calcium phosphate crystallization (Howard and Thomas, 1968) has largely waned. Recent studies emphasize differences in an as yet unidentified nonpeptide inhibitor anion (Thomas *et al.*, 1972). In studying a calcium oxalate system the Leeds group has described a high molecular weight substance "resembling a mucopolysaccharide" that is a potent inhibitor of crystal growth and aggregation (Robertson *et al.*, 1973; L. H. Smith, 1975). It appears to be deficient in certain stone formers. The degree of supersaturation of the urine for calcium oxalate as judged by the quantity of crystalluria and the risk for stone seemed to be best correlated with a simultaneous consideration of the calculated degree of supersaturation and the relative lack of inhibitory substance. For this analysis they coined the term "saturation-inhibition index" (Robertson *et al.*, 1976). However, as with the preceding inhibitor of the calcium phosphate system, this one too remains to be fully identified.

IV. PATHOGENESIS OF RECURRENT STONE DISEASE

From a practical clinical standpoint the pathogenesis of recurrent renal stone disease may be viewed under two major pathogenetic mechanisms: (1) increased urinary crystalloid content and (2) physicochemical changes in urine conducive to stone formation with normal crystalloid content. At the present time, the relative importance of these two mechanisms in the etiology of stone disease is unknown.

A. Stone Disease Secondary to Increased Urinary Crystalloid Content

A number of well-defined, acquired, and genetic conditions are associated with recurrent renal stone disease on the basis of increased urinary excretion of a number of important urinary crystalloids. These include primary hyperoxaluria, cystinuria, the hyperuricemic states associated with hyperuricosuria, xanthinuria, and the hypercalciuric states, particularly the syndrome of idiopathic hypercalciuria. Since the last group of conditions is the most frequent of this diverse collection, it will be discussed in some detail.

1. Hypercalciuria

No attempt will be made here to review the factors controlling calcium excretion in the urine, since these are discussed in detail in Chapter 2. Suffice it to say that any condition associated with persistent hypercalciuria, regardless of cause, will be associated with an increased incidence of renal stone disease. However, the definition of hypercalciuria has proved rather elusive. In any individual, the urinary calcium varies considerably from day to day and is a function of dietary calcium, carbohydrates, and sodium as well as exercise (Epstein, 1968), and seasonal variation (Robertson et al., 1974). The urinary calcium also varies between population groups and between different geographic areas. A generally acceptable working definition has been to assume that 90% of normal men excrete less than 300 mg/day and women less than 250 mg/day (Hodgkinson and Pyrah, 1958). This approximates 4 mg/kg of body weight. More recent evidence suggests that the upper limit may be somewhat higher (Nordin et al., 1972). Another problem with the definition of hypercalciuria is that its correlation with the stone-forming process is far from perfect. There are many recurrent calcium stone formers who do not have hypercalciuria, as well as those who continue to suffer recurrence even after their urine calcium excretions have been normalized. Finally, there are individuals who have hypercalciuria without a history of stones. Clearly, there are other factors operating in calcium stone disease. The calculi formed in these conditions are usually either pure calcium oxalate or mixed calcium oxalate and calcium phosphate, the latter in the form of hydroxyapatite. The most frequent hypercalciuric states associated with recurrent nephrolithiasis are hyperparathyroidism, renal tubular acidosis (type I or distal tubule type), and idiopathic hypercalciuria. Many of the remaining syndromes associated with hypercalciuria are discovered sufficiently early in their course to prevent stone disease from becoming a significant clinical problem.

Hyperparathyroidism has been recognized as a significant cause of calcium-containing renal stone disease since its description as a clinical syndrome. This diagnostic possibility must be considered carefully in all patients with recurrent calcium-containing renal stones (see Chapter 5). The incidence of renal calculi in patients with hyperparathyroidism has varied (50–80%), decreasing somewhat in recent years perhaps because of earlier diagnosis (Yendt and Gagne, 1968; Krementz et al., 1967). A recent summary of renal stone disease (Lavan *et al.*, 1971) documents the incidence of hyperparathyroidism as a cause of stone disease of approximately 4%. Other types of hyperparathyroidism, such as that secondary to chronic renal disease or to nonmetastatic malignancies that produce parathyroid-like peptides, are not generally associated with renal stone disease.

The stones in primary hyperparathyroidism are predominantly calcium oxalate with perhaps some increase in the frequency of mixed stones and pure calcium phosphate (apatite). However, there has been no large series of stone analyses from such patients. The mechanism for the high incidence of stone disease in hyperparathyroidism has been presumed to be hypercalciuria leading to supersaturation of urine with respect to calcium oxalate. It is interesting to note the disparity between the reported incidence of hypercalciuria (about 40%) and the incidence of stone disease in hyperparathyroidism (50–80%) suggesting that other factors may play a role in stone formation. This is also suggested by the very long history of stone disease in patients first diagnosed as having hyperparathyroidism, sometimes exceeding 20 years. Important solubilizers of calcium oxalate, such as pyrophosphate and the diphosphonates, need to be measured in a large series of patients with hyperparathyroidism to shed some light on this question.

Patients with hyperparathyroidism who form stones tend to have minimal evidence of bone disease (Lloyd, 1968). Conversely, patients with extensive bone disease rarely form stones, although nephrocalcinosis is seen equally in both groups. As pointed out by Lloyd (1968), patients with primarily bone disease tend to have higher serum calcium values and larger tumors, as well as higher concentrations of parathyroid hormone in the serum (Purnell *et al.*, 1971). Recently, Peacock (1975) has shown that the patients with stone disease have hyperabsorption of calcium from the intestine together with greater degrees of hypercalciuria. This hyperabsorption fell after parathyroidectomy. Of the hyperparathyroid patients without stone disease, calcium absorption was either normal or there was frank malabsorption of calcium. This latter group with subnormal calcium absorption had evidence of osteopenia or frank bone disease in spite of having the highest parathyroid hormone levels. It was postulated that in the patients with bone disease the action of parathyroid hormone on the intestine of increasing calcium absorption was blocked perhaps by a relative deficiency of vitamin D or its metabolites. Its action on bone remained intact.

Renal tubular acidosis of the distal or so-called "gradient" type (Morris, 1969) is associated with both hypercalciuria and recurrent calcium nephrolithiasis. In this familial syndrome, distal tubular acidification of urine is defective and leads to systemic acidosis, increased excretion of calcium ion secondary to the metabolic acidosis, and eventually nephrolithiasis and nephrocalcinosis in 73% of the patients (Wrong and Davies, 1959). The hypercalciuria, which is often associated with hypocalcemia and osteomalacia, seems directly related to the hyperchloremic acidosis since metabolic acidosis will induce hypercalciuria in man and in parathyroidectomized animals, and correction of acidosis in such patients with alkali therapy will reduce calcium excretion. An important associated phenomenon is reduced urinary citrate excretion resulting from systemic acidosis. Since the pK_3 of citric acid is 6.4, it is an important complexer for calcium only in relatively more alkaline urine (pH 6.5–8.0). It is precisely in renal tubular acidosis of the gradient type that the dual abnormalities of systemic acidosis (causing hypercalciuria and low urinary citrate) and relatively alkaline urine (where citrate would be expected to be a major calcium chelator) conspire to raise the urine supersaturation for calcium phosphate, resulting in apatite stones and nephrocalcinosis.

A similar situation exists with the renal tubular acidosis-like syndrome induced by acetazolamide (Diamox) therapy (Parfitt, 1969). Here the stones and nephrocalcinosis appear to be caused more by the low urinary citrate, as the hypercalciuria is inconstant and the alkaline urine is present only initially during the bicarbonate diuresis. In fact, since stones occur only in a minority of such patients, there is the clinical suspicion that they must have a second superimposed abnormality. Coincident idiopathic hypercalciuria or alkalinization therapy have been especially incriminated (Parfitt, 1970). It is paradoxical that acetazolamide induces a renal tubular acidosis of the so-called "proximal" type, and yet stones and nephrocalcinosis are not otherwise seen in this condition when caused by other diseases. The answer may reside in the likelihood that in the other forms of proximal renal tubular acidosis early renal failure may already have supervened and curtailed hypercalciuria. In addition, when urinary citrate has been measured, it has been normal. This may simply reflect the proximal leak of anions such as urate and phosphate. Plasma citrate may be similarly lost into the urine. Where the effect of acetazolamide has been studied in rats the additional finding of reduced urinary magnesium has been thought to be most important (Gyory et al., 1970).

Perhaps the most common syndrome of recurrent calcium oxalate stone disease due to hypercalciuria is "idiopathic hypercalciuria" (Henneman et al., 1958). This syndrome is characterized clinically by recurrent calcium oxalate nephrolithiasis and occurs after the age of 20 mostly in overweight men who often have a family history of stone disease in male relatives (Lavan et al., 1971). Persistent hypercalciuria with normal serum calcium, low serum phosphorus and low fecal calcium are characteristic features. The finding of reduced tubular reabsorption of phosphorus has suggested normocalcemic hyperparathyroidism in some of these patients, but exploration of the neck has usually revealed normal glands. Furthermore, the low serum phosphorus has been a very variable finding even in the same patient over short periods. Finally, in established hyperparathyroidism hypercalciuria is generally not manifest during normocalcemia. The recent finding of elevated plasma parathyroid hormone in some of these patients has been attributed to the hypercalciuria, since reversal of the increased calcium excretion with thiazide diuretics has reduced the parathyroid hormone level to normal (Coe *et al.*, 1973). Thus, if hyperparathyroidism is present it is "secondary" to calcium loss. Yendt has emphasized the diagnostic importance of hypercalciuria in women in that the hypercalciuric female has a 65% chance of having primary hyperparathyroidism while only 12% of hypercalciuric men are likely to have this diagnosis (Yendt and Gagne, 1968).

The pathogenesis of idiopathic hypercalciuria has been elusive and is still ardently debated. Recent work has clarified the mechanism considerably. It now appears that the majority of these patients have intestinal hyperabsorption of calcium (of unknown cause) as the primary disorder. As a consequence, they have hypercalciuria on normal or high dietary calcium intakes. These patients have normal 24 hour urinary calcium excretions on low calcium diets and normal morning urinary calcium/creatinine ratios after 14 hours of overnight fasting (Nordin *et al.*, 1972). This indicates that the source of the augmented urine calcium is dietary and not from the bones. This has been termed "absorptive" hypercalciuria.

It is equally clear that a minority of patients with idiopathic hypercalciuria (perhaps 10%) do not normalize their urinary calcium excretion on low calcium diets or their morning urinary calcium/creatinine ratios after 14 hours of fasting. This suggests that they have persistent loss of bone calcium. Such patients may be in negative calcium balance with secondary stimulation of their parathyroid glands and are at risk for bone disease. This has been termed "resorptive" (bone resorption) hypercalciuria. When other disorders of bone resorption, such as hyperparathyroidism, renal tubular acidosis, sarcoidosis, hyperthyroidism, and bony metastases, have been ruled out, then the term "renal" hypercalciuria is employed (Pak *et al.*, 1975). As with primary intestinal hyperabsorption the cause of the renal loss of calcium is unknown. It may be a primary renal problem or a renal response to some other factor such as a subtle form of bone disease. It is important to identify these patients with renal hypercalciuria and persistent negative calcium balance, as it needs to be rectified regardless of the severity of their stone disease. Thiazides appear to effectively curtail this form of resorptive hypercalciuria.

Both the existence and prevalence of renal hypercalciuria continue to be at issue. Those who deny its existence would maintain that the real diagnosis has been missed and that a conventional disorder of calcium metabolism is present and manifests itself as resorptive hypercalciuria. On the other hand, there is a study in which the majority of patients (26 out of 40) with idiopathic hypercalciuria had elevated levels of plasma parathyroid hormone that returned to normal when the hypercalciuria was curtailed with thiazides (Coe *et al.*, 1973). The implication is that they had a form of resorptive hypercalciuria and secondary hyperparathyroidism. It is hard to reconcile these results with those above, except to point out the difficulties in interpretation of current assays for parathyroid hormone. Furthermore, in the studies that demonstrate the relative infrequency of resorptive hypercalciuria, all patients were studied consecutively and calcium loaded so that no absorptive hypercalciurics were overlooked. In the conflicting study (Coe *et al.*, 1973) only patients who were hypercalciuric were consecutively studied while they were on their customary (low calcium) diet. It is likely that many absorptive hypercalciurics were not counted as they were not calcium loaded.

Finally, it should be reemphasized that disorders of calcium metabolism other than idiopathic hypercalciuria that manifest hypercalciuria with or without nephrolithiasis may show either absorptive or resorptive hypercalciuria or a combination of both. They must be diagnosed by other appropriate and customary studies. Also the failure to appreciate these other diagnoses may well result in hypercalcemia when thiazides are administered for what is presumed to be the renal form of resorptive hypercalciuria.

Before leaving the hypercalciuric states, a word about nephrocalcinosis will emphasize the diagnostic importance of this radiographic finding in patients with stone disease. Three radiographic types of nephrocalcinosis have been defined, and the diagnostic possibilities are often related to the recognition of the particular type (Black, 1967). Type I nephrocalcinosis is quite rare and is described as a fine diffuse calcification, chiefly cortical in location. Healed renal cortical necrosis and chronic glomerulonephritis usually cause this type of renal calcification. A coarse typical medullary calcification represents the pattern in type II, the most common form of nephrocalcinosis. Type II is most frequently associated with a metabolic cause and with nephrolithiasis. The three most common causes of type II are primary hyperparathyroidism, renal tubular acidosis, and chronic pyelonephritis. Many of the other causes of both hypercalcemia and hypercalciuria may also occasionally cause this form of nephrocalcinosis. Type III nephrocalcinosis refers to a localized coarse calcification in one or both kidneys and is caused by tuberculosis, cysts, malignancy, papillary necrosis, and medullary sponge kidney. For the most part, this type is not associated with nephrolithiasis except for medullary sponge kidney.

2. Hyperoxaluria

Since calcium oxalate is a common component of renal calculi, it seems important to consider briefly the chemistry and metabolism of oxalic acid. This simple dicarboxylic acid is a ubiquitous component of green leafy plants and vegetables, deriving its name from its source of origin in the meadow saffron or oxalis plant. It is a very strong acid with a K_{a_1} of 6.5×10^{-2} and K_{a_2} of 6.1×10^{-5}. It is extremely insoluble in water (8.7 gm free acid per 100 gm H_2O). At neutral or alkaline pH, the calcium salt demonstrates very low solubility (0.67 gm per 100 gm H_2O at pH 7, 13°C). This physiochemical feature alone accounts for its deleterious characteristics in man. Although present in many foodstuffs (tea, green leafy vegetables, cocoa, and others), it is poorly absorbed from the gastrointestinal tract in normal subjects (less than 13% of an oral load) (Earnest *et al.*, 1973).

The normal daily 24-hour urinary excretion of oxalate varies between 10 and 55 mg, most of it coming from endogenous production. It is not bound significantly to plasma proteins, is filtered freely by the glomerulus, and is both reabsorbed and secreted by the renal tubule, the renal clearance exceeding 150 ml/minute in man (Williams *et al.*, 1971).

Oxalate represents a metabolic end product of carbohydrate metabolism. Its two major precursors include glyoxylic acid and ascorbic acid. The latter compound accounts for approximately 35–50% of the oxalate excreted daily by normal man. Loading with oral ascorbate in large doses (4 gm) may raise urinary oxalate excretion (Baker *et al.*, 1966).

The more important precursor of oxalate is its reduced analogue, glyoxylic acid, which is in turn derived largely from glycine and glycolic acid. Glyoxylate itself is a reactive aldehyde with many reactions identified in mammalian species. It may be reduced to glycolate, transaminated to glycine (B_6-dependent), and converted to α-hydroxy-β-ketoadipate by a complicated carboligase reaction requiring thiamine pyrophosphate and utilizing α-ketoglutarate. Conversion of glyoxylate to formyl-S-CoA and α-keto-γ-hydroxyglutamate is probably quantitatively unimportant in man. Glyoxylate oxidation to oxalate is catalyzed by at least three different enzymes: lactic dehydrogenase, xanthine oxidase, and glycolic-acid oxidase. Recent evidence suggests that lactic dehydrogenase with NAD may be the most important enzyme controlling oxalate synthesis from glyoxylate (Gibbs and Watts, 1973).

Although approximately 65% of renal stones contain calcium oxalate, hyperoxaluria as a mechanism in the genesis of such stones seems to be at first glance a rather rare clinical event. This relates partly to a controversy over the upper limit of normal for urinary oxalate, estimated to be approximately 40 mg/day by enzymatic method and 50 mg/day by isotope dilution methods, a difference which at present cannot be reconciled other than by differences in methodology. Studies by the Leeds group (Robertson and Peacock, 1973) suggest that very small changes in oxalate excretion may have great effects on the state of saturation of calcium oxalate in urine. This further suggests that recurrent calcium oxalate stone disease could represent a disorder(s) of oxalate excretion in which only small changes in urinary oxalate may lead to stone disease, a phenomenon that would be aggravated in the presence of hypercalciuria. If this theory receives subsequent confirmation in future studies, treatment of recurrent calcium oxalate stone disease might best be directed toward attempts to lower urinary oxalate excretion.

Six definite causes of hyperoxaluria (Table II) are now recognized. This diverse group of acquired and genetic diseases which cause hyperoxaluria accounts for less than 5% of the patients with calcium oxalate stone disease. In the majority of patients with recurrent calcium oxalate nephrolithiasis, oxalate excretion does appear to be within the normal range, as measured by the isotope dilution method.

Hyperoxaluria has been noted after ingestion of abnormally large amounts of foodstuffs high in oxalate content, although this represents a distinctly unusual cause of hyperoxaluria. Ethylene glycol, a common component of antifreeze solutions, is metabolized *in vivo* to oxalate, and ingestion of this substance in attempted suicide has been associated with acute renal shutdown secondary to diffuse obstructive uropathy with calcium oxalate crystals plugging collecting ducts and distal tubules (Friedman *et al.,* 1962). Pyridoxine deficiency has been reported to produce hyperoxaluria in both man and laboratory animals because pyridoxine is an important cofactor in glyoxylate transamination to glycine (Runyan and Gershoff, 1965). Deficiency of this vitamin presumably leads to defective conversion of glyoxylate to glycine, glyoxylate accumulation, and subsequent increased synthesis and excretion of oxalate. It has not been possible to document hyperoxaluria as a result of thiamine deficiency in man, although this vitamin is a cofactor in the conversion of glyoxylate to α-hydroxy-β-ketoadipate. Intake of more than 4 gm/day of ascorbic acid

TABLE II

Causes of Hyperoxaluria

Ingestion of oxalate or precursor (ethylene glycol)
Pyridoxine deficiency
Primary hyperoxaluria, type I
Primary hyperoxaluria, type II
Small bowel disease or ileal resection
Methoxyflurane anesthesia

can raise urinary oxalate excretion, but it has not yet been possible to document an increased incidence of stone disease in patients regularly ingesting large amounts of this vitamin.

Primary hyperoxaluria types I and II represent two separate genetic disorders with a similar clinical picture and genetic mode of transmission (autosomal recessive), but with distinctly different pathophysiologic mechanisms (Williams and Smith, 1972). In both conditions, recurrent nephrolithiasis begins at an early age and leads to recurrent pyelonephritis and death from uremia before the age of 20 if untreated. In both conditions, hyperoxaluria in the range of 100–300 mg/24 hour is a constant feature and a *sine qua non* of the diagnosis. Oxalosis, a term referring to tissue deposits of calcium oxalate in several different organs, may occur late in the disease.

Patients with type I primary hyperoxaluria excrete excessive amounts of glyoxylic and glycolic acids, which is helpful in differentiating this type from type II. A deficiency of the soluble glyoxylate-α-ketoglutarate carboligase has been found in tissues from five patients, although one patient has been reported with normal activity of this enzyme in skeletal muscle (Bourke *et al.*, 1972). Deficiency of this cytoplasmic enzyme apparently leads to glyoxylate accumulation and increased synthesis and excretion of both oxalate and glycolate.

In patients with type II primary hyperoxaluria glycolic acid and glyoxylic acid excretion is normal and large amounts (up to 1000 mg/24 hour) of L-glyceric acid are found in the urine, a characteristic feature of this form of the disease. Deficiency of D-glyceric acid dehydrogenase has been documented in this disorder, accounting for both the L-glyceric aciduria as well as the hyperoxaluria. This enzyme controls the reduction of hydroxypyruvate to D-glyceric acid in the gluconeogenic pathway of serine. A defect in this metabolic step leads to hydroxypyruvate accumulation and increased reduction of hydroxypyruvate to L-glyceric acid in the presence of lactic dehydrogenase and reduced nicotine adenine dinucleotide.

An interesting mechanism has been postulated to explain the relationship of this enzyme defect in a pathway unrelated to that of oxalate metabolism to the impressive hyperoxaluria and normal glycolic acid excretion in patients with the type II syndrome. Since the conversion of glyoxylate to oxalate is catalyzed by lactic dehydrogenase and NAD, a linked reaction between hydroxpyruvate reduction to L-glycerate and glyoxylate oxidation to oxalate has been proposed to explain the increased diversion of glyoxylate into oxalate synthesis and away from glycolate formation (Williams and Smith, 1971). A diagram of this proposed mechanism is shown in Fig. 6.

Recently, Richardson and Liao (1973) demonstrated that [2-^{14}C]hydroxypyruvate is converted to oxalate in rat liver preparations. This has

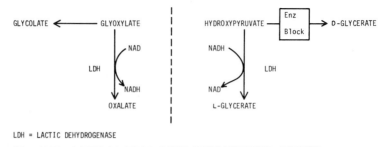

LDH = LACTIC DEHYDROGENASE

NAD and NADH = OXIDIZED AND REDUCED NICOTINE ADENINE DINUCLEOTIDE, RESPECTIVELY

Fig. 6. A proposed mechanism of hyperoxaluria in type II primary hyperoxaluria.

raised the possibility of a pathway connecting hydroxypyruvate and oxalate in man, which might explain the hyperoxaluria in type II primary hyperoxaluria. Studies with labeled hydroxypyruvate in normal human subjects and patients with the type II syndrome have not been reported to date.

The association of extensive small bowel disease or ileal resection with hyperoxaluria and recurrent calcium oxalate renal stones has been reported during the past 5 years (Dowling *et al.*, 1971; Admirand *et al.*, 1971; Smith *et al.*, 1972b). The relatively large numbers of patients reported in these series emphasize the frequency of the syndrome and suggest that it may represent the most common type of hyperoxaluria. Patients with the syndrome begin to develop recurrent stones shortly after the development of extensive inflammatory ileal disease or ileal resection. Hyperoxaluria of moderate to severe degree is unassociated with either glycolic aciduria or L-glyceric aciduria, differentiating these patients from those with the genetic forms of hyperoxaluria. Although the specific cause of the hyperoxaluria and its relationship to bowel disease are not known entirely, several facts suggest a possible mechanism.

When these patients are placed on an oxalate-free diet, urinary oxalate decreases into the normal range. Conversely, with a high oxalate intake, a marked increase in urinary oxalate excretion is observed (Fig. 7). These findings suggest hyperabsorption of dietary oxalate, a hypothesis confirmed by radioactive oxalate studies (Earnest *et al.*, 1973). Administration of [¹⁴C]oxalate by mouth to normal subjects reveals an excretion of approximately 13% of the administered isotope in urine. In patients with bowel disease or ileal resection, [¹⁴C]oxalate excretion in the urine after an oral dose exceeded 40%.

The mechanism for this hyperabsorption of oxalate has been defined by recent studies. The degree of hyperoxaluria and the increased oxalate absorption are directly proportional to the degree of fat malabsorption (Earnest *et al.*, 1974). Control of fat malabsorption and calcium supplementation both reduce oxalate excretion in these patients (Earnest *et al.,* 1975). These findings have led to the following postulate: Oxalate absorption in the small intestine is indirectly related to the availability of Ca^{2+} in the lumen of the intestine. Fat malabsorption leads to accumulation of fatty acids in the intestinal lumen, which then compete with oxalate for free calcium ion. The high affinity of fatty acids for calcium leads to a reduction in luminal calcium concentration allowing more oxalate to exist in a more soluble and more absorbable form. Therefore, hyperoxaluria in these patients can be reduced by appropriate methods to control fat malabsorption, reduce oxalate intake, and increase luminal calcium concentration.

Another recently recognized cause of hyperoxaluria and renal oxalosis has been identified in patients who have been anesthetized with methoxyflurane. In several patients from different medical centers (Paddock *et al.,* 1964; Frascino *et al.,* 1970), acute renal shutdown following anesthesia with this agent was associated with deposition of calcium oxalate crystals throughout the kidney and hyperoxaluria in the patients in whom it was measured. The mechanism for the hyperoxaluria has not as yet been identified, and no determinations of glycolic or L-glyceric acid have been reported. Since this anesthetic agent is a fluorinated two-carbon derivative it may be metabolized *in vivo* to oxalic acid. Regardless of the

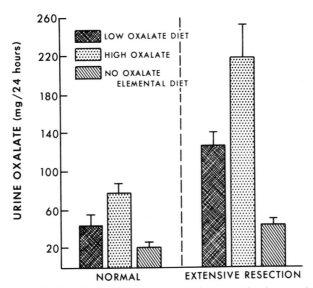

Fig. 7. Effect of oral oxalate intake on urinary oxalate excretion in normal subjects and patients with extensive small bowel resection. From L. H. Smith and H. E. Williams (1974). *In* "Heritable Disorders of Amino Acid Metabolism" (W. L. Nyhan, ed), pp. 343–358. Wiley, New York. Reproduced with permission of the publisher.

exact pathogenetic mechanism involved in this type of hyperoxaluria, the severity of this complication must be recognized and this anesthetic agent used carefully.

3. Uric Acid Stone Disease

Uric acid stones account for approximately 8% of renal calculi in this country. Numerous pathophysiologic mechanisms have been identified in this large group of stone formers (Atsmon *et al.,* 1963; Gutman and Yü, 1968), although they may be grouped under two major headings: (1) increased excretion of uric acid with or without hyperuricemia and (2) excretion of urine which favors the precipitation of uric acid in the absence of hyperuricosuria.

Increased excretion of uric acid results largely from overproduction of this organic acid as a result of myeloproliferative disorders, primary gout, or other overproduction hyperuricemia syndromes. The incidence of uric acid nephrolithiasis in the myeloproliferative disorders is generally higher (40%) than the incidence in primary gout (25%), perhaps because the total filtered load of uric acid tends to be much greater in the former. This problem may be particularly pronounced in the myeloproliferative states during periods of cytolytic therapy, sometimes leading to serum uric acid levels in excess of 50 mg per 100 ml.

In primary gout, the incidence of renal stone disease varies between 10 and 25%. In certain parts of the world where urinary concentration may also be a problem because of a very warm climate, the incidence of stone disease in gouty subjects may approach 75% (Wyngaarden, 1972). Uric acid nephrolithiasis may also occur in the rare Lesch–Nyhan syndrome. In those patients with idiopathic overproduction hyperuricemia, it is important to emphasize that uric acid stone disease may occur prior to the onset of clinical gouty arthritis.

Increased uric acid excretion may occur in the absence of hyperuricemia. This may be seen rarely after overconsumption of dietary purines and proteins, following the administration of uricosuric drugs, and with certain renal tubular disorders such as Wilson's disease, cystinosis, and the Fanconi syndrome. In addition, some patients with primary gout may have a period of hyperuricosuria without hyperuricemia generally early in their disease. In each of these instances, overexcretion of uric acid may lead to supersaturation of the urine with respect to uric acid, and stone disease may result. One exception to this is the renal tubular disorders where associated renal tubular acidosis leads to excessive alkalinity of the urine, increasing the solubility of the excreted uric acid.

Perhaps the most common mechanism for the development of uric acid stones is the excretion of urine that is conducive to uric acid precipitation in the absence of any hyperuricosuria. Excessive urinary concentration secondary to increased water loss by sweating in tropical climates may be a predisposing factor to uric acid stone formation. Loss of water through the gastrointestinal tract due to chronic diarrhea may similarly lead to excessive concentration of urinary uric acid. In addition to excessive urinary concentration secondary to decreased urine volume, many patients with normal uric acid excretion appear to form stones because of the excretion of persistently acid urine favoring uric acid precipitation. Patients with chronic diarrheal states, patients with ileostomy, and patients receiving medications that acidify the urine all have an increased incidence of uric acid stone disease. In addition to these groups, a number of patients with recurrent uric acid stones having neither gastrointestinal disease nor taking medications seem to have an abnormality causing a propensity to alkaline urine. In many series these patients with persistent acid urine make up the majority of uric acid stone formers. The exact physiologic mechanism for this abnormality is unknown although a defect in the renal production of ammonia has been documented in some (Yü and Gutman, 1973). A small number of patients with uric acid stone diathesis have neither hyperuricosuria nor a demonstrable abnormality in urine acidification at least at the time they are studied. The mechanism for the stone formation in these patients remains unexplained. It is important to realize that the finding of hyperuricemia in a patient with stones of unknown composition is of no diagnostic utility, as a small percentage (perhaps 20%) of calcium oxalate stone formers have hyperuricemia for unknown reasons (Smith and Boyce, 1969). The implications of this abnormality are unknown. However, in our experience, it is clear that these stones are pure calcium oxalate and do not contain uric acid nuclei, at least in the macroscopic sense.

4. Xanthinuria

Xanthine is an oxypurine precursor of uric acid with physiochemical characteristics similar to uric acid. Although normally excreted in very small amounts in the urine, its excretion increases in two clinical situations: (1) in patients with the very rare genetic disorder, hereditary xanthinuria (Wyngaarden, 1972), and (2) in patients receiving allopurinol therapy for hyperuricemia secondary to extensive lymphoproliferative disease (Ablin et al., 1972) or to the enzymatic defect seen in the Lesch–Nyhan syndrome (Greene et al., 1969). In each case, the enzymatic oxidation of xanthine to uric acid is blocked, leading to xanthine accumulation and its excessive excretion and subsequent precipitation in the urinary tract.

5. Cystinuria

Cystine is a component of renal stones found only in association with
the rare genetic disorder cystinuria. It is a recessively inherited abnormality of dibasic amino acid transport affecting the epithelial cells of the renal
tubules and the gastrointestinal tract. Increased amounts of cystine,
lysine, arginine, ornithine, and a mixed disulfide cystine-homocystine appear in the urine. If it were not for the insolubility of cystine and its
consequent precipitation, this disorder of amino acid transport would have
no clinical significance. In 1908 Garrod discussed this condition as one of
his original examples of diseases due to inborn errors of metabolism, in
this case cystine. This has not been borne out. The best postulation is that
of Dent and Rose (1951) based on the similarities in structure of the affected amino acids and the likelihood that they share a single renal transport mechanism that may be defective in cystinuria. The existence of
reduced intestinal absorption of dibasic amino acids was not appreciated
until much later, and has provided the basis for subdividing cystinuria into
three genetic classifications (Thier and Segal, 1972). The most common
type is type I, which is transmitted as a true recessive trait. Only the
homozygous family members have aminoaciduria. In types II and III the
heterozygous family members have excessive amounts of cystine and the
other dibasic amino acids except for arginine in their urine. The type II
heterozygotes have greater aminoaciduria than the type III, and yet none
of the type II heterozygotes apparently suffer the cystine stones of the
homozygous state. As there is considerable overlap in amino acid excretions between the various groups, the simplest way to differentiate
homozygotes from the incompletely recessive heterozygotes is by the
absence of increased arginine excretion in the latter subjects. The differentiation between the three types without the benefit of family studies can
only be done by the study of amino acid transport of intestinal biopsies *in vitro*.

Cystine stones are most frequently pure and have a honey-yellow color,
a fine crystallinity, and a waxy opalescence suggesting maple sugar. Occasionally, variable amounts of apatite are intermixed and often represent
a complication of alkalinization therapy. The stones occur almost exclusively in the homozygotes who excrete more than 250 mg of cystine per
day. The cyanide nitroprusside test will detect all homozygotes and an
occasional heterozygote. Contrary to early reports, the stones are
radioopaque, although somewhat less dense than a calcium stone of similar size. They have a homogeneous appearance on the roentgenogram.
They may occasionally form a staghorn configuration and should not be
confused with stones of mixed magnesium ammonium phosphate and apatite, which frequently have concentric layers of alternating radiodensity.

Although cystine is least soluble in acid urine, significant increases in solubility occur only at urinary pHs above 7.5. Consequently, adequate alkalinization is both difficult to achieve and risks superimposed precipitation of apatite. It should be pointed out that this unwanted complication may be especially encountered with the traditional regimen of alkalinization therapy, which employs alkali by day and acetazolamide (Diamox) by night. The effect of acetazolamide in reducing urinary citrate places such patients at risk for calcium phosphate stones.

6. Magnesium Ammonium Phosphate Stone Disease

Ammonia is a frequent constituent of renal stones particularly in the "triple phosphate" stones associated with chronic infection of the urinary tract. In this condition excessive amounts of ammonia are produced by urea-splitting microorganisms in the urinary tract, a process which also yields abnormally alkaline urine favoring precipitation of $MgNH_4PO_4$. Since urinary tract infection frequently complicates all forms of stone disease, it is often difficult to determine which event, infection or stone disease, is primary. In all cases of stones associated with urinary tract infection that are composed of mixed magnesium ammonium phosphate and apatite, a careful search for a possible stone nucleus of another composition should be made.

B. Physicochemical Changes in Urine Favoring Stone Formation at Normal Crystalloid Content

Although a great deal of investigative work has gone into the understanding of the conditions described above, it seems likely that they represent the minority of known causes of recurrent renal stone disease. Of more importance because of their frequency are those conditions in which stone disease occurs at normal crystalloid concentration because of changes in the physicochemical characteristics of the urine that favor the precipitation and growth of calculi.

Urinary pH is an important aspect of stone disease as has already been noted earlier in the case of uric acid, cystine, and $MgNH_4PO_4$ stones. Stasis anywhere in the urinary collecting system favors stone formation by mechanisms that are not clearly understood. This mechanism must be considered carefully when recurrent stone disease is limited to one kidney. Foreign bodies in the form of other calculi favor new stone formation, and this may account for the occasional stone found to be composed of more than one major urinary crystalloid.

One of the more exciting areas of research in recurrent stone disease has been the investigation into the role of certain protective substances in urine that normally inhibit crystal formation and growth. As discussed in Section III, absence of these factors could be of great importance in stone formation in patients with normal concentrations of urinary crystalloids. Unfortunately, it has been difficult to assign a primary role in stone disease to any of these factors, although relative decreases in urinary magnesium and citrate have been reported in some patients with recurrent renal stones. As noted, pyrophosphate is a potent inhibitor of calcium phosphate crystallization, but it has not been possible to demonstrate consistently reduced excretion of this compound in stone formers, although small groups of nonhypercalciuric men with recurrent stone disease have had reduced excretion of urinary pyrophosphate (Russell, 1973). Recently, several small molecular weight peptides, which are capable of inhibiting crystallization of both calcium phosphate and calcium oxalate in several *in vitro* systems, have been isolated from normal human urine. Since urine from patients with a stone diathesis often fails to inhibit calcification of rachitic rat cartilage *in vitro,* while urine from non-stone-formers shows nearly complete inhibition, it has been suspected, but not proved, that these stone formers may lack one or more of these urinary inhibitor peptides or perhaps other inhibitors of crystallization. Unfortunately, methods for isolation, characterization, and quantitative analysis of these inhibitors are extremely difficult to perform, and proof of this attractive hypothesis is not yet available.

Nevertheless, research into this area of pathogenetic mechanisms of stone disease continues to be promising. The possibility that reduced excretion of certain urinary mucopolysaccharides or compounds resembling the diphosphonates may explain recurrent nephrolithiasis is a very logical one, and preliminary evidence from laboratories engaged in this research supports this concept (Fleisch, 1973a; Smith and McCall, 1973). It seems likely that these types of studies will increase our understanding of mechanisms for recurrent stone disease in the very near future.

A new line of thought has issued from the association of hyperuricemia with calcium oxalate stones (Smith and Boyce, 1969). Although not appreciated in the initial report, a significant number of stone formers have relative hyperuricosuria of modest degree (800 to 1200 mg uric acid per 24 hours). The source of this excess uric acid appears to be dietary (Coe and Kavalach, 1974). This is not surprising as stone formers are heavy eaters in general. However, good therapeutic results have been reported employing allopurinol in calcium stone disease. Recently, the results of a 3 year double-blind controlled trial of allopurinol versus placebo was reported, and it clearly documented its effectiveness (M. J. V. Smith, 1975). In addition, it was also clear in the study that the placebo group faired better than before embarking on the program, a result which has long been suspected as patients naturally adhere to dietary restrictions and force more fluids when being followed closely by enthusiastic physicians. However, in this double-blind study both groups received sodium bicarbonate in addition. This substance can hardly be considered inert and detracts from any conclusions drawn from the placebo group.

The mechanism of the allopurinol effect is not readily apparent. It is rather uncommon for calcium oxalate stones to have uric acid nuclei in the macro- or microscopic sense. However, it is conceivable that submicroscopic crystals of uric acid or sodium acid urate could be nucleating calcium oxalate stones from urines that are only modestly supersaturated (metastable). The detection of the presence of such uric acid in stones must await more sensitive methods of analysis, and studies should be persued only on small stones (less than 0.5 cm in diameter). Although both substances can nucleate supersaturated solutions of calcium oxalate, sodium acid urate is so soluble in urine that it is an unlikely candidate for this role. Uric acid can exceed its capacity for supersaturation and form crystals spontaneously, especially in acid urines. This phenomenon could explain the improvement in the above-mentioned placebo group who received sodium bicarbonate along with their placebo pill. However, it is just as conceivable that allopurinol exerts its effect through some other mechanism than simply lowering urine uric acid excretion. Xanthine oxidase is one of three enzymes involved in the conversion of glyoxalate to oxalate. But this pathway appears to be of minor importance, and the administration of allopurinol does not reduce urinary oxalate (Gibbs and Watts, 1966). Finally, this drug may have some effect on the urinary inhibitors of crystallization. Robertson (1976) has recently reported that uric acid (perhaps in colloidal form) interferes with the natural urinary inhibitor for the calcium oxalate system. Allopurinol may reduce urine uric acid and restore the potency of the inhibitory substance.

V. SPECIFIC BONE DISEASES ASSOCIATED WITH NEPHROLITHIASIS

Because of the nature of this treatise it seems important to emphasize those disorders of bone which are associated with an increased incidence of renal stones. The more common diseases of bone associated with nephrolithiasis are listed in Table III. The division into two major groups is an arbitrary one based on the clinical severity of the bone disease. In category A hyperparathyroidism, malignant disease, and renal tubular acidosis represent the most common associations. Paget's disease and osteoporosis

TABLE III

Disorders of Bone Associated with Nephrolithiasis

A. Severe clinically significant bone disease
    Hyperparathyroidism
    Metastatic malignancy
    Multiple myeloma
    Renal tubular acidosis
    Paget's disease
    Osteoporosis

B. Mild clinically insignificant bone disease
    Sarcoidosis
    Hyperthyroidism
    Vitamin D intoxication
    Gout
    Hyperoxaluria

are associated with stone disease only during periods of prolonged inactivity for the patient, during which urinary calcium excretion increases. In category B a variety of bony lesions rarely produce any significant clinical symptoms. Patients with any form of stone disease may develop chronic pyelonephritis and subsequent renal damage, leading to chronic renal failure and renal osteodystrophy. Once chronic renal failure supervenes in the patient with recurrent renal stone disease, new stone formation usually ceases and clinical symptoms are dominated by those of uremia.

VI. TREATMENT OF RENAL STONE DISEASE

The treatment of recurrent renal stone disease has been rather empirical, and specific treatment programs, although highly touted, often lack sound evidence for objective success. This is undoubtedly related in part to the natural variability in the course of renal stone disease and to the difficulty in evaluating the criteria for clinical success. Proof of interruption of the formation of new stones requires careful repeated radiographic evaluations, often with tomography, and then minor changes can be missed easily. Carefully controlled prospective studies carried out over many years are still needed to prove the efficacy of most of the following therapeutic modalities.

General methods of therapy applicable to all types of renal stone disease include high fluid intake, treatment of infection, and surgical intervention. Increased fluid intake to reduce urinary crystalloid concentration is an extremely important aspect of therapy, regardless of the specific cause of the stone disease. This should be stressed repeatedly to all stone formers. Preferably the fluid intake should be spread throughout the day and particularly at night when urinary concentration usually reaches its peak. Urinary tract infection, which often complicates stone disease, should be treated using tests of antibiotic sensitivity as a guide. Surgical intervention is necessary for acute ureteral obstruction that does not respond to fluid loading and for correction of congenital anomalies of the urinary tract that favor stasis and stone formation.

More specific therapeutic measures are based on the particular type of stone disease. Since calcium oxalate or mixed calcium oxalate and calcium phosphate stones are the most common urinary calculi, their therapy is particularly important. Calcium oxalate solubility is not significantly affected by changes in urinary pH between 4.5 and 7.5. Therefore, manipulations designed to change urinary pH are usually of no benefit in recurrent calcium oxalate stone formers. If calcium phosphate either in the form of apatite or brushite is the nidus for calcium oxalate precipitation and stone growth, acidification of the urine may be of benefit. Except in patients with "absorptive" hypercalciuria, diets low in calcium generally do not greatly affect the urinary excretion of calcium or the incidence of new stone formation. Avoidance of large calcium loads is advisable in all patients with calcium-containing stones, but strict low calcium diets are probably of significant clinical benefit only in patients with idiopathic hypercalciuria.

A number of specific agents have been used to lower calcium excretion and interfere with the solubility of calcium oxalate and calcium phosphate in urine. In the former category, thiazide diuretics have received the most encouraging and extensive support (Yendt, 1970). The dose of hydrochlorothiazide is 50 to 150 mg per day in divided doses. Modest sodium restriction is also required. If significant diuresis is induced, these agents will produce a fall in urine calcium excretion by mechanisms that are not well understood (Epstein, 1968). Long-term studies of the use of the diuretics in the prevention of recurrent stone disease have not yet appeared, and toxicity needs to be evaluated further. In a few patients treated with thiazide diuretics, significant hypercalcemia has developed, but these may represent patients with underlying parathyroid disease or unrecognized metabolic bone disease. Dietary sodium restriction can produce a fall in urine calcium probably by mechanisms similar to those attributed to the thiazide diuretics, but efficacy is probably less because of the difficulties in maintaining rigid adherence to such diets.

Orthophosphate therapy in the form of neutral mixtures of mono- and dibasic sodium phosphate salts or as potassium acid phosphate (1–2 gm phosphorus per day) can lower urinary calcium excretion somewhat, although gastrointestinal absorption of calcium does not appear to be reduced. It is more likely that these agents are effective in stone disease through their ability to increase calcium oxalate and calcium phosphate solubility in urine, an effect that may be mediated by the increase in urinary pyrophosphate induced by these compounds (Ettinger and Kolb, 1973). Cellulose phosphate has also been used in the treatment of calcium stones (Dent *et al.*, 1964; Pak *et al.*, 1974). This compound appears to lower calcium excretion by decreasing gastrointestinal absorption and by decreasing the state of saturation of urine with respect to brushite. Whatever the mechanism, this form of treatment does seem effective in reducing stone recurrence, although potential toxicity does exist. While it seems ideal for patients with absorptive hypercalciuria, it is not clear whether orthophosphate therapy is safe for the normocalciuric stone former. It certainly should not be used in resorptive hypercalciuria. It has not been released for use in the United States. Some magnesium supplementation is also required. Although tissue deposits of calcium phosphate have been reported in patients on oral phosphate therapy, most of these patients have had hypercalcemia before treatment and reports of large numbers of patients with stone disease treated with oral orthophosphate for several years fail to mention any significant toxicity.

Magnesium oxide (200–400 mg/day) used either alone or in conjunction with pyridoxine (100–200 mg/day) has been introduced in the therapy for recurrent calcium-containing stones (Melnick *et al.*, 1971; Prien and Gershoff, 1974). In 1929, Hammarsten demonstrated the solubilizing effect of magnesium on calcium oxalate and subsequently reported that it prevented experimentally induced stone formation in rats. Subsequently, it has been shown that the level of vitamin B_6 is inversely related to the urinary oxalate excretion and that its administration may reduce oxalate excretion somewhat in man. The ultimate efficacy of this form of therapy remains to be defined.

Allopurinol is also effective as alluded to above. The presumption is that the patients should have relatively high uric acid excretions in the range of 600 to 1000 mg/day. However, since the mechanism of action is uncertain, this requirement may be irrelevant. The doses used have been surprisingly small. In the controlled trial, it was 100 mg three times a day for 1 week and then only 100 mg/day thereafter. Others have used 150 to 200 mg/day (Coe *et al.*, 1973). Of course, dietary restriction of purines might be just as effective.

An important adjunct to therapy is weight reduction in the obese subject. This will curtail the occult sources of dietary calcium as in breads and pastries and the glutinous meat eating that contributed to hyperuricosuria.

The recent studies with the diphosphonates emphasize the potential usefulness of these compounds in the treatment of recurrent renal stone disease (Fleisch, 1973b). These stable compounds with a P–C–P bond structure are very potent inhibitors of calcium phosphate and calcium oxalate crystal formation from metastable solutions. They also inhibit the transformation of amorphous calcium phosphate into crystalline form, and they disperse aggregates of microcrystals of calcium phosphate. Their effectiveness in reducing calcium oxalate and calcium phosphate bladder stone formation in rats has strongly emphasized their potential usefulness in man. No reports of clinical trials of these compounds in patients with recurrent stone disease have yet appeared. Several controlled trials are being conducted.

In patients with hyperoxaluria, the measures described earlier are useful and may be efficacious in preventing new stone formation. Pyridoxine in massive doses (200–400 mg/day) has partially reduced oxalate excretion in some patients with primary hyperoxaluria, perhaps by increasing transamination of glyoxylate to glycine (Smith and Williams, 1967). Pyridoxine therapy is, of course, indicated in patients who are deficient in this vitamin. Search for a safe and useful inhibitor of oxalate synthesis has generally been unsuccessful, although *in vitro* studies have been encouraging (Williams and Smith, 1972; Smith *et al.*, 1972a). The recent report of successful reduction of oxalate excretion with succinamide therapy (Thomas *et al.*, 1973) is intriguing, but will require further confirmation on large series of patients to assess efficacy and toxicity over long periods of time. Studies in rat liver preparations demonstrating inhibition of oxalate synthesis from glyoxylate with DL-phenyllactate will also require further study in man (Liao and Richardson, 1973). Taurine and cholestyramine have both been effective in reducing the hyperoxaluria associated with small bowel disease in some but not all patients with this syndrome (see above). In these patients, a low oxalate diet may be useful in reducing urinary oxalate excretion.

Patients with recurrent uric acid stones usually respond well to a modest increase in urine pH. Generally, the urine pH should be maintained in the range of 6.0–6.5, particularly in overnight urine samples. If hyperuricemia is present, allopurinol therapy will reduce both serum and urine uric acid by inhibition of xanthine oxidase and reduction in uric acid synthesis and excretion. In patients with the Lesch–Nyhan syndrome or in patients with lymphoproliferative disorders receiving chemotherapy and allopurinol, alkali therapy is essential to avoid xanthine nephropathy Ablin *et al.*, 1972). Uricosuric agents should be avoided in patients with uric acid stones. As with other forms of stone disease, adequate hydration is important to maintain urine uric acid concentration as low as possible.

In the patient with uric acid calculi and normal serum uric acid concentrations, hydration and alkali therapy to maintain urine pH between 6.0 and 6.5 are often sufficient to reduce the incidence of stone formation. If this is ineffective, allopurinol may be added to reduce the total uric acid load excreted.

In cystinuria, the solubility of cystine can be increased by alkalinization of the urine above a pH of 7.0, but this is frequently difficult and impractical for long-term therapy; consequently, the forcing of fluid is the *sine qua non* of successful therapy. Since methionine is a major metabolic precursor of cystine, low methionine diets have been utilized with variable success in reducing urinary cystine excretion (Earll and Kolb, 1967). D-Penicillamine therapy, which leads to the formation of soluble mixed disulfides of cystine and penicillamine, does decrease total cystine excretion, but the high incidence of toxic reactions, such as serum sickness and the nephrotic syndrome, has limited the clinical usefulness of this compound (Crawhall and Watts, 1968).

Treatment of triple phosphate stones, commonly forming in alkaline urine infected with urea-splitting organisms, has depended largely on acidification of the urine with compounds such as ascorbic acid and cranberry juice and on the use of appropriate antibiotic drugs.

The large number of therapeutic modalities used in the treatment of recurrent nephrolithiasis is indicative of continued efforts to improve clinical effectiveness. As the intimate pathogenetic details of stone disease are uncovered, rational forms of preventive therapy will undoubtedly be developed and nephrolithiasis may eventually achieve historic significance as a disease of the past.

ACKNOWLEDGMENT

This work was supported in part by United States Public Health Service Grants AM-13672, GM-19527, AM-03564, and AM-04501.

REFERENCES

Ablin, A., Stephens, B., Hirata, T., Wilson, K., and Williams, H. (1972). *Metabolism* **21,** 771.

Admirand, W. H., Earnest, D. L., and Williams, H. E. (1971). *Trans. Assoc. Am. Physicans* **84,** 307.

Atsmon, A., DeVries, A., and Frank, M. (1963). "Uric Acid Lithiasis." Elsevier, Amsterdam.

Baker, E. M., Saari, J. C., and Tolbert, B. M. (1966). *Am. J. Clin. Nutr.* **19,** 371.

Beeler, M. F., Veith, D. A., Morriss, R. H., and Biskind, G. R. (1964). *Am. J. Clin. Pathol.* **41,** 553.

Black, D. A. K. (1967). "Renal Disease," 2nd ed., pp. 421–445. Davis, Philadelphia, Pennsylvania.

Bourke, E., Frindt, G., Flynn, P., and Schreiner, G. E. (1972). *Ann. Intern. Med.* **76,** 279.

Boyce, W. H. (1968). *Am. J. Med.* **45,** 673.

Chambers, A., Hodgkinson, A., and Hornung, G. (1972). *Invest. Urol.* **9,** 376.

Coe, F. L., Canterbury, J. M., and Reiss, E. (1973). *J. Clin. Invest.* **52,** 134.

Coe, F. L., and Kavalach, A. G. (1974). *N. Engl. J. Med.* **291,** 1344.

Crawhall, J. C., and Watts, R. W. E. (1968). *Am. J. Med.* **45,** 736.

Dent, C. E., and Rose, G. A. (1951). *Q. J. Med.* **20,** 205.

Dent, C. E., Harper, C. M. and Parfitt, A. M. (1964). *Clin. Sci.* **27,** 417.

Dowling, R. H., Rose, G. A., and Sutor, D. J. (1971). *Lancet* **1,** 1103.

Earll, J. M., and Kolb, F. O. (1967). *Mod. Treat.* **4,** 539.

Earnest, D. L., Williams, H. E., and Admirand, W. H. (1973). *Gastroenterology* **64,** 723.

Earnest, D. L., Johnson, G., Williams, H. E., and Admirand, W. H. (1974). *Gastroenterology* **66,** 1114.

Earnest, D. L., Williams, H. E., and Admirand, W. H. (1975). *Trans. Assoc. Am. Physicians* **88,** 224.

Elliot, J. S. (1973). *J. Urol.* **109,** 82.

Epstein, F. H. (1968). *Am. J. Med* **45,** 700.

Ettinger, B., and Kolb, F. O. (1973). *Am. J. Med.* **55,** 32.

Finlayson, B. (1972). *Invest. Urol.* **9,** 258.

Fleisch, H. (1973a). *In* "International Symposium of Renal Stones Research" (L. Cifuentes Delatte, A. Rapado, and A. Hodgkinson, eds.). pp. 53–56. Karger, Basel.

Fleisch, H. (1973b). *In* "International Symposium on Renal Stone Research" (L. Cifuentes Delatte, A. Rapado, and A. Hodgkinson, eds.), pp. 296–301. Karger, Basel.

Frascino, J. A., Vanamee, P., and Rosen, P. P. (1970). *N. Engl. J. Med.* **283,** 676.

Friedman, E. A., Greenberg, J. B., Merrill, J. P., and Dammin, G. J. (1962). *Am. J. Med.* **32,** 891.

Garrod, A. E. (1908). *Lancet* **2,** 1, 73, 142, and 214.

Gershoff, S. N., and Prien, E. L. (1967). *Am. J. Clin. Nutr.* **20,** 393.

Gibbs, D. A., and Watts, R. W. E. (1966). *Clin. Sci.* **31,** 285.

Gibbs, D. A., and Watts, R. W. E. (1973). *Clin. Sci.* **44,** 227.

Greene, M. L., Fujimoto, W. Y., and Seegmiller, J. E. (1969). *N. Engl. J. Med.* **280,** 426.

Gutman, A. B., and Yü, T.-F. (1968). *Am. J. Med.* **45,** 756.

Gutman, A. B., and Yü, T.-F. (1973). *In* "International Symposium on Renal Stone Research" (L. Cifuentes Delatte, A. Rapado, and A. Hodgkinson, eds.). Karger, Basel (in press).

Györy, A. Z., Edwards, K. D. G., Robinson, J., and Palmer, A. A. (1970). *Clin. Sci.* **39,** 605.

Haggitt, R. C., and Pitcock, J. A. (1971). *J. Urol.* **106,** 342.

Hammarsten, G. (1929). *C. R. Trav. Lab. Carlsberg* **17,** 1.

Hauschka, P. V., Lian, J. B., and Gallop, P. M. (1975). *Proc. Nat. Acad. Sci. U.S.A.* **72,** 3925.

Henneman, P. H., Benedict, P. H., Forbes, A. P., and Dudley, H. R. (1958). *N. Engl. J. Med* **259,** 802.

Hodgkinson, A., and Pyrah, L. N. (1958). *Br. J. Surg.* **46,** 10.

Howard, J. E., and Thomas, W. C., Jr. (1968). *Am. J. Med.* **45,** 693.

Jensen, A. T. (1941). *Acta Chir. Scand.* **84,** 207.

Keutel, H. J., and King, J. S., Jr. (1964). *Invest. Urol.* **2,** 115.

Krementz, E. T., Race, J. L., Sternberg, W. H., and Hawley, W. D. (1967). *Ann. Surg.* **165,** 681.

Lavan, J. N., Neale, F. C., and Posen, S. (1971). *Med. J. Aust.* **2**, 1049.
Lemann, J., Jr. Donor, D. W., Jr., and Kelly, A. O. (1971). *Abstr. 5th Annu. Meet. Am. Soc. Nephrol.* Vol. 5, p. 44.
Lewis, A. M., Thomas, W. C., Jr., and Tomita, A. (1966). *Clin. Sci.* **30**, 389.
Lian, J. B., and Prien, E. L., Jr. (1976). *Fed. Proc.* (Abst) **35**, 1763.
Liao, L. L., and Richardson, K. E. (1973). *Arch. Biochem. Biophys.* **154**, 68.
Lloyd, H. M. (1968). *Medicine (Baltimore)* **47**, 53.
Melnick, I., Landes, R. R., Hoffman, A. A., and Burch, J. F. (1971). *J. Urol.* **105**, 119.
Meyer, J. L., Bergert, J. H., and Smith, L. H. (1975). *Clin. Sci.* **49**, 369.
Morris, R. C., Jr. (1969). *N. Engl. J. Med.* **281**, 1405.
Nordin, B. E. C., Peacock, M., and Wilkinson, R. (1972). *In* "Clinics in Endocrinology and Metabolism" (I. MacIntyre, ed.), Vol. 1, No. 1, pp. 169–183. Saunders, Philadelphia, Pennsylvania.
Paddock, R. B., Parker, J. W., and Guadagni, N. P. (1964). *Anesthesiology* **25**, 707.
Pak, C. Y. C. (1969). *J. Clin. Invest.* **48**, 1914.
Pak, C. Y. C. (1972). *Metab., Clin. Exp.* **21**, 447.
Pak, C. Y. C., Eanes, E. D., and Ruskin, B. (1971). *Proc. Natl. Acad. Sci. U.S.A.* **68**, 1456.
Pak, C. Y. C., Delea, C. S., and Bartter, F. C. (1974). *N. Eng. J. Med.* **290**, 175.
Pak, C. Y. C., Kaplan, R., Bone, H., Townsend, J., and Waters, O. (1975). *N. Engl. J. Med.* **292**, 497.
Parfitt, A. M. (1969). *Arch. Intern. Med.* **124**, 736.
Parfitt, A. M. (1970). *Lancet* ii, 153.
Peacock, M. (1975). *In* "Calcium Regulating Hormones" (R. V. Talmage, M. Owen and J. A. Parsons, eds.) pp. 78–81. Excerpta Medica, Amsterdam.
Pinto, B. (1973). *In* "International Symposium of Renal Stone Research" (L. Cifuentes Delatte, A. Rapado, and A. Hodgkinson, eds.), pp. 46–52. Karger, Basel.
Prien, E. L. (1949). *J. Urol.* **61**, 821.
Prien, E. L. (1955). *J. Urol.* **73**, 633.
Prien, E. L. (1975). *J. Urol.* **114**, 500.
Prien, E. L., and Frondel, C. (1947). *J. Urol.* **57**, 949.
Prien, E. L., and Gershoff, S. F. (1974). *J. Urol.* **112**, 509.
Purnell, D. C., Smith, L. H., Scholz, D. A., Elveback, L. R., and Arnaud, D. C. (1971). *Am. J. Med.* **50**, 670.
Randall, A. (1939). *Int. Soc. Urol. Congr. Rep.* **7**, 186.
Richardson, K. E., and Liao, L. L. (1973). *Fed. Proc., Fed. Am. Soc. Exp. Biol.* **32**, 565.
Robertson, W. G. (1976). Presented at the International Symposium on Urolithiasis Research, Davos, Switzerland.
Robertson, W. G., and Peacock, M. (1973). *In* "International Symposium on Renal Stone Research" (L. Cifuentes Delatte, A. Rapado, and A. Hodgkinson, eds.), pp. 302–306. Karger, Basel.
Robertson, W. G., Peacock, M., and Nordin, B. E. C. (1969). *Lancet* **2**, 21.
Robertson, W. G., Peacock, M., and Nordin, B. E. C. (1971). *Clin. Sci.* **40**, 365.
Robertson, W. G. and Peacock, M., and Nordin, B. E. C. (1973). *Clin. Chim. Acta.* **43**, 31.
Robertson, W. G., Gallagher, J. C., Marshall, D. H., Peacock, M., and Nordin, B. E. C. (1974). *Br. Med. J.* **4**, 436.
Robertson, W. G., Peacock, M., Marshall, R. W., Marshall, D. H., and Nordin, B. E. C. (1976). *N. Engl. J. Med.* **294**, 249.
Runyan, T. J., and Gershoff, S. N. (1965). *J. Biol. Chem.* **240**, 1889.
Russell, R. G. G. (1973). *In* "International Symposium on Renal Stone Research" (L. Cifuentes Delatte, A. Rapado, and A. Hodgkinson, eds.), pp. 307–312. Karger, Basel.

Smith, L. H. (1975). Presented at International Colloquium on Renal Lithiasis, Gainesville, Florida.

Smith, L. H., Jr., and McCall, J. T. (1973). *In* "International Symposium on Renal Stone Research" (L. Cifuentes Delatte, A. Rapado, and A. Hodgkinson, eds.), pp. 318–327. Karger, Basel.

Smith, L. H., Jr., and Williams, H. E. (1967). *Mod. Treat.* **4**, 522.

Smith, L. H., Jr., Bauer, R. L., Craig, J. C., Chan, R. P. K., and Williams, H. E. (1972a). *Biochem. Med.* **6**, 317.

Smith, L. H., Jr., Fromm, H., and Hofmann, A. F. (1972b). *N. Engl. J. Med.* **286**, 1371.

Smith, M. J. V. (1975). Presented at International Colloquium on Renal Lithiasis, Gainesville, Florida.

Smith, M. J. V., and Boyce, W. H. (1969). *J. Urol.* **102**, 750.

Spector, A. R., Gray, A., and Prien, E. L., Jr. (1976). *Invest. Urol.* **13**, 387.

Sutor, D. J. (1968). *Br. J. Urol.* **40**, 29.

Sutor, D. J., Wooley, S. E., MacKenzie, K. R., Wilson, R., Scott, R., and Morgan, H. G. (1971). *Br. J. Urol.* **43**, 149.

Thier, S. O., and Segal, S. (1972). *In* "The Metabolic Basis of Inherited Disease" (J. B. Stanbury, J. B. Wyngaarden, and D. S. Fredrickson, eds.), 3rd ed., pp. 1504–1519. McGraw-Hill, New York.

Thomas, J., Melon, J. M., Steg, E., Thomas, E., and Aboulker, P. (1973). *In* "International Symposium on Renal Stone Research" (L. Cifuentes Delatte, A. Rapado, and A. Hodgkinson, eds.), pp. 57–66. Karger, Basel.

Thomas, W. C., Tilden, M. T., and Baskin, A. D. (1972). *In* "Urolithiasis: Physical Aspects. Proceedings of a Conference" (B. Finlayson, L. L. Hench, and L. H. Smith, eds.), pp. 145–156. Nat. Acad. Sci., Washington, D.C.

Tsay, Y. C. (1961). *J. Urol.* **86**, 838.

Vermeulen, C. W., and Lyon, E. S. (1968). *Am. J. Med.* **45**, 684.

Vermeulen, C. W., Ellis, J. E., and Hsu, T.-C. (1966). *J. Urol.* **95**, 681.

Williams, H. E., and Smith, L. H., Jr. (1971). *Science* **171**, 390.

Williams, H. E., and Smith, L. H., Jr. (1972). *In* "The Metabolic Basis of Inherited Disease" (J. B. Stanbury, J. B. Wyngaarden, and D. S. Fredrickson, eds.), 3rd ed., pp. 196–219. McGraw-Hill, New York.

Williams, H. E., Johnson, G. A., and Smith, L. H., Jr. (1971). *Clin. Sci.* **41**, 213.

Wrong, O., and Davies, H. E. F. (1959). *Q. J. Med.* **28**, 259.

Wyngaarden, J. B. (1972). *In* "The Metabolic Basis of Inherited Disease" (J. B. Stanbury, J. B. Wyngaarden, and D. S. Fredrickson, eds.), 3rd ed., pp. 992–1002. McGraw-Hill, New York.

Yendt, E. R. (1970). *Can. Med. Assoc. J.* **102**, 479.

Yendt, E. R., and Gagne, R. S. A. (1968). *Can. Med. Assoc. J.* **98**, 331.

Yü, T. F., and Gutman, A. B. (1973). *In* "International Symposium on Renal Stone Research" (L. Cifuentes Delatte, A. Rapado, and A. Hodgkinson, eds.), pp. 101–104. Karger, Basel.

Index